Comprehensive Manuals of Surgical Specialties

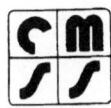

Richard H. Egdahl, editor

Anthony J. Edis   Clive S. Grant   Richard H. Egdahl

MANUAL OF ENDOCRINE SURGERY

SECOND EDITION

With 305 illustrations in full color
and 32 in black and white

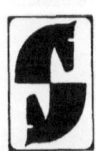

Springer Science+Business Media, LLC

SERIES EDITOR   Richard H. Egdahl M.D., Ph.D., Professor of Surgery, Boston University Medical Center, Boston, Massachusetts 02118, U.S.A.

AUTHORS   Anthony J. Edis M.D., Associate Professor, University Department of Surgery, Royal Perth Hospital, Victoria Square, Perth, Western Australia
Clive S. Grant, M.D., Department of Surgery, Mayo Clinic, Rochester, Minnesota 55901, U.S.A.
Richard H. Egdahl M.D., Ph.D., Boston University Medical Center, 720 Harrison Avenue, Boston, Massachusetts 02118, U.S.A.

MEDICAL ILLUSTRATORS   David J. Mascaro, Assistant Professor, School of Medical Illustration, Medical College of Georgia, Augusta, Georgia 30902; Jerome T. Glickman, Team Administrator, Educational Media Support Center, Boston University Medical Center, Boston, Massachusetts 02118; Karen Waldo, Office of Biomedical Communications, Dartmouth–Hitchcock Medical Center, Hanover, New Hampshire 03755; Judy M. Glick, Educational Media Support Center, Boston University Medical Center, Boston, Massachusetts 02118; Charles H. Boyter, Educational Media Support Center, Boston University Medical Center, Boston, Massachusetts 02118

GRAPHIC ILLUSTRATORS   Douglas P. Russell, Educational Media Support Center, Boston University Medical Center, Boston, Massachusetts 02118; Eric Hieber, Technical Art—Studio One, New York, New York

Library of Congress Cataloging in Publication Data

Edis, Anthony J.
  Manual of endocrine surgery

  (Comprehensive manuals of surgical specialties)
  Bibliography: p.
  Includes index.
    1. Endocrine glands—Surgery.   I. Grant, Clive S.
II. Egdahl, Richard H., 1926–   .   III. Title.
IV. Series.   [DNLM: 1. Endocrine Glands—surgery.
WK 100 E23m]
RD599.E34   1984   617′.44   84-13929

Composition by Bi-Comp, Inc., York Pennsylvania, U.S.A.

9 8 7 6 5 4 3 2 1

ISBN 978-1-4612-9744-4   ISBN 978-1-4612-5222-1 (eBook)
DOI 10.1007/978-1-4612-5222-1

To Our Wives

Editor's Note

Comprehensive Manuals of Surgical Specialties is a series of surgical manuals designed to present current operative techniques and to explore various aspects of diagnosis and treatment. The series features a unique format with emphasis on large, detailed, full-color illustrations, schematic charts, and photographs to demonstrate integral steps in surgical procedures.

Each manual focuses on a specific region or topic and describes surgical anatomy, physiology, pathology, diagnosis, and operative treatment. Operative techniques and stratagems for dealing with surgically correctable disorders are described in detail. Illustrations are primarily depicted from the surgeon's viewpoint to enhance clarity and comprehension.

Other volumes in the series:

Published:

Manual of Endocrine Surgery
Manual of Burns
*Manual of Surgery of the Gallbladder, Bile Ducts,
  and Exocrine Pancreas*
Manual of Gynecologic Surgery
Manual of Urologic Surgery
Manual of Lower Gastrointestinal Surgery
Manual of Vascular Surgery, Volume I
Manual of Cardiac Surgery, Volume I
Manual of Cardiac Surgery, Volume II
Manual of Liver Surgery
Manual of Ambulatory Surgery
Manual of Pulmonary Surgery
Manual of Soft-Tissue Tumor Surgery
*Manual of Vascular Access, Organ Donation, and
  Transplantation*

In Preparation:

Manual of Vascular Surgery, Volume II
Manual of Orthopedic Surgery
Manual of Upper Gastrointestinal Surgery
Manual of Trauma Surgery
Manual of Sports Surgery
Manual of Aesthetic Surgery

Richard H. Egdahl

Contents

Preface

This book, as originally conceived, was an attempt to create a different kind of surgical atlas by adopting the use of full color illustrations to provide a greater sense of operative realism. The primary emphasis was to be on high visual impact for quick ready reference by the practicing general surgeon. As the project evolved, however, the limited concept of a surgical atlas was superseded by a plan to provide a comprehensive and fully referenced *manual* covering all pertinent aspects of surgical anatomy, pathophysiology, principles of diagnosis and perioperative management of those endocrine diseases encountered by the general surgeon. It was in this format that the first edition of the *Manual of Endocrine Surgery* appeared in 1975.

The recipe remains unchanged for the second edition—although the text has been entirely rewritten to bring it up to date and many new photographs and schematics illustrating the pathology and diagnosis of the various endocrine disease entities have supplanted those used in the first edition. As before, the manual deals in a systematic way with those endocrine diseases affecting the parathyroids, thyroid, adrenals and pancreas. Pituitary disease is dealt with *en passant* in relation to Cushing's disease and no attempt has been made to deal with reproductive endocrinology—these are facets outside the scope of general surgery. As an addition to the introduction, our contributing coauthors discuss some of the basic theoretic concepts of the origin, structure, and function of the endocrine system and speculate on future developments in endocrine surgery.

Many of the operative illustrations have been upgraded and new plates have been added in Chapter 4, Surgery of the Pancreas. As in the first edition, particular attention has been devoted to presenting the operative techniques with sufficient detail and clarity so that the surgeon can visualize the operation step by step. The orientation of the operative field is shown as the surgeon himself would see it, not as an illustrator or photographer might see it over the surgeon's shoulder or from an observation point overhead.

Endocrine surgery is undergoing constant evolution. Since the publication of the first edition of the *Manual of Endocrine Surgery* in 1975 such significant changes have occurred as to warrant a major revision. For example, parathyroid surgery has become much more common owing to the increasingly frequent diagnosis of primary hyperparathyroidism by routine automated biochemical screening of hospitalized and clinic patients. On the other hand, we are now undertaking far fewer adrenalectomies—pituitary microadenectomy has supplanted bilateral adrenalectomy as the treatment of choice in adult Cushing's disease, and various hormonal manipulations have been substituted for adrenalectomy in the treatment of metastatic breast cancer. An interesting phenomenon of the last 10 years in the United States has been the adoption and increasing popularity of fine needle aspiration biopsy in the evaluation of thyroid nodules. This has had the salutary effect of refining the selection of patients for surgery to exclude malignancy and reducing the number of unnecessary operations on benign thyroid nodules.

Perhaps the most striking developments since 1975 have been those which have taken place in endocrine gland imaging and tumor localization. Computerized tomography has come into its own as a localizing tool *par excellence* in adrenal disease and it has also proved valuable in the identification of mediastinal parathyroid tumors and some pancreatic lesions. Newer radionuclide scanning agents, especially NP59 and ^{131}I MIBG, have provided a quantum leap in the localization of hyperfunctioning adrenal cortical and medullary tissue, respectively. High resolution ultrasonography has now proved its ability to identify the majority of parathyroid tumors preoperatively and new applications for this technology are currently being explored—such as the intraoperative localization of pancreatic islet cell tumors. Such has been the pace of change in diagnostic radiology that any recommendation concerning imaging techniques made one year may be rendered obsolete the next. In this context, one can envisage nuclear magnetic resonance perhaps rivalling computerized tomography as an imaging tool in certain areas of endocrine surgery in the very near future.

The recognition and description of several new endocrine diseases (somatostatinoma and 'CCK-oma') and the elucidation of the basic pathophysiology of glucagonoma and vipoma have all occurred in the 9 years since the publication of the first edition. There has been further evolution of A.G.E. Pearse's prescient APUD hypothesis, which seeks to explain the integration and overlapping homeostatic functions of the nervous and endocrine systems. In fact, at the urging of 1977 Nobel laureate Roger Guillemin, it has now become fashionable to describe the endocrine system as the *neuro*endocrine system and to think of it as the third main division of the nervous system, along with the somatic and autonomic divisions.

These observations, which are discussed below, demand that the modern surgeon adopt a more holistic approach to disorders of the endocrine system. It is no longer reasonable to confine one's interest to just the adrenal glands (as part of urologic surgery) or just the thyroid gland (as part of head and neck surgery). Surgical endocrinology has truly come of age as a discipline in its own right.

COMMON DENOMINATORS IN ENDOCRINE NEOPLASIA

The traditional belief that the endocrine and nervous systems are separable but interacting entities has ceased to exist. Pathologic alterations in both endocrine and nervous systems are often observed in the same clinical syndrome, suggesting that few biologic processes are controlled exclusively by either system. Most clinicians now agree that these two systems are so interdependent that it is more accurate to consider them as a single unit, the *neuroendocrine system*.

The neuroendocrine system is composed of a number of specialized tissues organized in a central and peripheral manner. It has been argued that the neuroendocrine system should be considered the third division of the nervous system—the first being the somatic (motor and sensory neurons) and the second the autonomic (sympathetic and parasympathetic neurons). Within the neuroendocrine system, much of the central (brain–pituitary) component is related developmentally, anatomically, and/or functionally to the peripheral endocrine component in a variety of ways. Central and peripheral feedback mechanisms are quite similar in a number of systems. Developmentally, a group of peripheral endocrine structures is derived in early fetal life from neural crest tissue and consequently shares certain structural, histologic, and biochemical characteristics with central nervous system endocrine tissue. In 1966, it was proposed that the name APUD (amine precursor, uptake and decarboxylation) be given to this system of cells derived from common embryonic neuroectoderm. The "diffuse neuroendocrine system" (DNES), named in 1979, is now considered to comprise two divisions: the central division contains neuroendocrine and endocrine cells of the hypothalamic–pituitary axis and pineal gland; and the peripheral division contains all APUD cells outside these regions (the majority of which are situated in the gastrointestinal tract and pancreas).

For the endocrine surgeon, a working understanding of the theory of a common embryonic denominator in endocrine neoplasia is critical to present-day considerations regarding "ectopic" hormone production. The number of cells now included in the APUD group has increased steadily from an original 6 to well over 40 different peptide-secreting cell types. The concept of the neuroectodermal origin linking all cell types has been supplanted by a new theory in which all cells are "neuroendocrine-programed" and arise in the embryonic epiblast or one of its principal descendants. The APUD concept originally provided a means of explaining the multipotentiality of many endocrine cells as more and more clinical "ectopic" syndromes were observed and reported in the literature. The ability of nonendocrine neoplasias to secrete hormones and the ability of endocrine tumors to secrete several different peptides can be explained using the APUD hypothesis. This concept of multipotentiality based on embryonic differentiation may, if proved valid, make the concept of "ectopic" hormone production obsolete. These "apudomas" have been classified as tumors arising from the neural crest, capable of sequentially or simultaneously secreting various peptide hormones and/or their putative biosynthetic precursors.

Although an interesting hypothesis, the APUD concept has evoked considerable controversy. One problem inherent in the theory is that the ectoblastic origin concept is virtually untestable. Another criticism maintains that the APUD concept is applied inconsistently—cell types that do not possess the required biochemical characteristics are included in the system (parathyroid chief cells and gonadotrophs), while other cells possessing appropriate biochemical characteristics are excluded (basophils and mast cells). In addition, many cell groups long considered endodermal in origin have been reported to be of neuroectodermal origin to fit the theory, and it has been argued that neoplastic processes associated with peptide hormone production should not automatically be considered neuroectodermally derived "apudomas." To this end, the APUD concept has vigorously been challenged. Many reports have been compiled of "APUD" activity by endodermally and mesodermally derived tumors and have suggested that "apudomas" do exist that have endodermal microscopic features.

Although the APUD concept has been embraced by many researchers and clinicians, the controversy concerning its validity remains unresolved. It has been alternatively hypothesized that malignant forms of cells may be fixed at a level of differentiation at which random gene sequences may be activated, leading to the production of oncofetal proteins or peptide hormones. Within this theory, the presence of double minute chromosomes has been suggested to be a cytologic marker of gene amplification and cellular production of peptides. It may indeed be possible that cancer cells have the capacity to synthesize a wide variety of hormonal products regardless of their embryonic derivation.

The observation that neural and endocrine tissue may elaborate and secrete more than one type of hormone has expanded present-day surgical concepts concerning the functional potentiality of the neuroendocrine system. Intra- or extraneuronal enzymes such as peptidases may be missing or defective in malignant tumors, resulting in the elaboration of abnormally large precursor molecules that have extraordinary physiologic activity (proopiomelanocortin, proinsulin). Certain endocrine neoplasias, such as pancreatic, thyroid, or adrenal adenoma, may result in the elaboration or hypersecretion of a number of peptide or aminergic moieties. If secreted in sufficient quantities and in biologically active forms, these peptides may cause paraendocrine syndromes with metabolic and clinical features. Since many of these peptides have been implicated as putative central and peripheral neurotransmitters, central nervous system changes may accompany endocrine dysfunction in clinical disease states.

The peptide secreted most commonly by tumors probably arising from DNES cells is adrenocorticotropic hormone (ACTH). Causative tumors in approximate order of frequency are oat cell carcinoma of the bronchus, carcinoid tumor, epithelial carcinoma of the thymus, islet cell tumor of the pancreas, medullary carcinoma of the thyroid, pheochromocytoma, and other miscellaneous tumors. It is well known that these tumors may secrete other peptides in addition to ACTH, including gastrin, vasopressin, glucagon, norepinephrine, and serotonin. In addition, the recently discovered pituitary precursor of ACTH, proopiomelanocortin, may be secreted by ACTH-producing tumors along with other biologically active fragments including β-lipotrophin, β-endorphin, enkephalin, and corticotropinlike intermediate lobe peptide (CLIP).

Additional peptide-secreting tumors have been isolated in other unexpected peripheral sites. Recently, leukemic marrow cells have been shown to produce ACTH, renal adenocarcinomas have been reported to produce massive amounts of insulin and glucagon, and squamous cell carcinoma of the cervix and burn scars have been shown to produce insulin and parathyroid hormone, respectively. The peptide-producing tumors that have been fully characterized in the adrenal, lung, and pancreas include vipoma, glucagonoma, pancreatic polypeptidoma, somatostatinoma, neurotensinoma, gastrinoma, insulinoma, and bombesinoma. In addition, somatostatin has been found to be produced in thyroid C cells, thyrotropin-releasing hormone–like peptides in gut endocrine cells, and human growth hormone–releasing hormone in pancreatic cells. Indeed, it has become evident that the multipotentiality of these hormone-producing sites may partially explain why surgical treatment for certain endocrinopathies is sometimes ineffective. Surgical management of these peptide-producing tumors is also complicated by the fact that selective venous sampling and computerized tomographic scanning are frequently ineffective in localizing tumors. With the development of refined immunoassays and high-performance liquid chromatography techniques, the measurement of circulating peptides may become an important diagnostic tool in the surgical management of endocrine disease.

VISTAS FOR THE FUTURE IN ENDOCRINE SURGERY

It has become apparent over the past decade that progress will continue to be made in endocrine surgery as new syndromes are described, previously recognized ones are diagnosed with greater certainty, and more definitive therapy is developed. For example, advances in ultrasound and computerized tomography make possible the delineation of the adrenal areas with a degree of accuracy that can lead to the virtual exclusion of an adrenal tumor. By combining this information with knowledge about the periaortic and bladder areas, it is now possible to rather confidently rule out the presence of bilateral adrenal tumors, especially pheochromocytomas—thereby permitting the surgeon to operate from the approach that provides the least morbidity to the patient. In our experience, the posterior approach is turning out to be a very adequate one for many large adrenal tumors (including pheochromocytomas) that previously would have had to be removed from the front because of uncertainty about the presence of other adrenal tumors. This is made possible by refined radiologic diagnosis, which permits a high degree of confidence that a contralateral adrenal tumor or other intraabdominal tumors in ectopic sites are not present.

There appears to be a rather high incidence of hyperparathyroidism in elderly people who are considered to be senile or depressed solely as a result of their advanced age. We have had experience with many of these individuals over the past decade, and the return of an elderly and incapacitated individual to an active and happy family life has been a rewarding therapeutic experience. The importance of screening for parathyroid disease in patients in whom the disease is suspected, at whatever age symptoms appear, has been established.

Certainly, thyroid needle biopsy of solitary thyroid tumors has the potential for markedly decreasing the number of patients with thyroid nodules who go to surgery. Many factors account for the resistance of senior surgeons to this procedure, including lack of experience, fear of hemorrhage, and lack of availability of an experienced pathologist. However, like all major therapeutic advances, thyroid needle biopsy has already been shown to have the potential for greatly decreasing unnecessary surgery of the thyroid, and it should rapidly become a key component of the armamentarium of all endocrine surgeons.

Great advances in radiologic procedures involving selective catheterization of veins and arteries, and sampling of blood for hormones, now permit a quite precise pinpointing of pancreatic tumors of various sorts and of parathyroid tumors in aberrant locations. These procedures should not become routine in endocrine cases being operated on for the first time, since they carry their own morbidity and cost, but they are extremely important adjuvants in patients who need reoperation for clearly present surgical endocrinopathies.

The complex interaction of a variety of hormones, coupled with the constant interplay between neural and endocrine systems, enables the individual to respond to emergency demands such as starvation, infection, trauma, and psychologic stress. In the perioperative period, a complex mixture of hormones conditions the physiologic response of the individual to anesthetic agents, chemotherapeutic drugs, vasoactive and psychoactive drugs, and total parenteral nutrition. Over the past few years, circadian variations in endocrine function have received increasing attention from surgeons. Alterations in hormonal circadian rhythms may be involved in the etiology of certain endocrinopathies, and recent studies have revealed that the internal timing of endocrine rhythms in relation to one another can be adjusted, altered, or completely disrupted by factors associated with the surgical experience.

The inherent resistance of an individual's hormone rhythms to desynchronization may play an important role in susceptibility to endocrine dysfunction and surgical outcome. Since alterations in plasma rhythms of certain hormones are known to be associated with various affective disorders, a goal for the future will be to determine how these circadian rhythm changes relate to the affect of the surgical patient, the stress of anesthesia and surgery, and the response of the patient to both exogenous agents and other circulating hormones.

The second edition of the *Comprehensive Manual of Surgical Specialties: Manual of Endocrine Surgery* can only provide a snapshot of the specialty at a given point in time; but it includes some major changes from the first edition, and it is hoped it will be of value to surgeons and other physicians who wish to get an overview of the diagnostic and surgical aspects of endocrine disorders.

Surgery of the Parathyroids

General Introduction

Primary hyperparathyroidism (HPT), hitherto characterized as a rare disease with severe, progressive skeletal, gastrointestinal, and renal manifestations, is now recognized as a relatively common condition that is frequently mild and symptomless. The increase in frequency of diagnosis can be attributed mainly to the detection of a large group of relatively asymptomatic patients by the increasingly popular use of multichannel biochemical screening as part of the general medical examination (1–4). The prevalence of primary HPT in clinic and hospital populations has been reported to vary between 100 and 200 cases per 100,000 (1,3). According to two recent population-based studies, the incidence in the general population is at least 25–28 cases per 100,000 population per year (5,6), with the highest frequency occurring in postmenopausal women.

This plethora of new cases has resulted in cervical exploration for primary HPT becoming common; the operation is no longer restricted to a few major institutions with a special interest in the disease. Frequently, the operation is so easy that the uninitiated surgeon wonders what all the fuss is about. However, there are many potential pitfalls and an unsuccessful exploration may have serious and far-reaching consequences. Reexploration of the neck to find a missed parathyroid tumor may be difficult due to scarring, bleeding, and anatomic distortion and is fraught with hazard to the recurrent laryngeal nerves and any remaining normal parathyroid glands. Therefore, it is important that anyone undertaking parathyroid surgery be thoroughly familiar with the embryology and pathology of the parathyroids and with the many nuances of operative technique which may make the difference between success and failure.

SURGICAL ANATOMY

Notwithstanding opinions to the contrary, a normal parathyroid gland is usually easily recognizable at operation (7–10).

Parathyroid glands may have various *shapes:* when suspended in loose areolar tissue, fat, or thymus, they may be oval, spherical, pyriform, or leaflike; when situated deep to the surgical capsule of the thyroid, they are frequently flattened or stretched to resemble a disk or pancake. The normal *weight* of a parathyroid gland is 30–40 mg (11–14);

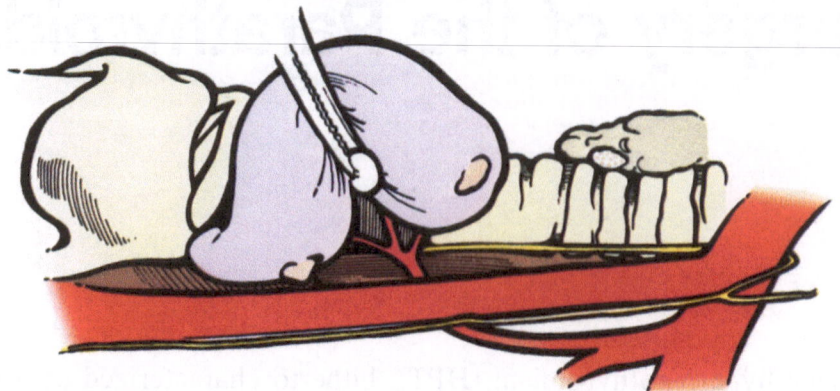

A

Fig. 1-1. **Normal locations of the parathyroid glands.** **A.** Lateral view. **B.** Posterior view. The *superior parathyroid gland* on each side is almost always located on the dorsal surface of the thyroid gland at the proximate level of the cricoid cartilage (7,12). When not in its usual location, the superior gland may be found in a retroesophageal or retropharyngeal position; less often it is alongside the superior thyroid vessels, above the upper pole of the thyroid gland. The *inferior parathyroid gland* is more variable in location. In approximately 50% of patients it lies on the lateral surface at the lower pole of the thyroid, near the point of attachment of the thyrothymic ligament (7,12). In the other 50% the inferior parathyroids are intimately associated with the thymus (hence the term ''parathymus glands''), either in the neck or in the superior mediastinum (7,12); most of these glands are found embedded in, or adjacent to a cervical tongue of thymic tissue that extends up from the chest behind the suprasternal notch to reach the inferior pole of the thyroid gland. The thymus is recognized by its smooth, pale gray-white appearance, its transparent fascial envelope, and the fact that it is not adherent to surrounding fat. By gentle probing of the thymus,

however, normal glands weighing up to 70 mg have been described at autopsy (12,13), and, on occasion, we have encountered even larger normal glands while performing thyroidectomies in eucalcemic patients (7,15).

A normal parathyroid gland has a soft *consistency* and a characteristic tan-yellow *color*. Thyroid nodules are firmer and more red in color; lymph nodes are likewise firm and have an opalescent gray color; and thymic tissue is characteristically a pale gray-yellow color. So-called ''brown'' fat, and ordinary lobules of yellow fat that have become blood stained, closely resemble parathyroid tissue in color and texture. As a general rule, however, a biopsy of parathyroid tissue sinks in normal saline, whereas fat floats (12); the cut surface of a parathyroid bleeds freely, whereas fat bleeds little, if at all.

Quite often one finds tiny, subcapsular cysts or bubbles in normal parathyroid glands. These structures are epithelial vesicles known as Kürsteiner's canals. They are of unknown origin and significance (16), but their distinctive appearance may be of help to the surgeon in identifying parathyroids that are partially obscured by fat or thymus.

The usual *number* of parathyroids is four, however, five and some-

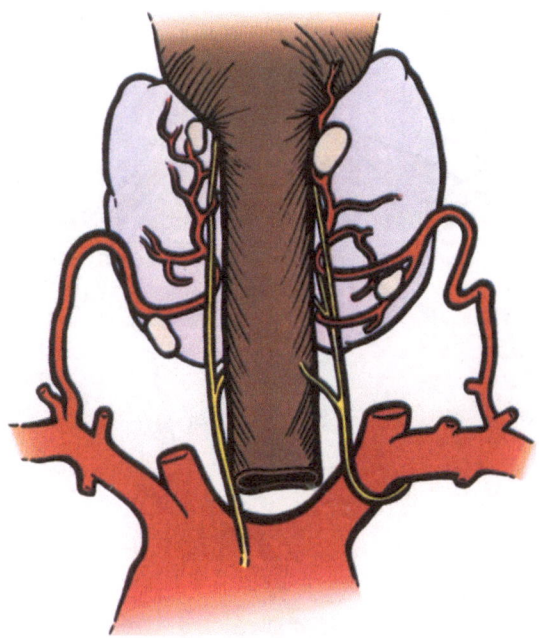

B

the parathyroid gland can be manipulated to the surface, where it can be seen just beneath the thymic capsule as a darker tan body immersed in the lighter thymic tissue. Very occasionally, (in approximately 1% of all patients with primary HPT), the inferior parathyroid gland descends with the thymus all the way into the mediastinum (19,20). Even more rarely, it may be left stranded high in the neck as a result of early developmental arrest; the identity of one of these so-called "undescended parathymus glands" (19) is often suggested by the presence of a closely associated thymic remnant (12,19,20).

times six glands are found in approximately 5% of careful postmortem examinations (11). Given the inherent limitations of postmortem dissection, it is probable that the true frequency of supernumerary glands is higher than 5%. Boyd (17) found either five or six parathyroid glands in 5 (14%) of 36 human embryos subjected to serial sectioning.

It is extremely unusual to encounter fewer than four parathyroids. In his detailed study of 352 postmortem cases, Alveryd (13) found only 1 case in which fewer than four parathyroids were identified and the combined weight of the glands suggested that none had been overlooked. Likewise, Norris (16) found at least four parathyroids in each of 109 human embryos studied by serial section. Thus, when one is exploring a patient with primary HPT it can be reasonably assumed that at least four parathyroids should be found.

The anatomic distribution of the parathyroids is reasonably constant and one finds a rough topographical symmetry on opposite sides of the neck in most cases. The normal anatomic location of the parathyroid glands is shown in Figure 1-1. Unusual or ectopic locations are the result of developmental aberrations or of displacement of glands after they have become enlarged (Fig. 1-2).

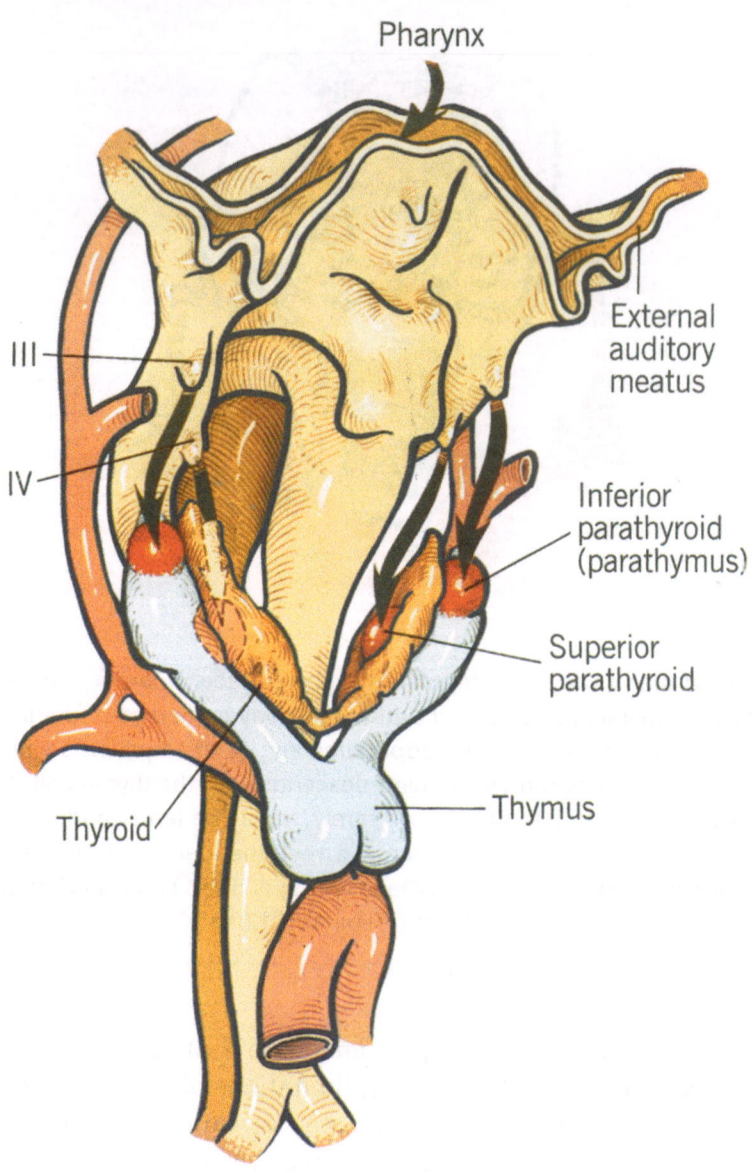

A

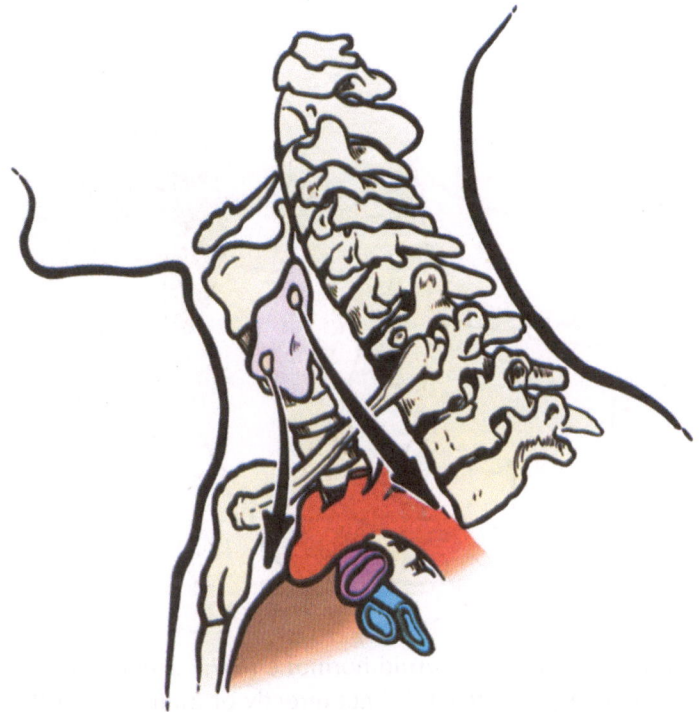

B

Ectopic locations of parathyroid glands. **A.** Developmental aberrations. **Fig. 1-2.**
The superior parathyroid gland on each side develops from the fourth branchial
pouch. From the embryologic standpoint, therefore, the upper glands should
not be found outside the zone bounded by the upper border of the larynx and
the lower pole of the thyroid. The inferior pair of parathyroids develop with the
thymus from the third branchial pouch and may be found anywhere from the
angle of the jaw to the pericardium (12,16,19–22). (After Westwood and
Didusch.) **B.** Displacement of enlarged glands (*arrows*). Parathyroid glands,
when enlarged, may be displaced caudally, in much the same manner as a low-
lying adenoma of the thyroid that eventually becomes substernal (20,21). Tumors of the upper glands are usually displaced down the tracheoesophageal
groove into the posterior mediastinum. Tumors of lower glands are usually displaced into the anterior mediastinum.

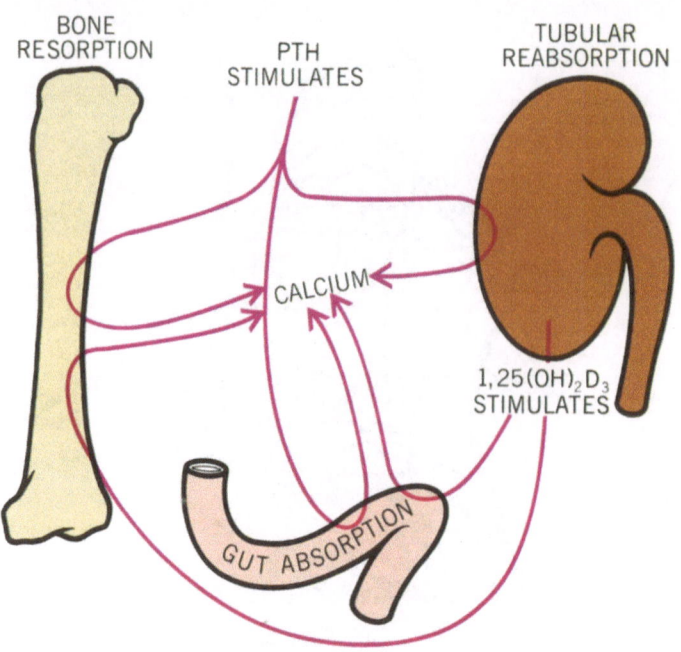

BONE RESORPTION

PTH STIMULATES

TUBULAR REABSORPTION

CALCIUM

$1,25(OH)_2D_3$ STIMULATES

GUT ABSORPTION

Fig. 1-3. **Parathyroid physiology.** Parathyroid hormone (*PTH*), calcitonin (*CT*), and 1,25-dihydroxyvitamin D_3 [*1,25(OH)$_2$D$_3$*] act directly or indirectly on the intestine, kidney, and bone to regulate extracellular fluid calcium homeostasis (23–26). *Vitamin D_3*, a sterol hormone, is obtained from dietary sources and by the action of ultraviolet light on precursors in the skin. This substance is transported to the liver, where it undergoes 25-hydroxylation. Full metabolic activation occurs with a second hydroxylation step in the kidney to form 1,25-dihydroxyvitamin D_3. This process is enhanced by increased levels of PTH and low plasma phosphorus concentrations. 1,25-Dihydroxyvitamin D_3 increases intestinal calcium and phosphorus absorption and enhances calcium and phosphorus mobilization from bone. *Calcitonin* is a polypeptide hormone that is secreted by the parafollicular cells of the thyroid. We still do not know whether this hormone has an important physiologic function in humans, but it is thought to inhibit bone resorption and thus can be considered a counterregulator of PTH. *PTH* is also a polypeptide hormone that is secreted by the parathyroid glands in response to a decrease in the serum ionic calcium concentration. PTH acts to increase the translocation of calcium from bone into plasma, both by enhancing transport of a soluble calcium fraction originating from bone fluid and by stimulating resorption of bone matrix by osteoclasts. The latter action appears to be mediated via cyclic adenosine 3′,5′ monophosphate (cyclic AMP). In the kidney, PTH also acts via cyclic AMP to increase the renal reabsorption of calcium and to inhibit the reabsorption of phosphate (so-called phosphaturic effect). PTH increases the intestinal absorption of calcium, both by a direct action on the gastrointestinal cells and indirectly through stimulating renal synthesis of 1,25-dihydroxyvitamin D_3. Thus, PTH and 1,25-dihydroxyvitamin D_3 are closely coupled, and together they serve to regulate serum calcium levels within a narrow physiologic range. The PTH parent molecule is cleaved into carboxyl(C)-terminal and amino (N)-terminal fragments in the parathyroid gland itself and also peripherally in the liver and kidney. The N-terminal fragment has a very short half-life (less than 10 minutes) and is fully biologically active. The C-terminal fragment has a longer half-life (1–2 hours) and has no known biologic activity. Both the C- and N-terminal fragments are cleared from the plasma by renal excretion.

6

PATHOLOGY

Primary HPT may be caused by an *adenoma,* which is almost always solitary, although on occasion there may be two (27) (Fig. 1-4); by *hyperplasia,* usually involving all four glands (Figs. 1-5 and 1-6); or, rarely, by *parathyroid carcinoma* (Fig. 1-7). The relative incidence of adenoma and hyperplasia was considerably debated during the past decade, but the matter has now been largely resolved. The consensus of opinion is that adenomas are encountered in approximately 80% of cases, chief cell hyperplasia in approximately 20% of cases, and water-clear cell hyperplasia and carcinoma in less than 1% of all cases.

Most experienced pathologists acknowledge that it may be extremely difficult to distinguish histologically between chief cell hyperplasia and adenoma (15,32–35). Likewise, there are no reliable histologic criteria to separate early hyperplasia from normal (15,32,34). Adenomas typically exhibit a compressed rim of normal tissue outside the tumor capsule, but this appearance is also encountered in cases in which the other glands are clearly enlarged and hyperplastic (34).

In the past, it was conventional to describe normal parathyroids as comprising approximately 50% parenchyma and 50% stromal fat. Thus, a decreased amount of stromal fat was equated with hypercellularity and hence hyperfunction. However, a number of anatomic studies have

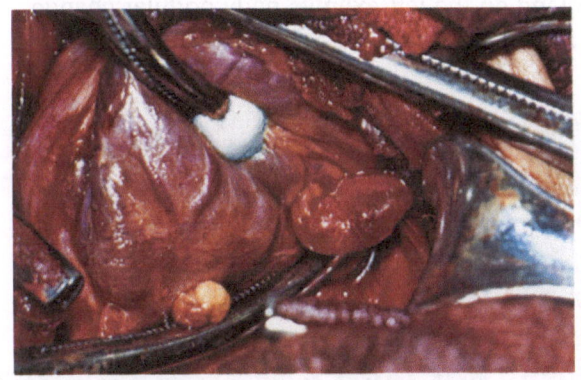
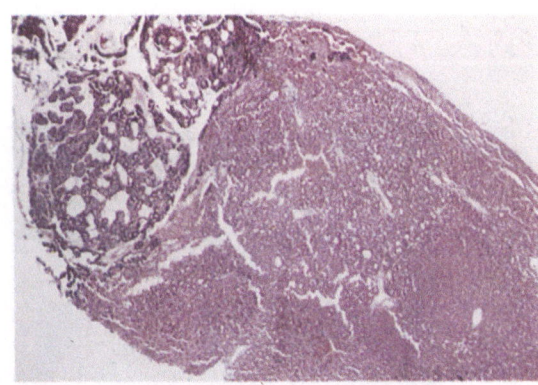

A   B

Parathyroid adenoma. **A.** Adenoma of right inferior gland with a normal superior gland (strap muscles divided). Parathyroid adenomas usually are reddish brown and have a smooth capsule. In general, they are not adherent to surrounding tissues. Most often, they have a soft consistency, although when large, areas of secondary calcification, cystic change, hemorrhage, or necrosis may be seen. They range in size from slightly larger than a normal gland to 20 g or more. Nonadenomatous parathyroid glands, found in association with adenomas, are not atrophic; grossly and histologically they do not differ significantly from normal glands (28). **B.** Microscopic appearance of a typical chief cell adenoma (other adenomas have water-clear cells or oxyphils at the predominant cell type). The cells are closely packed with a diffuse rather than a nodular distribution, and there is little or no fat (lipoadenoma is a rare exception) (29). Note the compressed rim of normal parathyroid tissue seen outside the tumor capsule to the left.   **Fig. 1-4.**

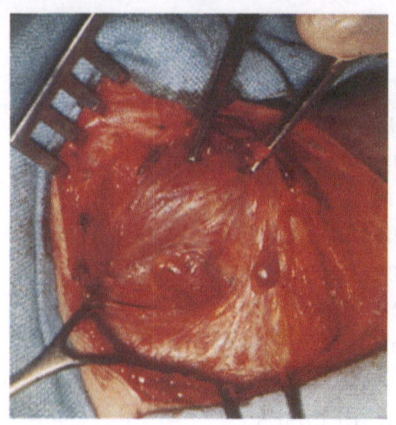
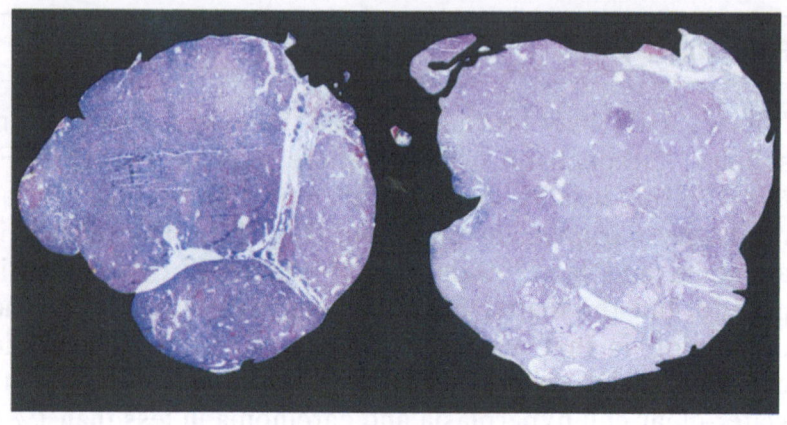

A   B

Fig. 1-5.   Chief cell hyperplasia.   A. Hyperplastic parathyroid glands on the left.
In chief cell hyperplasia the glands may be tan to reddish brown and
either smooth and globular (as in this case) or somewhat nodular. A single hyperplastic gland is indistinguishable from a chief cell adenoma both grossly and
on microscopic examination. Even the rim of compressed normal glandular
tissue outside an adenoma can be simulated in cases of nodular chief cell hyperplasia that has affected only part of the parathyroid. The two conditions are
differentiated by the fact that in hyperplasia more than one gland (usually all
four) is enlarged. Often, the glands are asymmetrically enlarged. Chief cell hyperplasia is usually encountered in the context of familial HPT or MEN.   **B.**
Cross sections of two hyperplastic parathyroid glands (left ×3, right ×2) from
the same patient. The histologic appearance is one of compact increased cellularity and practically no fat. The gland on the left exhibits early nodular change,
whereas that on the right shows a diffuse pattern.

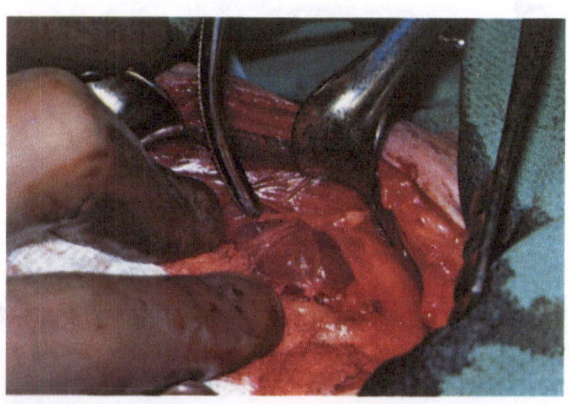
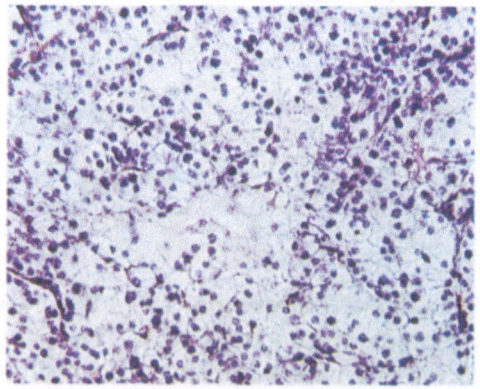

A   B

Fig. 1-6.   Water-clear cell hyperplasia.   A. Hyperplastic right inferior gland with
branches of the recurrent laryngeal nerve stretched across it. In water-clear cell
hyperplasia the glands are distinctively chocolate brown, are often markedly enlarged, and have a notable lobulated contour, often with pseudopods. For some
unknown reason, the upper pair of parathyroids in this condition are usually
much bigger than the lower pair.   **B.** Histology. The glands are composed of
large clear cells arranged uniformly in alveolar pattern.

now documented great variation in the gross and microscopic structure of normal parathyroids (15,18,36) (Fig. 1-8). It is apparent that some normal glands are almost totally devoid of fat (especially those from children and from adults suffering from nutritional depletion), whereas others have an abundant amount of stromal fat (typically, those glands from elderly or obese individuals) (15,18,33). Even within the same gland, it is quite common to find considerable variation in the distribution of parenchymal and fat cells (15,18,36). Thus, to describe properly the microscopic anatomy of a parathyroid, it is necessary to examine several sections from different levels (36). A number of novel methods have been devised to help distinguish between normal, adenomatous, and hyperplastic parathyroid glands. These include density measurements (15,37), estimation of cellular DNA content (38), detection of ABO (H) cell surface antigens (39), and quantitation of intracytoplasmic fat content (40). However, there is not yet proof of the practical value of these techniques by correlation with long-term results of operative treatment.

From a practical point of view, all that the pathologist should be asked to do at the time of operation for HPT is to confirm the identity of biopsied or excised parathyroid glands. Any further attempt to characterize the underlying pathology may only serve to confuse the situation and direct the surgeon to take an inappropriate course of action. The gross findings at operation, coupled with information derived from the clinical history and laboratory data, should dictate the extent of resection (see the section Operative Strategy).

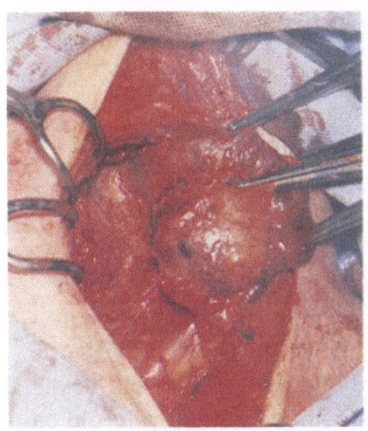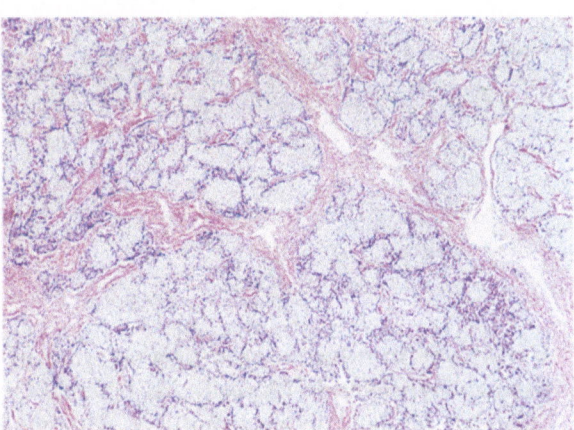

A   B

Parathyroid carcinoma. A. Locally invasive parathyroid carcinoma. Typically, cancerous glands are large and considerably firmer than adenomatous glands. They may be grayish white in color and are often difficult to dissect from adjacent tissues because of local tumor invasion or because of the desmoplastic reaction they incite. Metastasis occurs late in the course, mainly to regional lymph nodes; distant sites of predilection are lungs and bone. **B.** Photomicrograph showing monotonous cell proliferation with thick, fibrous bands separating lobules of tumor. The principal histologic features that distinguish parathyroid carcinoma from adenoma are a trabecular pattern, mitotic figures, thick fibrous bands, and capsular and blood vessel invasion (30,31).

Fig. 1-7.

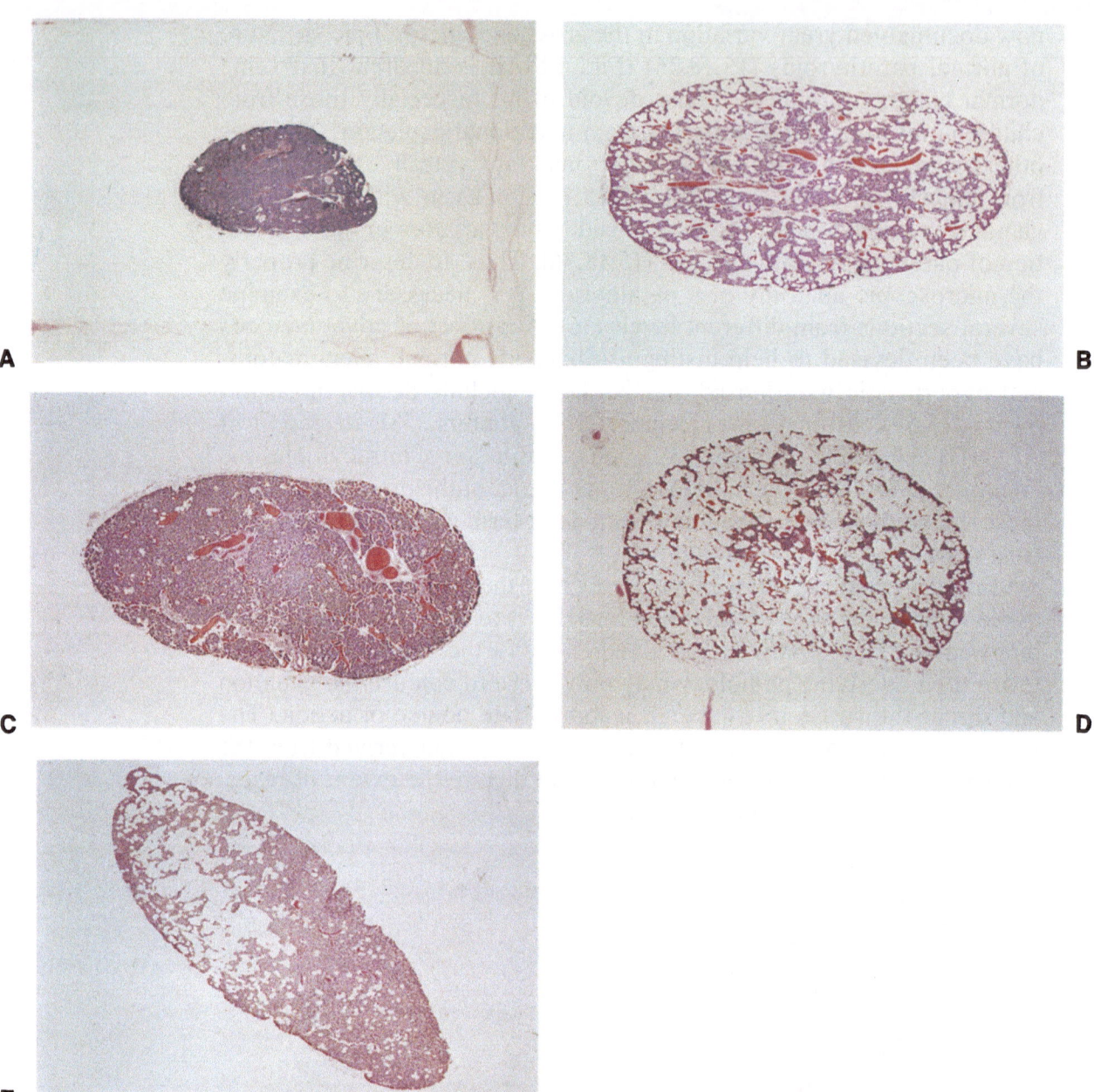

Fig. 1-8. **Variations in microscopic appearance of normal parathyroids (from euparathyroid individuals).** **A.** Minimal fat cell content (2-year-old boy). **B.** "Normal" fat cell content (adult). **C.** Minimal fat cell content (60-year-old cachectic man). **D.** Large number of fat cells (60-year-old obese woman). **E.** Markedly uneven fat cell distribution throughout the gland. (Reprinted by permission from Grimelius L, et al: Pathology Annual, Part II, 1981, pp 1–24. Courtesy of Dr. Henry Johansson, Academic Hospital, Uppsala, Sweden.)

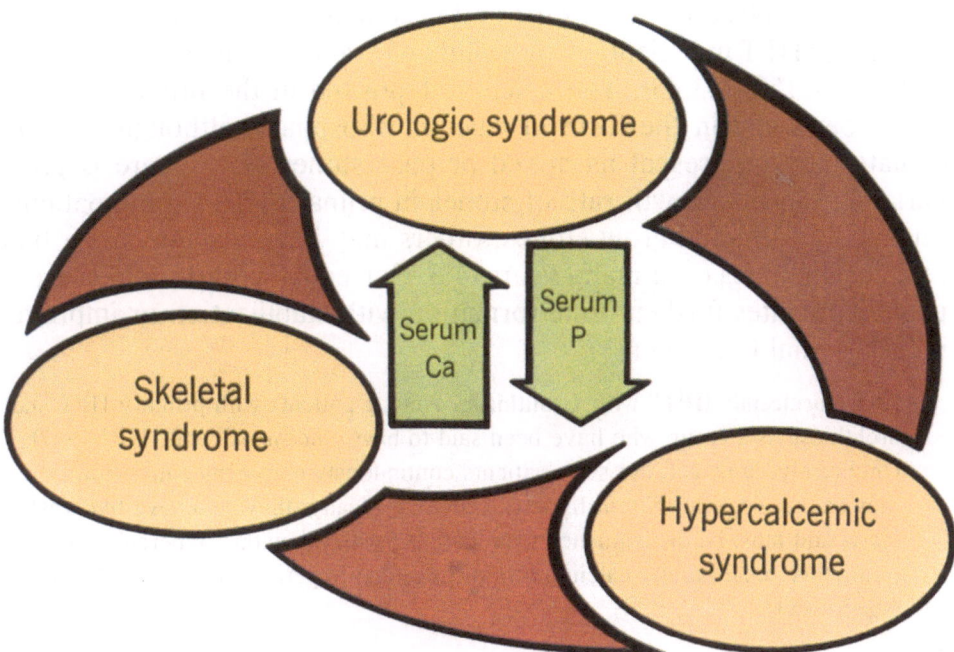

Manifestation of primary HPT. Increased levels of circulating PTH elevate the serum calcium by several actions: bone resorption is increased over bone formation; absorption of calcium from the distal renal tubules is stimulated; and hydroxylation of 25-hydroxyvitamin D_3 to 1,25-dihydroxyvitamin D_3 is stimulated—thus adding the effects of vitamin D to other actions of parathyroid hormone in altering calcium metabolism. The serum phosphorus level is decreased in 50% of cases. The signs and symptoms of primary HPT fall into three categories: those associated with the skeleton, with the urinary tract, or with hypercalcemia per se.

Fig. 1-9.

DIAGNOSIS

CLINICAL FEATURES

The most common mode of clinical presentation today is the serendipitous detection of hypercalcemia by routine, automated biochemical screening of hospital and clinic patients. A recent review of 500 consecutive patients undergoing neck exploration for primary hyperparathyroidism revealed that 60% were picked up in this fashion (41). It is important to note, however, that nearly one-third of these patients had unsuspected complications of their disease—primarily, asymptomatic renal stones. When symptoms are present they are referable to the skeletal or urologic complications of HPT or to hypercalcemia per se (Fig. 1-9) (42–44).

Urologic Syndrome. When complications occur in primary HPT, the most common site is the urinary tract. Urolithiasis and/or nephrocalcinosis (renal parenchymal calcification) was present in approximately one-third of 500 cases in the series referred to above (41). The incidence of primary HPT in patients with urolithiasis ranges from less than 5% to as high as 15% (43,45). The calcium deposited in the urinary tract is most commonly in the form of calcium phosphate, although calcium oxalate may be present as mixed or pure stones (45). There is great variability in the growth rate of stones in primary HPT: some patients repeatedly form and grow stones; others may have a single stone that remains unchanged for many years (46). Corrective parathyroid surgery usually obviates further stone formation with stabilization or improvement of renal function (43).

"Normocalcemic HPT" with Urolithiasis. Among patients with primary HPT and urolithiasis is a group who have been said to have "normocalcemic HPT" (47). Only rarely, however, are such patients continuously normocalcemic—rather, they have mild, intermittent hypercalcemia. Typically, they also have hypercalciuria and must be distinguished from patients with idiopathic hypercalciuria due to primary renal tubular calcium loss or intestinal hyperabsorption of calcium (see below).

Skeletal Syndrome. Diffuse osteitis fibrosa cystica, with bone cysts and pathologic fractures, characterized the first few cases of primary HPT described around the turn of the century. Today, however, this condition is so rare that it is considered a medical curiosity. Conventional x-ray examination of the skeleton disclosed obvious abnormalities in only 10% of 500 surgical cases in our recent experience (41). However, the use of more sensitive techniques such as bone histologic study, radiocalcium measurements, and photon beam densitometry reveals a much greater degree of skeletal involvement (as evidenced by decreased bone mineral content or increased bone turnover) than is visible on standard skeletal x-rays (44). Milder degrees of skeletal involvement may be evident symptomatically as vague aches or bone pains and also as arthralgias.

Hypercalcemic Syndrome. Vague symptoms such as lethargy, fatigue, depression, polyuria, polydipsia, and nonspecific gastrointestinal upset have been ascribed directly to the hypercalcemia of primary HPT. These symptoms may represent the only clinical evidence of HPT and may be so mild and nondescript that the patient recalls them only in retrospect, after successful parathyroid surgery (6,49,50). On occasion, some patients present with marked hypercalcemia and with symptoms so severe that their treatment constitutes a medical and surgical emergency (51–53).

Acute Hypercalcemic Crisis. The crisis is usually due to either primary HPT or malignant disease with or without bone metastases. Anorexia, nausea, vomiting, polyuria, and abdominal pain are the usual presenting symptoms (Fig. 1-10). Within days or even hours, the patient develops dehydration, oliguria, and renal failure. Bone pain, profound muscular weakness, and delerium are sometimes prominent features, and fever, cardiac arrhythmias, and acute pancreatitis have

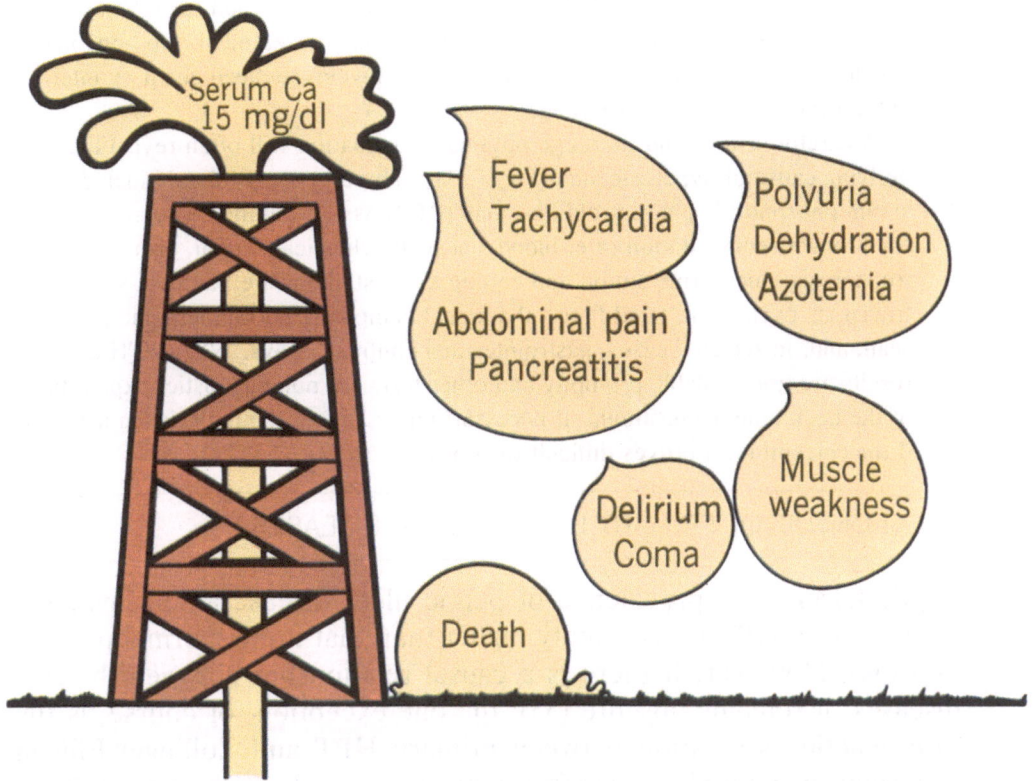

Acute hypercalcemic crisis. When the serum calcium level exceeds 15 mg/
dl, serious complications usually ensue. This catastrophic syndrome is most often caused by disseminated carcinoma with bone metastases (usually breast
carcinoma); however, primary HPT can produce the same picture. Early exploration of the neck is indicated as soon as the diagnosis of primary HPT is confirmed.

Fig. 1-10.

all been described. Without treatment, coma and death will supervene. Serum
calcium levels exceeding 15 mg/dl (3.7 mmol/L)* are critical and urgent treatment is required.

The immediate goals of management are (a) rapid rehydration; (b) concurrent
investigation to determine the cause of hypercalcemia; and (c) restoration of normocalcemia. The standard therapy in the past was to rapidly infuse normal saline intravenously, and then to promote a vigorous diuresis with furosemide (20
mg IV at hourly intervals). Once a diuresis began, the normal saline solution was
infused at a rate equal to the urine output in order to maintain fluid balance. Of
course, potassium depletion had to be anticipated with this regimen and
promptly corrected.

Because there is an inherent danger of potassium depletion with vigorous diuretic therapy, this treatment has been superseded in recent years by therapy
with mithramycin. While hydration is being restored with saline, mithramycin is
given as an intravenous infusion of 25 μg/kg body weight in dextrose or saline
solution over 4 hours. This single dose usually effects a return of the calcium

* To convert mg/dl to mmol/L, multiply by 0.2495.

level to near normal within 24 hours and maintains suppression for several days or more, thereby allowing time to plan more definitive treatment. No bone marrow toxicity has been encountered when mithramycin has been given by intermittent injection in this dose range.

A careful history and thorough physical examination will often reveal the underlying cause of hypercalcemia (Fig. 1-11). Laboratory tests should include a serum phosphorus, parathyroid hormone (PTH) assay, routine hemogram and erythrocyte sedimentation rate, blood smear, biochemical screen, protein electrophoresis, microurine study, and certain x-ray studies—i.e., a chest x-ray, intravenous pyelogram, hand films, abdominal computerized tomographic (CT) scan, and, in selected cases, gastrointestinal contrast x-rays. When PTH assay results are not available promptly and other tests are nondiagnostic, exploration of the neck (and mediastinum, if necessary) may have to be undertaken urgently if the calcium level proves difficult to control.

RELATIONSHIP OF PRIMARY HPT TO OTHER DISEASES

Peptic Ulcer. The prevalence of peptic ulcer disease among patients with primary HPT is reportedly higher than that in the normal population (54). However, if there is a causal relationship between the two diseases, it remains obscure (55); the one exception, of course, is the rare genetic association between primary HPT and Zollinger-Ellison syndrome in multiple endocrine neoplasia type I syndrome (multiple endocrine adenopathy syndrome). Experimentally induced hypercalcemia has been shown to stimulate gastric acid secretion (56), but a definitive clinical study by Wilson and co-workers (57) failed to show any significant increase in either basal or stimulated gastric acid secretion or in serum gastrin levels in patients with HPT. Moreover, parathyroidectomy in these patients did not produce any consistent change in either serum gastrin or gastric acid secretion.

Pancreatitis. Evidence linking pancreatitis to HPT is largely anecdotal, and if such a relationship exists the mechanism is unclear (58,59). The prevalence of pancreatitis in most recent large series of surgically confirmed HPT has been extremely low (1.5% or less), and often other etiologic factors, such as alcoholism or biliary calculi, are present in such patients (10,41,58,59). It remains to be resolved whether or not there is any true causal link between HPT and pancreatitis. From a practical point of view, it is worth emphasizing that the coexistence of these two diseases in the clinical setting does not absolve the physician from making a careful search for other etiologic factors (such as gallstones) that may require treatment to control pancreatitis.

Hypertension. Hypertension is very common among hyperparathyroid patients, occurring in 20%–50% (60). It is also common among persons in the general population of comparable age group. However, a recent age- and sex-matched control study documented a small but statistically

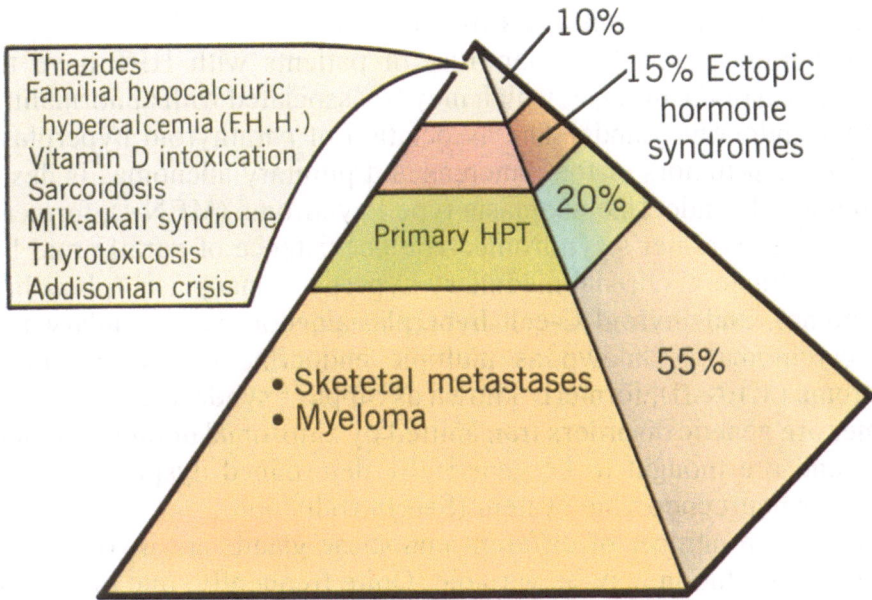

Causes of hypercalcemia: relative frequency. The most common cause of   **Fig. 1-11.**
hypercalcemia *in hospitalized patients* is malignancy—especially multiple
myeloma, breast tumors, and bronchial tumors. Most of these patients (75%)
have obvious metastatic disease at the time of clinical presentation. Malignant
tumors cause hypercalcemia either by bone destruction due to metastases, or
by secreting substances into the general circulation that cause bone resorption.
These substances include a native PTH (so-called ectopic HPT), prostaglandin
E_2, osteoclast activating factor, and an as yet poorly characterized peptide that
mimics some of the physiologic actions of PTH but fails to react with antisera
that recognize PTH (48). It is now thought that most cases of ectopic, humoral,
cancer-associated hypercalcemia are due to this factor. Primary HPT accounts
for about 20% of all cases of hypercalcemia.

significant increase in the risk of definite hypertension in patients with
HPT (5). Surgical correction of HPT did not consistently lower the
blood pressure in these patients.

Thiazides and related diuretics (chlorthalidone) are commonly used as first-time
treatment for hypertension. These drugs may actually produce hypercalcemia,
possibly by decreasing urinary excretion of calcium or by potentiating the action
of PTH.

In normal individuals, any increase in the serum calcium level produced by
thiazide ingestion rarely exceeds 1.0 mg/dl above normal. Moreover, the normal
levels usually return within 1 month after cessation of the treatment. Thus, if the
serum calcium level is higher than 11–11.5 mg/dl or it fails to normalize after
thiazide withdrawal, the patient is likely to have primary HPT (43).

Under these circumstances, parathyroid exploration is usually advised, although the patient may be otherwise asymptomatic with respect to HPT. Even if
restoration of a eucalcemic state is unsuccessful in lowering the blood pressure
in such patients, it will be safe to use thiazides or related diuretics in the treatment of the hypertension postoperatively.

Multiple Endocrine Neoplasia (MEN) Syndromes. In the authors' recent experience (41), less than 10% of patients with HPT have the familial form of the disease, which may be associated with abnormalities of other endocrine glands. The association of parathyroid hyperplasia with islet cell tumors of the pancreas and pituitary adenomas is designated multiple endocrine neoplasia type I syndrome (MEN-I), formerly described as Wermer's syndrome. The coexistence of parathyroid hyperplasia, bilateral adrenal medullary hyperplasia/neoplasia (pheochromocytoma), and thyroid C-cell hyperplasia/neoplasia (medullary thyroid carcinoma) is known as multiple endocrine neoplasia type II syndrome (MEN-II), formerly known as Sipple's syndrome. These syndromes are genetic disorders transmitted by autosomal dominant inheritance and are thought to be genetically determined dysplasias of the APUD or neuroendocrine system (See Introduction).

Because a number of different endocrine glands are involved, the clinical presentation may be variable. Quite frequently, one or another endocrine component is subclinical. When a patient is found to have familial HPT or one of the MEN syndromes it is important to screen other family members for associated endocrinopathies.

It is important in surgical management to recognize that HPT occurring in the context of familial HPT or MEN syndrome is virtually always due to hyperplasia—even though the gross findings at operation may reveal only one or two obviously enlarged glands. If less than a subtotal parathyroidectomy is performed, the disease will probably eventually recur.

Other Purported Associations. Several reports have tried to link various forms of inflammatory joint disease (gout, pseudogout, ankylosing spondylitis, and chondrocalcinosis) with primary HPT. The most common of these joint involvements appears to be chondrocalcinosis, a condition in which there is deposition of calcium pyrophosphate dihydrate and related crystals in articular hyaline and fibrocartilage. It has been described in up to 20%–30% of patients with primary HPT. However, there appears to be no correlation between the serum calcium level and the development of chondrocalcinosis, and successful parathyroid surgery has no predictable effect on this condition.

An increased prevalence of cholelithiasis has also been reported in patients with primary HPT; however, one recent well-controlled study noted the same prevalence of gallstones in normocalcemic age- and sex-matched subjects (61). The purported association between these two common diseases is probably yet another example of the well-known "Berkson bias," whereby selection factors tend to increase the probability that multiple diseases will be found in hospitalized patients when compared with the general population (62).

An association between primary HPT and prior therapeutic irradiation of the neck has been established (62,63); however, it probably accounts for no more than a small proportion of all cases (less than 1%).

LABORATORY STUDIES

The following protocol has proved reliable at the Mayo Clinic in confirming hypercalcemia and establishing the provisional diagnosis of primary HPT (Table 1-1).

Serum Calcium. Hypercalcemia is still the most reliable biochemical sign of primary HPT, although the degree of hypercalcemia may sometimes be trivial or only intermittent. Therefore, at least three blood samples for calcium on three separate days should be obtained in patients suspected of having primary HPT before the diagnosis is excluded (65,66). This is especially important in patients with recurrent nephrolithiasis, in whom borderline or intermittent hypercalcemia is encountered fairly frequently.

The diagnosis of primary HPT in patients with minimal or borderline elevation of serum calcium constitutes a fairly common and difficult problem. Good quality control in the determination of serum calcium and the importance of defining the normal range within narrow confidence limits have long been recognized as essential prerequisites for the reliable diagnosis of HPT.

Oral Calcium Tolerance Test. Broadus et al. (67) recently described a simple oral calcium tolerance test as a means of diagnosing primary HPT in patients with borderline or intermittent hypercalcemia and recurrent nephrolithiasis. These patients with subtle primary HPT display a characteristic pattern of responses following a loading dose of 1000 mg oral calcium—namely, induced hypercalcemia, calciuria, and abnormal parathyroid suppressability as determined by nephrogenous cyclic 3′,5′-adenosine monophosphate (cyclic AMP) activity.

According to Broadus, this test enables one to distinguish between the various forms of hypercalciuria. In patients with renal hypercalciuria there is no hypercalcemic response to an oral calcium load. Approximately 20% of patients with absorptive hypercalciuria display some induced hypercalcemia following the

Laboratory Studies to Establish Primary HPT.   **Table 1·1.**

Serum	Calcium,* phosphorus,* protein electrophoresis, uric acid, alkaline phosphatase, creatinine, PTH (method of Arnaud et al.)
Blood	Erythrocyte sedimentation rate, complete blood count
Urine	Routine analysis, bacteriologic culture (when pyuria, renal lithiasis, or nephrocalcinosis is encountered), calcium, creatinine clearance by 24-hour collection
Roentgenography	Chest, hands (industrial film), skull, excretory urogram (intravenous pyelogram).

From Purnell et al. (65).
* At least three determinations.

oral calcium load, but they show a striking and appropriate suppression of urinary nephrogenous cyclic AMP—in contrast to patients with primary HPT, who show little or no suppression of cyclic AMP.

Primary HPT is only one of a number of different causes of hypercalcemia (see Fig. 1-11). In the past, the diagnosis of primary HPT was made by excluding all other causes of hypercalcemia. Often this involved a long, drawn-out process of diagnostic evaluation. Now that reliable PTH radioimmunoassays are available, the diagnostic process can be substantially shortened by documenting an inappropriate increase in the serum PTH level. There are only three known conditions in which the serum calcium level is elevated and the serum PTH level is simultaneously increased (either absolutely or relative to the calcium level): (a) primary HPT; (b) ectopic HPT, due to elaboration of a PTH-like polypeptide by a nonparathyroid neoplasm; and (c) familial hypocalciuric hypercalcemia (FHH).

Ectopic HPT. Nonparathyroid malignant neoplasms may produce PTH (perhaps as a result of the process of genetic derepression) and thus cause hypercalcemia; this condition is described as "ectopic or pseudo-HPT" (68). Subtle immunologic differences in the serum PTH of patients with true primary HPT and those with ectopic HPT permit differentiation between the two conditions by PTH immunoassay: the latter patients tend to have lower measures levels of PTH at the same level of serum calcium. It would appear from a review of the recent literature, however, that true ectopic secretion of PTH is relatively rare. Most cases of cancer-associated hypercalcemia which were formerly thought to be due to ectopic HPT are now attributed to secretion of another, as yet poorly characterized peptide that resembles PTH in some of its physiologic actions but is not detectable by PTH assay.

Familial Hypocalciuric Hypercalcemia. (familial benign hypercalcemia). This condition was first described by Foley et al. in 1972 (69) and was recently further characterized by Marx (70). It is a genetic disorder transmitted by autosomal dominant inheritance and is characterized by uncomplicated hypercalcemia, inappropriately normal levels of immunoassayable PTH, normal to low serum phosphorus levels, and relative hypocalciuria. The parathyroid glands are grossly and histologically normal in some cases, whereas in others they have been described as hyperplastic. Subtotal parathyroidectomy has no effect on the hypercalcemia, however, total parathyroidectomy produces hypocalcemia. Thus, although the cause of the hypercalcemia in FHH is not known, it is presumably PTH dependent. It has been postulated that the disorder represents a generalized insensitivity to calcium ion (70).

Unlike primary HPT, hypercalcemia in FHH generally begins before age 10 years. The two conditions usually may be distinguished by measuring the ratio of renal calcium clearance to creatinine clearance: a value below 0.01 suggests FHH; above 0.01 primary HPT is more likely. If hypocalciuric hypercalcemia is also found in several relatives, particularly if they are young, the diagnosis of FHH is strongly suggested. The current recommendation is that such patients should be observed rather than undergo cervical exploration.

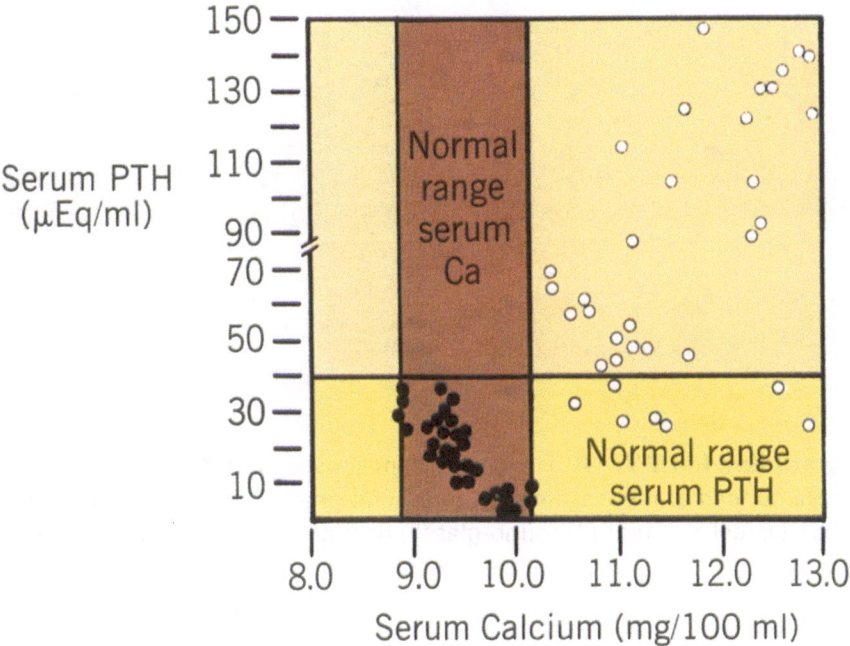

Relationship between serum PTH (C-terminal fragment assay) and serum calcium in normal subjects (●) and patients with surgically proved HPT (○). In normal subjects the concentration of PTH varies inversely with serum calcium, as one would expect in a simple negative-feedback control system. In patients with primary HPT, the serum PTH is *inappropriately* elevated at any given concentration of serum calcium above the normal range. There is a significant positive relationship between the two variables, indicating semiautonomous PTH secretion. (Adapted from Arnaud CD, Tsao HS, Littledike EF: Radioimmunoassay of human PTH in serum. J Clin Invest 50:21–34, 1971.)

Fig. 1-12.

Radioimmunoassay of PTH. As discussed previously, PTH is present in the circulation as several immunologically distinct fragments. It has been empirically demonstrated that assays that are specific for the carboxyl (C)-terminal region of the PTH molecule are far superior to those that are specific for the amino (N)-terminal region in separating normal subjects from patients with primary HPT (23). The greater utility of the anti-C assay may be related to the fact that C-terminal fragments are present in greater quantities than N-terminal fragments or intact PTH in the peripheral circulation of patients with primary HPT. The greater pool size of the C-terminal fragments is probably a function of both their longer half-time of survival and their preferential secretion by some parathyroid tumors.

When the best anti-C PTH assay systems are used, approximately 90% of patients with primary HPT are found to have an absolute increase in their serum PTH level (Fig. 1-12) (71). Even the 10% of patients whose values overlap into the normal range do not present a

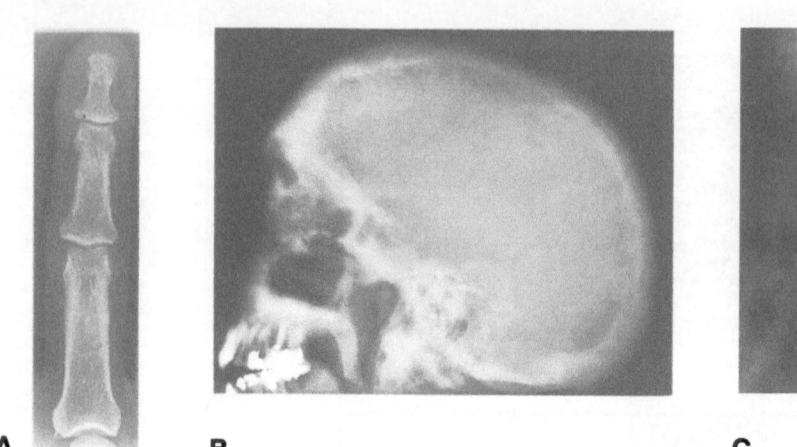
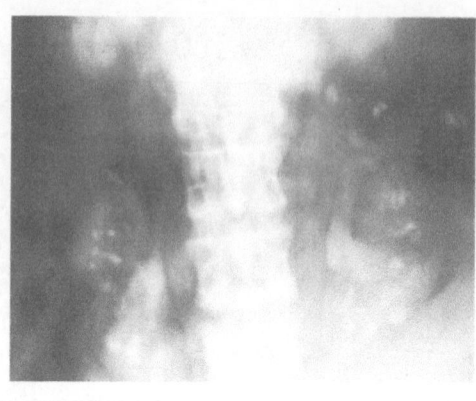

A   B   C

Fig. 1-13.   **X-Ray studies in HPT.**   **A.** Hand x-ray film showing subperiostal resorption most pronounced at the margins of the second phalange.   **B.** Skull x-ray film depicting typical granular ("ground-glass") demineralization.   **C.** Intravenous pyelogram showing advanced bilateral nephrocalcinosis.

major diagnostic problem because *normal levels of PTH in the presence of hypercalcemia represent an inappropriate increase in PTH level* and, as such, are indicative of excess, semiautonomous PTH secretion.

X-Ray Studies. Minimal changes of osteitis fibrosa cystica are best demonstrated by magnified hand x-rays taken on an industrial-grade film (65) (Fig. 1-13A). Fraying of distal phalangeal tufts, subperiosteal resorption of the margins of the phalanges, cysts of the carpal bones, and chondrocalcinosis of the triangular fibrocartilage of the wrist occurred in various combinations in 7.5% of surgical cases in the authors' recent experience (41). Granular "ground-glass" demineralization of the skull usually occurs only in the presence of extensive skeletal demineralization (Fig. 1-13B). Occasionally, the only skeletal x-ray finding may be a solitary bone cyst. Special dental x-ray films may reveal thinning or focal loss of the lamina dura in some patients.

Intravenous pyelography should be performed in all patients being investigated for hypercalcemia unless contraindicated by allergy to contrast dye or heavy proteinuria in a patient suspected to have multiple myeloma. A plain abdominal x-ray is less satisfactory because it does not demonstrate nonopaque oxalate stones and one is more likely to miss a hypernephroma using this technique rather than an intravenous pyelogram (65). Since about one-third of malignant tumors producing PTH-like peptides are hypernephromas, rarely should a patient undergo surgery for suspected primary HPT until adequate x-rays of the kidneys are obtained (65). An additional one-third of patients with ectopic HPT have carcinoma of the lung, usually of the squamous cell type. Thus, a chest x-ray is another essential prerequisite to cervical exploration for suspected HPT. Patients with various malignancies, originating in the gastrointestinal, reproductive, or hematopoietic system, make up the remainder of those with ectopic HPT.

Serum Phosphorus. Although the serum phosphorus level is generally low in patients with primary HPT, true hypophosphatemia (i.e., less than 2.5 mg/dl) is encountered in only 50% of patients (65,66). An elevated serum phosphorus in the presence of hypercalcemia and normal renal function suggests bony metastases or vitamin D intoxication.

Calculating the chloride to phosphorus ratio may be useful, since most patients with primary HPT have serum chloride levels above 102 mEq/liter (due to PTH-induced renal bicarbonate loss). A chloride to phosphorus ratio greater than 33 favors the diagnosis of primary HPT; a ratio less than 30 usually indicates that the hypercalcemia is due to another cause (72).

Ionized Calcium. The determination of serum ionized calcium may be of special value in the diagnosis of primary HPT in patients with recurrent renal calculi and borderline elevations of total serum calcium (72,73). Routine diagnostic use of ionized calcium determinations, however, is not feasible because the laboratory procedure tends to be somewhat tedious and slow and the electrode flow-through system requires frequent servicing. There are also problems with the accurate analysis of frozen serum or serum stored for more than several days.

Urinary Cyclic AMP. Urinary cyclic AMP values expressed in terms of urinary creatinine secretion are capable of separating 70%–80% of patients with primary HPT from normal subjects (74). This diagnostic yield is very similar to that of many serum PTH assays, so that in the absence of a satisfactory C-terminal–specific PTH radioimmunoassay, the measurement of cyclic AMP is helpful. In general, patients with nonparathyroid hypercalcemia (excluding malignancy) have low values of urinary cyclic AMP; in hypercalcemia of malignancy, the available results indicate that cyclic AMP excretion is frequently increased.

Urinary Calcium Excretion. When renal function is normal, hypercalcemia usually results in hypercalciuria due to an increase in the amount of calcium filtered by the kidney. PTH facilitates renal tubular reabsorption of calcium and thereby acts to minimize hypercalciuria in primary HPT. Therefore, hypercalciuria in excess of 500 mg/24 hr is unusual in HPT. In various other hypercalcemic disorders, however, where there is suppression of PTH secretion, comparable levels of serum calcium are often associated with appreciably greater levels of hypercalciuria. The diagnostic usefulness of hypercalciuria is limited by the frequency with which it is observed in renal stone formers who do not have HPT. A relatively low urine calcium output (less than 200 mg/24 hr) despite hypercalcemia is a hallmark of FHH; the importance of the renal calcium clearance to creatinine clearance ratio as a means of distinguishing this entity from primary HPT was discussed above.

Other Tests. Other metabolic tests have been used in the past to help establish the diagnosis of HPT—for example, the tubular reabsorption of phosphate and the cortisone suppression test (Dent test). Serum calcium levels rarely decrease in response to glucocorticoids in patients with primary HPT; they do decrease in about one-half of the patients with malignancy and in virtually all of the patients with sarcoidosis and vitamin D intoxication (75). The usefulness of these tests, however, is limited by false-negative and false-positive results.

PREOPERATIVE LOCALIZATION STUDIES

The surgical treatment of HPT may be complicated by difficulty in locating the parathyroid glands. Even abnormal glands may be small or atypical in appearance and vary in location. The problem is compounded in patients undergoing reexploration of the neck for persistent or recurrent HPT, when scar tissue, anatomic distortion, and bleeding all serve to frustrate the surgeon.

A number of different tests have been devised to help localize parathyroid tumors either preoperatively or intraoperatively. Preoperative studies such as cine esophagography, thermography, and seleomethionine scanning have uniformly proved of little help in the authors' experience because these studies have failed to detect all but the largest of parathyroid tumors (greater than 2 g). The intraoperative use of methylene blue (given as an intravenous infusion over 30 minutes, in a dose of 5 mg/kg body weight diluted in 500 ml normal saline) stains the parathyroids and may possibly assist the inexperienced parathyroid surgeon to identify these glands. However, methylene blue is unlikely to identify tissue that might be overlooked by an experienced surgeon. Moreover, identification of stained glands requires that they be visible. This means that parathyroids that are hidden from view in the mediastinum, within the thyroid, or tucked away in some recess of the neck are not revealed by this technique.

From a practical point of view, there are currently four useful means of preoperative parathyroid tumor localization: selective arteriography and selective thyroid venous sampling for PTH, both of which are invasive studies; and ultrasonography and CT, which are noninvasive.

Arteriography. Studies of the superior and inferior thyroid and internal mammary arteries may demonstrate a parathyroid tumor blush (Fig. 1-4). Because parathyroid tissue is intimately related to thyroid tissue in the neck, arteriography cannot always distinguish the staining of an enlarged parathyroid gland from that of a thyroid nodule. Despite the use of high-resolution magnification techniques, subtraction, and preliminary thyroid scans, arteriography provides accurate prospective localizing information in only 50% of cases (76). This study has proved of greatest value in the localization of mediastinal parathyroid tumors because there is less ambiguity in the interpretation of the stain arising from a branch of the internal mammary artery.

Complications that have been reported with parathyroid arteriography include tetraplegia, hemiplegia, cortical blindness, homonymous hemianopsia, and even death (77–82). The overall risk of complications in experienced hands is very low but the sequelae may be catastrophic. Therefore, the authors believe that arteriography should be reserved for selected cases, as discussed below.

Selective Venous Sampling for PTH. This test is able to lateralize hyperfunctioning parathyroid glands by detecting a localized step-up in hormone concentration in the venous effluent from such glands (Fig. 1-15). The study involves transfemoral, retrograde catheterization of the superior, middle, and inferior thyroid, vertebral, and thymic veins as well as the internal jugular and innominate veins; blood samples for PTH assay are taken from these multiple sites. Usually 15–20 samples are obtained. It requires great skill and patience to catheterize and sample blood from small thyroid veins. The temptation to withdraw the catheter from the small veins (where aspiration of blood is difficult) into larger veins must be avoided because the results of large-vein catheterization studies have proved almost worthless.

Selective venous sampling has proved highly accurate in lateralizing hyperfunctioning parathyroid glands in patients who have not been previously explored (83). However, when there has been previous neck surgery, the venous anatomy and patterns of drainage may be thoroughly distorted, and the study may actually provide misleading information. In order to rationally interpret the venous sampling data in such patients, selective arteriography should be performed prior to venous sampling to identify abnormal venous drainage (81,84). This means, of course, exposing the patient to the potential risks of arteriography and it adds additional cost to what is already an expensive undertaking. The prospective localizing accuracy of selective venous sampling when performed alone in reoperative cases is no better than 40%–50%; when interpreted in the light of a preceding arteriogram, however, it will provide correct localizing or lateralizing information in 70% or more of cases (76,81).

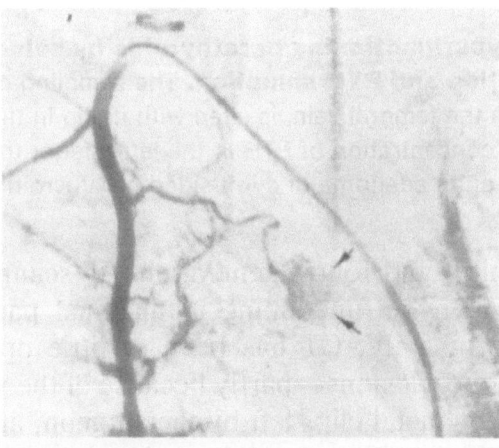

Demonstration of mediastinal parathyroid tumor (arrows) **by selective right internal mammary arteriography.**　　　　**Fig. 1-14.**

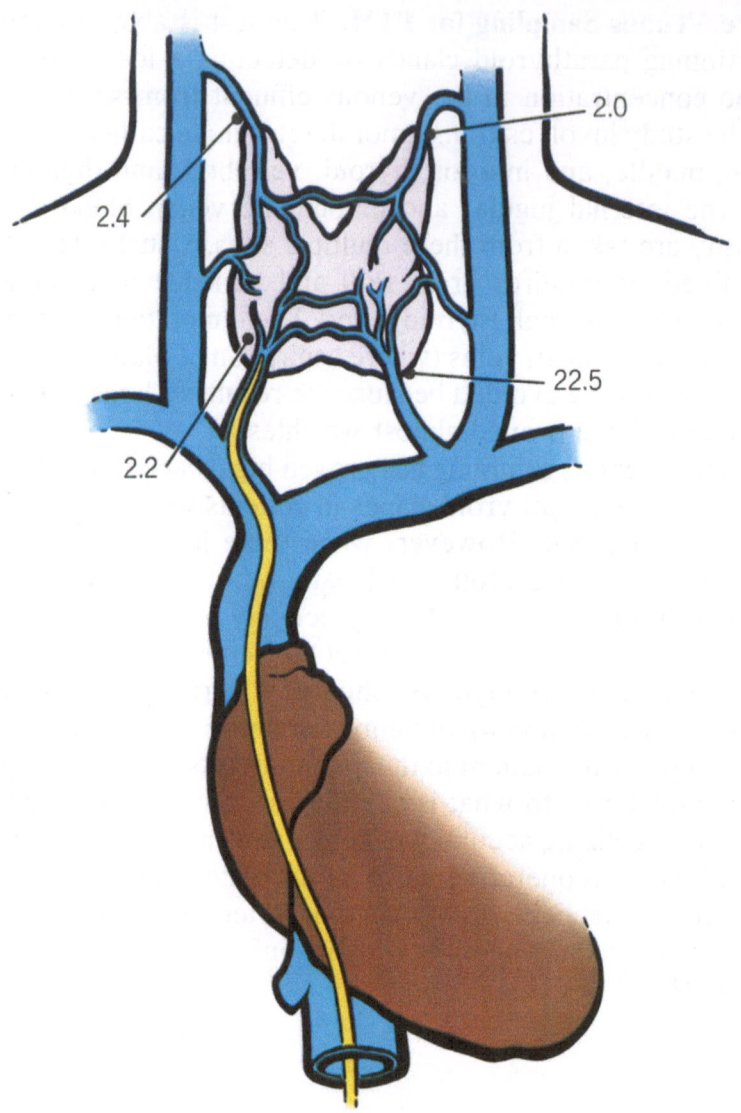

Peripheral level 1.7 ng/ml PTH

Fig. 1-15. Localization of hyperfunctioning parathyroids by selective thyroid venous catheterization and PTH sampling. The sampling catheter, which has been introduced via the femoral vein, is sited with its tip in the right inferior thyroid vein. The high concentration of PTH in the left inferior thyroid vein indicates the presence of an adenoma of a left-sided parathyroid gland.

CT Scanning. Third- and fourth-generation CT scanners have proved useful in detecting hyperfunctioning mediastinal parathyroid tumors (Fig. 1-16). Unfortunately, CT has been of little or no value in the localization of cervical lesions—partly because of the so-called sparkler artifact produced by metal clips left by the surgeon, and partly because the x-ray attenuation coefficients of thyroid and parathyroid tissues are too similar.

CT scanning for the detection of mediastinal tumors should be performed using a state-of-the-art fast scanner with 1-cm serial sequential

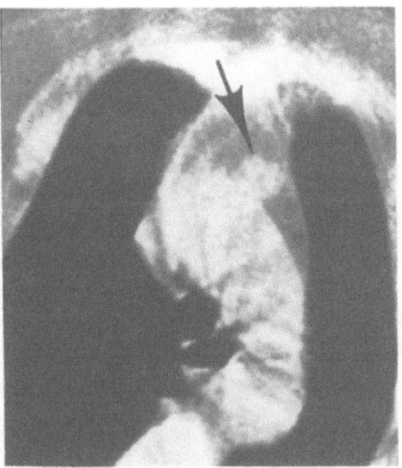

Positive mediastinal CT scan showing a parathyroid adenoma embedded in the thymus gland just anterior to the aortic arch (*arrow*). **Fig. 1-16.**

overlapping scans extending from low in the neck to the tracheal bifurcation. Scans should be obtained before and during the intravenous infusion of contrast material into both arms; this improves the definition of some glands and permits the separation of soft tissue and vascular structures.

In a recent prospective review of 56 mediastinal CT scans performed in 54 patients undergoing reoperation for persistent or recurrent primary HPT, 10 of 20 mediastinal parathyroid tumors were identified, for an overall accuracy of 50% (85); the smallest tumor was 1.5 cm in diameter. There were 4 false-positive scans: tumors that were thought to have been seen in the mediastinum were discovered at operation to be in the neck. In view of the significant number of false-positive scans, the authors are reluctant to proceed directly with median sternotomy unless they can be sure that the neck has been thoroughly and systematically explored at the previous operation.

Ultrasonography. Conventional B-mode, gray-scale ultrasonography of the neck can identify large parathyroid tumors (greater than 1 cm in diameter) with fair accuracy. However, a significant proportion of abnormal glands encountered in most contemporary surgical series are smaller than 1 cm in diameter and would therefore escape detection with conventional ultrasonic scanning. Of course, ultrasound cannot detect retrosternal glands. The new generation of high-resolution, real-time ultrasound instruments (10 MHz) are able to identify parathyroid tumors as small as 3 mm (86,87) (Fig. 1-17). Thus it can be expected that the great majority of parathyroid adenomas will be suitable for detection by means of high-resolution ultrasonography.

This technique has some obvious advantages over other preoperative localizing tools in that it is safe, simple, noninvasive, and relatively inexpensive, and operation of the equipment requires no special skills.

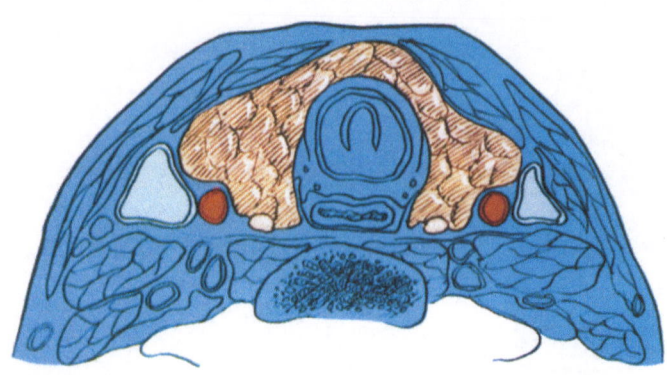
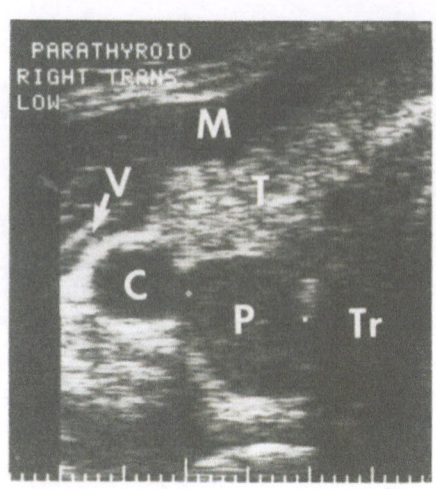

A

B

Fig. 1-17. **High resolution real-time ultrasonography.** **A.** Cross-sectional cervical anatomy demonstrates normal relationships of muscles, thyroid, vessels, trachea, and parathyroids. **B.** Parasaggital sonogram shows a 1-cm parathyroid adenoma (*P*), thyroid (*T*), strap muscle (*M*), trachea (*Tr*), jugular vein (*V*), and carotid artery (*C*). (From Grant CS, vanHeerden JA, Goellner JR: New diagnostic techniques in endocrine surgery. In Farnell MB, McIlrath DC (eds): Problems in General Surgery 1:141–153, 1984.)

Real-time, high-resolution scanners are now commercially available and it is expected that these instruments will find widespread future application in the preoperative localization of parathyroid tumors.

An experienced parathyroid surgeon will be able to identify and remove abnormal glands for cure in 90%–95% of cases of primary HPT at the *initial cervical exploration* without any assistance from preoperative tumor localization studies. Given the success of real-time ultrasonography in several studies, however, one might anticipate future routine use of this inexpensive and noninvasive localizing technique in this setting. CT scanning of the mediastinum prior to initial cervical exploration cannot be justified. Hyperfunctioning mediastinal parathyroid tumors are very rare (less than 1% of all patients with primary HPT); consequently, the cost–benefit ratio of routine CT scanning would be extremely high. There is also the problem of false-positive scans. Certainly, invasive methods, such as arteriography or venous sampling, have no place prior to the initial exploration of the neck.

In the patient who has *previously undergone an unsuccessful neck exploration* for primary HPT, real-time ultrasonography of the neck and CT scanning of the mediastinum should be done. The authors do not perform arteriography and venous sampling unless they can be certain from a careful study of the prior operative findings and pathology reports that the patient has already had a thorough and systemic exploration of the neck (see the section, Operative Strategy).

Obviously, the investigation and treatment of patients with persistent or recurrent hypercalcemia following unsuccessful parathyroid surgery should be carried out in those referral centers equipped with the necessary radiographic and surgical expertise.

TREATMENT

The only effective treatment of primary HPT is surgical. Pharmacologic treatment has been tried—with inorganic phosphate, calcitonin and recently with cimetidine (88) and with propranolol (89)—but has not proved satisfactory in the long term.

INDICATIONS FOR OPERATION

Surgery is recommended for all patients with *symptomatic or complicated disease* and for those patients whose *serum calcium levels exceed 11 mg/dl.* It may be difficult to evaluate nonspecific hypercalcemic symptoms such as lethargy, fatigue, and depression (90); this is especially true in the elderly patient, in whom such symptoms are frequently interpreted by indicating other disease or senile dementia. Several authors, however, have drawn attention to the fact that surgical correction of HPT in the elderly patient often leads to a remarkable improvement in mental and neuromuscular complaints and they have little hesitation in recommending operation in such patients (50,91).

There seems to be general agreement that parathyroid exploration should be recommended for hypertensive patients with primary HPT—even if they are otherwise asymptomatic with respect to their parathyroid disease. Their hypertension may be cured or ameliorated and, in those cases where the blood pressure does not return to normal, thiazides can be safely used postoperatively in the treatment of any residual hypertension.

For patients with *asymptomatic, uncomplicated primary HPT, in whom the serum calcium level is less than 11 mg/dl*—that is, so-called "biochemical HPT"—there are two management choices: surgery, which is curative; or careful surveillance, which is not. The results of a 10-year prospective follow-up study of 147 patients with untreated biochemical HPT were recently published (46,92). The study was designed to determine the frequency with which asymptomatic disease became symptomatic and to identify those patients most likely to experience later complications. After 10 years, 35 patients (24.6%) had come to surgical exploration, 24 (16%) of these because they had developed renal or skeletal complications of their disease. There were difficulties in determining the precise status of the disease in many of the remaining patients, but the authors could detect no obvious trends toward the late development of progressive renal failure or urolithiasis. Moreover, they were not able to identify any factors at the time of the patient's initial presentation that would enable them to predict the ultimate need for surgical intervention.

From this study we can conclude that many patients with the provisional diagnosis of primary HPT do not have a clinically progressive form of the disease and can be observed safely without surgical treatment. However, it is also clear that some 15%–20% of patients develop clinically evident renal or bone disease within 5–10 years of diagnosis. Furthermore, careful medical follow-up of patients with untreated HPT is often time consuming and frustrating, because patient interest and cooperation are difficult to sustain. Many patients are simply not willing to commit themselves to a carefully supervised medical follow-up program.

There are also economic considerations. According to Hodgson and Heath (93), adequate medical follow-up should include the following: an annual assessment of the patient's general health; measurement of serum calcium, phosphorus, and alkaline phosphatase; determination of renal function; x-ray evaluation for metabolic stone disease; and measurement of urinary calcium excretion. The annual cost of these tests is approximately 20% of initial diagnostic studies and surgical treatment (5,93). One might seriously question the cost-effectiveness of such a follow-up program.

In the authors' opinion, surgical therapy for patients with asymptomatic, uncomplicated primary HPT is recommended for the following reasons: (a) It offers safe, definitive treatment and a precise diagnosis. In the hands of an experienced parathyroid surgeon the cure rate is approximately 95% (41,94–96). (b) It would appear to be more cost-effective than long-term follow-up (93) and is more practicable and acceptable to most patients (92,93). (c) Renal damage and progressive bone disease occur in about 15%–20% of patients who are left untreated (92,97). There is also now considerable evidence that most patients with asymptomatic HPT are losing bone and are consequently at risk of developing osteoporosis in the long term (94,98,99). Successful parathyroidectomy normalizes bone turnover in these patients, just as it does in symptomatic patients (94).

Of course, patients who choose not to have surgery or who have serious medical contraindications to surgery must have careful long-term follow-up.

OPERATIVE STRATEGY

In view of the uncertainty surrounding the histologic diagnosis of parathyroid disease, the surgeon must depend ultimately upon the gross findings at operation, correlated with knowledge of the clinical history and laboratory data, to distinguish between single-gland and multiple-gland disease and to make a decision regarding specific surgical treatment (7,32,41).

The authors employ the following operative strategy:

A reasonable effort is first made to *identify all four parathyroid glands* in every case. Biopsy of normal-sized glands is performed only if there is some doubt as to their identity.

If only *one or two glands are grossly enlarged* (estimated weight of each greater than 70 mg), and the patient does not have familial HPT or MEN syndrome, then only the enlarged glands are removed.

If *three or more glands are grossly enlarged,* or the patient has familial HPT or MEN syndrome, a subtotal parathyroidectomy is done to remove all but 50 mg of viable parathyroid tissue.

Total Parathyroidectomy with Heterotopic Autotransplantation. Wells et al. (14) have advocated total parathyroidectomy with autotransplantation of a portion of one gland to the muscles of the forearm rather than subtotal parathyroidectomy in cases of multiple-gland disease. They cite a high rate of recurrent HPT after conventional subtotal parathyroidectomy. Their rationale for autotransplantation is that if recurrent HPT does occur in these patients, it can be dealt with simply by removal of a portion of the graft from the forearm under local anesthesia. However, in our experience (100) and that of others (101,102), true recurrent HPT is extremely uncommon following subtotal parathyroidectomy for chief cell hyperplasia. There would appear, therefore, to be no advantage in performing total parathyroidectomy and autotransplantation for primary chief cell hyperplasia. There may even be significant disadvantages, such as a higher incidence of postoperative hypoparathyroidism while waiting for the grafts to function; there also appears to be an unusual propensity for subsequent overgrowth of grafted parathyroid tissue to cause recurrent hypercalcemia. Wells et al. (103) reported recurrent HPT due to graft overgrowth in as many as 60% of patients with familial HPT and up to 11% of patients with nonfamilial HPT within 5 years of autotransplantation; these figures are much higher than those reported after conventional subtotal parathyroidectomy (100,101,102).

At the present time, we would resort to parathyroid autotransplantation in cases of primary HPT only as a means of preserving a parathyroid remnant that was devitalized in the course of subtotal parathyroidectomy. This should be a rare occurrence if proper precautions are taken to prepare a suitable remnant prior to removal of any of the parathyroids. If the first attempt to secure a viable remnant is unsuccessful, the surgeon will then have several more chances at it. The remnant is tagged with a long silk suture to facilitate its identification should subsequent operation ever be required.

If preliminary bilateral dissection fails to reveal any abnormal parathyroid glands, biopsies are taken from all normal-sized glands to confirm their identity and the exploration is systematically widened to look for the missing glands. The dissection is extended as far as possible under direct vision into the anterior and posterior mediastinum and the thymus is removed for careful sectioning. The retroesophageal and retropharyngeal space is examined next, and then the region alongside the larynx above the upper pole of the thyroid reaching up as far as the angle of the jaw. The carotid sheath is also opened and explored. Finally, the authors recommend subtotal resection of the thyroid gland on the side of the missing gland to look for an intrathyroid parathyroid tumor. Formal mediastinal exploration via a median sternotomy should not be performed at the initial operation unless the patient is in parathyroid crisis.

If four normal-sized glands are found, their identity is confirmed by biopsy and an adenoma of a supernumerary parathyroid gland is sought. If none is found, the normal-sized glands are left in situ and marked with long silk sutures for future identification. Should subsequent study confirm the diagnosis of primary HPT, efforts are then made to localize the missing tumor prior to reoperation.

> Roth et al. (104) advocated that if initial exploration of one side of the neck reveals an enlarged gland and a normal-sized parathyroid it is not necessary to explore the opposite side. However, we have encountered "double adenomas" in up to 5% of our patients (27), and very often the second tumor was found on the contralateral side of the neck. Bruining et al. (95) carefully charted the location of enlarged parathyroid glands at operation in 615 patients explored for primary HPT: had Roth's principle been followed in this particular surgical series, up to 15% of the multiple parathyroid tumors encountered would have been overlooked because they were situated on the opposite side of the neck.

POSTOPERATIVE MANAGEMENT

In most patients the postoperative care is straightforward. The serum calcium level usually returns to normal within 12–36 hours; subsequently, temporary hypocalcemia (rarely symptomatic) may occur, but by the morning of the third postoperative day the serum calcium is usually returning to the normal range and the patient can be discharged from the hospital.

The risk of death from this operation is essentially no higher than that for the associated general anesthetic. Morbidity due to injury to the recurrent laryngeal nerves should be entirely avoidable except in those rare incidences where local invasion by parathyroid carcinoma requires sacrifice of the nerve. It should be mentioned however, that transient vocal cord dysfunction will be encountered from time to time after a straightforward cervical exploration (less than 3% of all patients). This is probably due to some edema of one or another recurrent nerve secondary to minor operative trauma. Complete recovery can be expected within 4–6 weeks (41). The only other significant complication that may be encountered is symptomatic hypocalcemia. This is usually transient, but in 1%–2% of patients it may be permanent.

POSTOPERATIVE HYPOCALCEMIA

A certain degree of hypocalcemia after parathyroidectomy is not entirely unwelcome because it gives some assurance of cure. However, hypocalcemia that is sufficient to cause symptoms represents significant morbidity and should be avoided if at all possible. Hypocalcemia after parathyroidectomy is caused either by hypoparathyroidism (when the level of serum phosphorus is high) or "bone hunger" (when the serum phosphorus level is low)—the rapid accretion of calcium into demineralized bone after correction of the hyperparathyroid state. Bone hunger is most likely to occur in the 5% of patients who have obvious radiologic evidence of osteitis cystica.

In general, treatment of hypocalcemia is not indicated unless symptoms are present. Apprehension, anxiety, hyperventilation, and circumoral and acral paresthesias are the earliest symptoms; Chvostek's sign is positive at this stage. (Remember, however, that 10% of the normal population have a positive Chvostek's sign; this should be checked before operation.) Treatment should be initiated before Trousseau's sign becomes positive because this tends to occur late and is usually an indication of severe hypocalcemia with impending carpopedal spasm, laryngeal stridor, and convulsions. A blood sample should always be drawn to check the serum calcium level before any calcium treatment is administered (the same clinical picture may be produced by alkalosis due to hyperventilation). It is reasonable, of course, to embark on therapy while awaiting the laboratory result.

The *mild symptoms* of hypocalcemia usually respond well to oral calcium, either calcium carbonate or calcium lactate, administered every 6 hours. Calciferol (50,000 IU daily), dihydrotachysterol (1.25 mg daily), or 1,25-dihydroxyvitamin D_3 (0.25-1 μg daily) may be added to enhance calcium absorption if oral calcium alone is not sufficient to maintain a normal serum level. 1,25-Dihydroxyvitamin D_3 has the advantage of rapid onset and offset of its biologic effects; however, it is expensive.

Urgent intervention is required for *severe symptoms* with cramps and carpopedal spasm. Immediate relief is afforded by an intravenous bolus infusion over 10 minutes of a 10% solution of calcium gluconate, with the pulse monitored all the time; repeated injections may be required to relieve the crisis. Subsequent calcium needs over the next 6 hours or so can best be met by a continuous infusion of calcium (15 mg elemental calcium/kg body weight) (53).

> Each 10-ml ampule of 10% solution of calcium gluconate contains approximately 100 mg elemental calcium. Thus, for a patient weighing 60 kg, nine ampules should be added to 500 ml normal saline to be infused over 6 hours.

The serum calcium level can be monitored throughout the infusion and appropriate adjustments can be made to the rate of infusion. Oral calcium and vitamin D therapy can be started at the same time. Since hypomagnesemia can delay the therapeutic response to calcium in tetany, serum magnesium levels should be checked and corrected if low.

It is usual to discontinue the use of the vitamin D preparation after normocalcemia has been maintained for several weeks. Ultimately, the oral calcium supplement can also be stopped if parathyroid function returns.

PERSISTENT OR RECURRENT HYPERCALCEMIA

Persistent hypercalcemia usually results from the failure to find a single parathyroid adenoma, most often located somewhere in the neck (14,105–108). Most authors blame such failures on the surgeon's lack of familiarity with the anatomy and topography of the parathyroids and stress the importance of centralizing the treatment of HPT to clinics where there are surgeons experienced in parathyroidectomy and pathologists accustomed to the histology of the parathyroid glands. Other, less frequent causes of persistent hypercalcemia include the following: unusual, ectopic locations of parathyroid glands, including supernumerary glands (109,110) either in the neck or in the mediastinum (82,111); failure to recognize and adequately treat multiglandular disease; and preoperative misdiagnosis (i.e., hypercalcemia due to a nonparathyroid cause, such as malignancy or FHH).

Hypercalcemia recurring after a normocalcemic postoperative period of at least 6 months (112) implies enlargement and hyperfunction of a parathyroid gland or glands identified at operation as normal. Usually hyperplasia is the culprit, and the patients frequently have the familial form of HPT or one of the MEN syndromes (102). Alternatively, the problem may be one of locally recurrent or metastatic parathyroid carcinoma. Recurrence from heterotopic parathyroid autotransplants has also been described (as discussed above). The authors' experience, as well as that of others (105–108), underscores the fact that persistent rather than recurrent HPT is the major indication for reoperation.

Strategy and Technique of Reoperative Parathyroid Surgery for Persistent or Recurrent HPT (20,112–114). The first step is to confirm the diagnosis of primary HPT. The decision to pursue any further treatment is based on an assessment of the severity of the disease and any associated operative risk factors.

If reexploration is warranted, the next step is to review all of the previous operative notes, pathology reports, and histologic sections; one can generally ascertain the nature of the underlying parathyroid pathology.

If this review of all the available information indicates that the *patient has had a thorough and systematic cervical exploration,* an ultrasound study of the neck and CT scan of the mediastinum should be performed. Invasive localizing studies, such as arteriography and selective venous sampling, should be considered only if the noninvasive studies are not revealing.

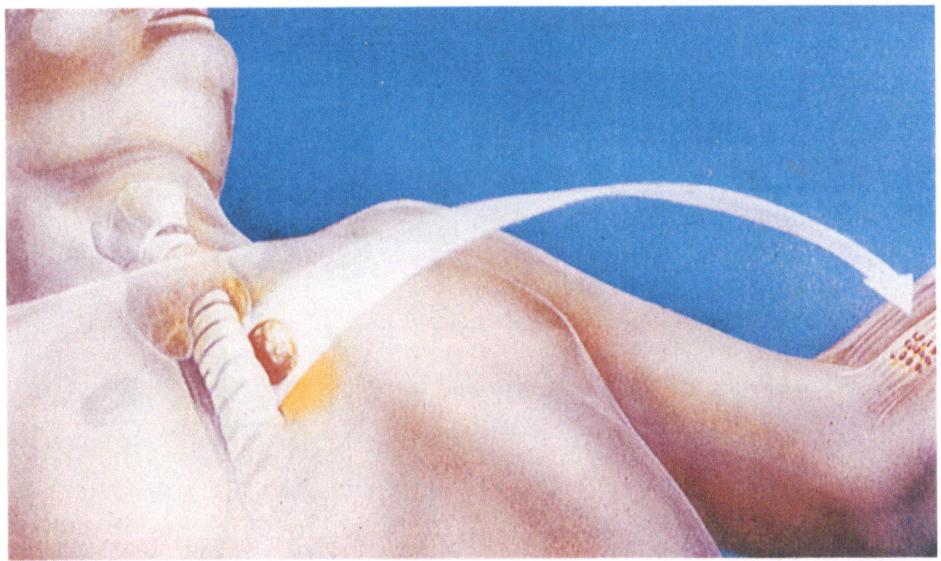

A

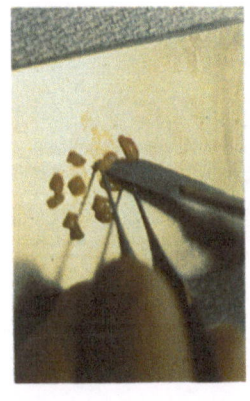

B

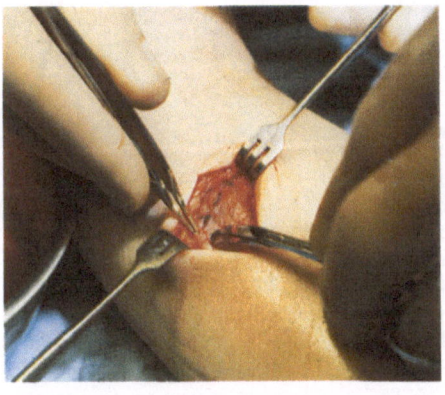

C

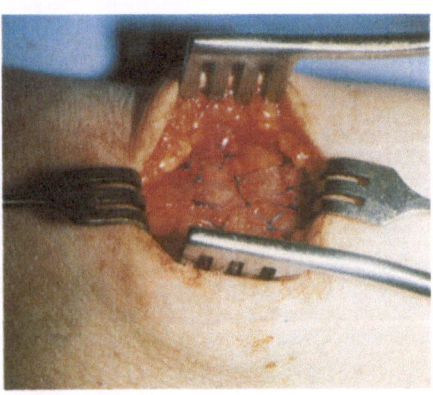

D

Heterotopic parathyroid autotransplantation. This technique has been
employed in conjunction with total parathyroidectomy in the treatment of primary and secondary chief cell hyperplasia (see text). Another useful application
has been in the prevention and treatment of postoperative hypoparathyroidism
which may follow successful reoperation for persistent or recurrent primary HPT
when the normal parathyroid glands have been destroyed or removed at previous operation.   **A.** Schema of immediate autotransplantation of portion of hyperfunctioning mediastinal parathyroid adenoma to the forearm musculature if
three normal parathyroid glands have been removed at a previous operation.
B. Portion of parathyroid is diced into 10–15 pieces measuring 1 × 1 × 3 mm.
C. A series of individual pockets are created in the exposed flexor muscle bel-
lies of the forearm to receive the pieces.   **D.** Sutures of nonabsorbable suture
material are used to close the mouth of each pocket so as to prevent extrusion
of the graft and to mark its position in the event that subsequent removal is ne-
cessitated by graft-dependent hypercalcemia. (Parts A–D from Edis AJ, Beart
RW Jr: Parathyroid autotransplantation: An innovative approach. Hosp Pract Jan
1979, pp 78–84. Part A by Carol Donner.) (*Cont.*)

Fig. 1-18.

DEMONSTRATION OF
PARATHYROID GRAFT FUNCTION

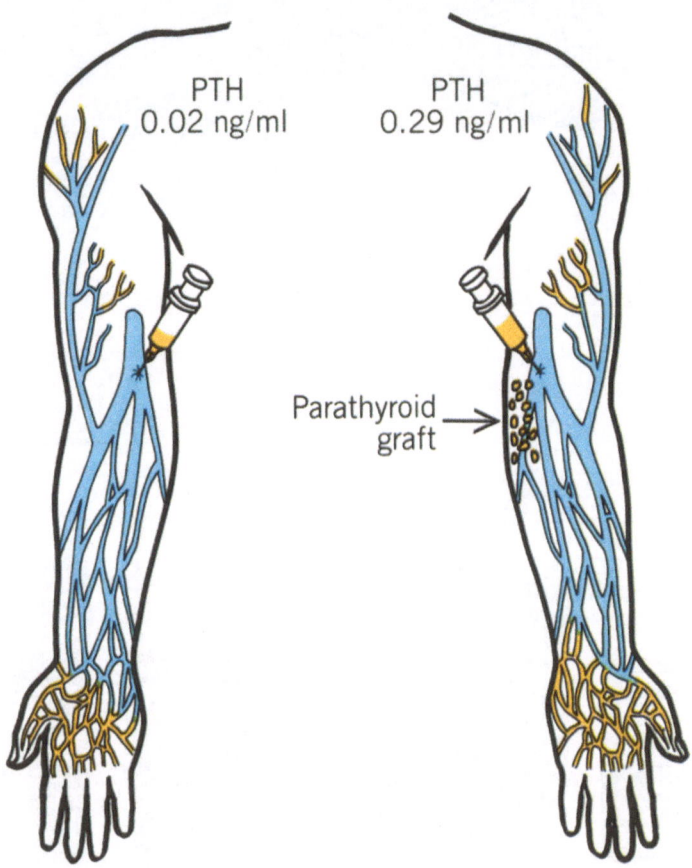

Fig. 1-18. **E.** Function of the parathyroid autotransplants is confirmed by detecting a
(Cont.) higher PTH concentration in the effluent venous blood sampled from the ante-
cubital vein on the grafted side compared with the nongrafted side.

When it is felt that the *patient has had a less than adequate initial
cervical exploration,* invasive localizing studies are not undertaken but
an ultrasound and CT scans are obtained. A clearly positive mediastinal
CT scan would lead directly to a median sternotomy. Otherwise, one
proceeds initially with reexploration of the neck, being prepared to
extend the dissection into the chest via a median sternotomy should the
neck exploration prove fruitless.

After the missing hyperfunctioning gland(s) have been found and
removed, consideration must be given to parathyroid transplantation.
The best course is to cryopreserve the resected gland and observe the
postoperative serum calcium response. Autotransplantation of portion
of the abnormal gland can be performed subsequently should postoperative hypoparathyroidism develop and persist longer than 6 months (115)
(Fig. 1-18). Brennan and Brown (116) and Saxe and Brennan (117) have
further refined this protocol by testing the cryopreserved tissue in vitro

for evidence of autonomous function. When they find that PTH secretion by the tissue cannot be suppressed by increasing the ambient calcium concentration of the culture medium, they do not transplant the tissue for fear that it might proliferate locally and cause graft-dependent hypercalcemia. According to these workers, only suppressible parathyroid tissue should be autotransplanted.

Obviously, the evaluation and treatment of this special group of patients with recurrent or persistent HPT should be undertaken only by an experienced team in a large referral center that is equipped with facilities for tumor localization, tissue cryopreservation, and tissue culture. Under these circumstances, reoperative parathyroid surgery is successful in approximately 85%–90% of cases.

Secondary Hyperparathyroidism

In most, if not all, patients with chronic renal failure, hyperplasia of the parathyroid glands develops to some degree. The stimulus to hyperplasia of the parathyroids appears to be hypocalcemia, which is due to several factors (118–121): (a) phosphate retention resulting from the inability of the diseased kidneys to excrete the phosphate load (hyperphosphatemia leads to a reciprocal fall in the ionized serum calcium); (b) decreased gut absorption of the calcium, due to decreased production of 1,25-dihydroxyvitamin D_3 (a function of the decreased renal mass and high blood phosphate levels). There is excessive secretion of PTH by the hyperplastic glands and, as renal failure progresses, there is also decreased renal clearance of the hormone, which contributes to the hyperparathyroidism (119). The combination of hypocalcemia, hyperphosphatemia, and markedly elevated PTH in chronic renal failure is known as secondary HPT.

SIGNS, SYMPTOMS, COMPLICATIONS

As a result of the increased levels of PTH and deficiency of 1,25-dihydroxyvitamin D_3, there is excessive bone resorption and defective bone mineralization that can eventually lead to disabling symptoms of bone pain and pathologic fractures, so-called renal osteodystrophy. The radiologic features of uremic bone disease may include the following: subperiosteal resorption and bone cysts due to osteitis fibrosa; areas of increased radiolucency of bone (i.e., pseudofractures) due to osteomalacia; aseptic necrosis of the femoral heads; and, in children, slipped epiphyses, metaphyseal fractures, and sometimes osteosclerosis ("rugger-jersey spine") (118,121–124).

Soft tissue calcification is a common complication of secondary HPT and is particularly likely to occur when the calcium–phosphate (mg/dl) product exceeds 70. Vascular calcification may be associated with the rare complication of ischemic necrosis of the skin. Periarticular calcification may cause rheumatolgic problems with tendonitis, tendon rupture, and limitation of joint movement. Ocular calcification is occasionally symptomatic, causing conjunctival irritability.

Other manifestations attributed to secondary HPT include psychoneurologic disorders, muscle weakness (proximal myopathy), headaches, weight loss, easy fatigability, decreased myocardial contractility, and anemia. Many of these complications can be prevented and often reversed by proper medical management (118,121).

CLINICAL MANAGEMENT

Management should first be directed at prevention by trying to maintain the serum calcium and phosphate levels within the normal range. If secondary HPT develops despite all preventive measures (and renal transplantation is not feasible for one reason or another), then parathyroidectomy may be indicated. Approximately 5% of patients require parathyroidectomy and most can be expected to benefit from the procedure (121).

NONSURGICAL

Phosphate intake and absorption is restricted by a low-phosphate diet and the use of phosphate binders (usually antacids containing aluminum hydroxide, such as Alucaps or Basaljel). The dose is individually adjusted to keep the serum phosphate levels normal. Hypophosphatemia must be avoided because it may result in osteomalacia and a potentially life-threatening myopathy.

Once the serum phosphate level is maintained below 5 mg/dl, measures can be taken to increase the serum calcium concentration with due care not to induce soft tissue calcification by exceeding the critical calcium–phosphate product. The active form of vitamin D, 1,25-dihydroxyvitamin D_3, may be used to enhance calcium absorption from the gut. It should be prescribed in small amounts (0.5 μg/day or less), however, because of its great potency and potential for inducing a high calcium–phosphate product (115). In patients receiving dialysis, the best approach is to increase the calcium concentration in the dialysate (120). A dialysate calcium concentration of 3.1–3.8 mEq/liter is recommended: lower levels result in a negative calcium balance with osteoporosis and progressive HPT, whereas higher levels cause metastatic calcification (121).

SURGICAL

Indications for Operation. The current indications for parathyroid surgery and secondary HPT are (118,121–124):

1. Severe bone disease (bone pain, spontaneous fractures) not responsive to medical therapy
2. Severe pruritis

3. Extensive soft tissue calcification
4. Other indications: calcium–phosphate product consistently greater than 70; persistent hypercalcemia; soft tissue necrosis and skin ulceration; psychoneurologic disorders.

After parathyroidectomy there is usually early and dramatic relief of pruritis and bone pain. Reversal of the radiologic signs of bone disease is seen within 2–3 months of surgery in most cases; however, improvement does not always occur. Vascular calcifications do not resolve, although metastatic calcification in other soft tissues frequently disappears (118, 122–124).

Operative Strategy. There are two current options for surgical treatment: subtotal parathyroidectomy, or total parathyroidectomy with heterotopic parathyroid transplantation into the forearm musculature. The rationale for the latter approach is easier access to the transplanted parathyroid tissue in the event of recurrent disease. However, symptomatic postoperative hypoparathyroidism is more of a problem after parathyroidectomy and autotransplantation, and a period of calcium and vitamin D supplementation is usually necessary for a variable period of time before the grafted tissue functions well enough to sustain the serum calcium level. A reasonable policy is to perform subtotal parathyroidectomy in those cases in which a well-vascularized, 50-mg remnant of parathyroid gland can be preserved in situ and subsequent renal transplantation is likely. If a remnant cannot be preserved with a good blood supply, or if future kidney transplantation is not feasible, then total parathyroidectomy with autotransplantation is a reasonable alternative.

Tertiary Hyperparathyroidism

Some patients with chronic renal failure and longstanding secondary HPT go on to develop hypercalcemia with aggravation of their hyperphosphatemia and are said to have "tertiary hyperparathyroidism". A similar situation may be encountered when hypercalcemia develops after otherwise successful renal transplantation.

These patients were initially thought to have autonomous parathyroid hyperfunction, and support for this view was provided by the occasional demonstration of a single parathyroid adenoma (although the usual pathologic finding in these cases is marked parathyroid hyperplasia). In fact, true autonomous PTH secretion does not occur in these cases because the parathyroid glands remain responsive to variations in serum calcium level (125). It appears that the combined activity of the excessive number of parathyroid cells encountered in these cases simply resembles autonomy.

> Transplantation of many isologous normal parathyroid glands into the peritoneal cavity of a single rat uniformly results in hypercalcemia. Thus, even though individual parathyroid cells may be normally responsive to negative-feedback con-

trol from the plasma calcium, the mass of cells in the aggregate behaves in a manner resembling autonomy (126). The occasional occurrence of parathyroid adenomas in patients with chronic renal failure is not unexpected, given their known prevalence in the general population.

Persistence of parathyroid hyperplasia following successful renal transplantation is associated with increased levels of serum PTH and hypercalcemia in as many as one-third of patients, and PTH levels often remain elevated for several years (125,127). Significant hypercalcemia (greater than 11.5 mg/dl) that persists for 6 months or more after renal transplantation and is not responsive to medical treatment (in this case, administration of oral phosphate supplements) should be treated by parathyroidectomy to circumvent kidney and skeletal damage (118,121,125,127).

Operative Technique   The initial steps in exposing the parathyroids are shown in Figures 1-19 to 1-26.

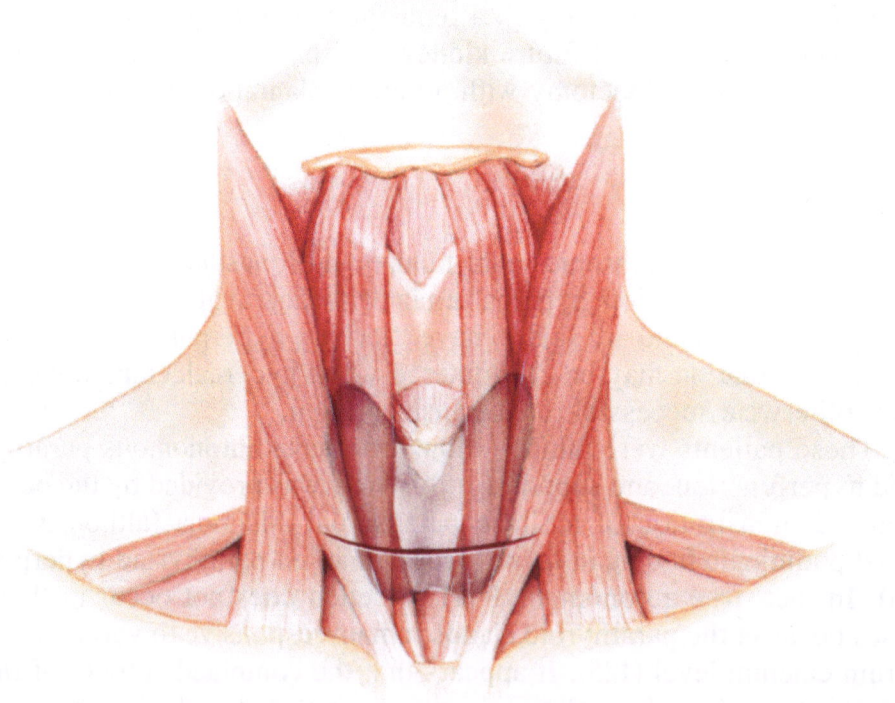

Fig. 1-19.   Surface anatomy. Midline structures of the neck are shown in relation to the conventional Kocher collar incision.

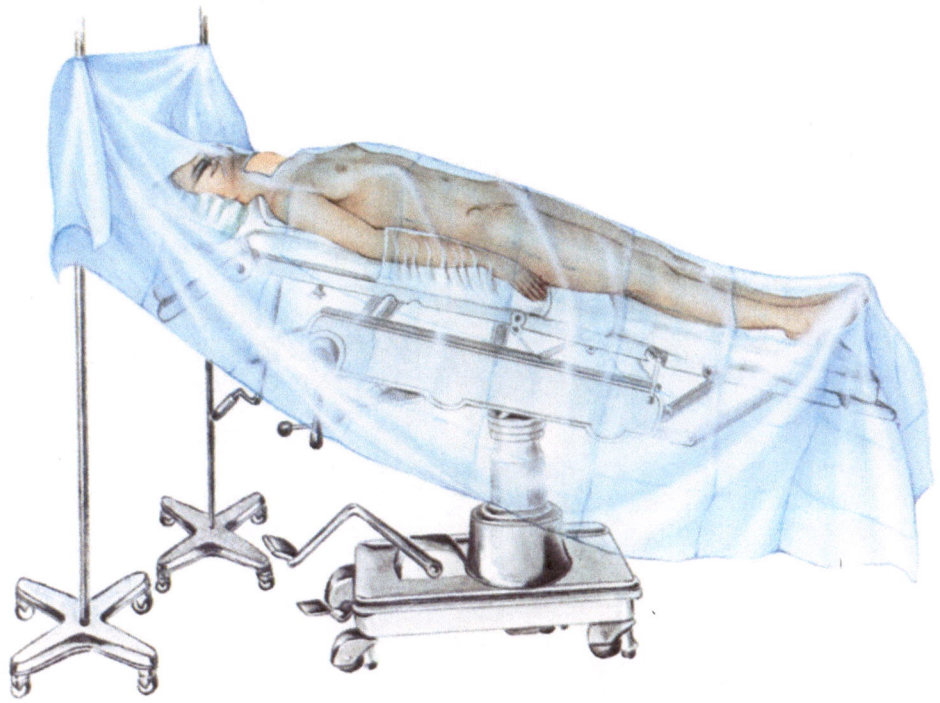

A

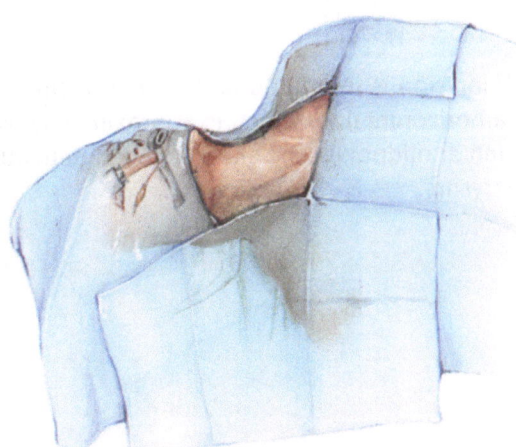

B

Position and drape. **A.** The table is tilted at 15° to the horizontal to diminish bleeding. A small pillow is placed beneath the shoulders and the head rest is adjusted to provide optimal extension of the neck. **B.** The skin of the operative area is prepared in the usual manner and the neck is draped out with four towels. The drape is completed with a thyroid sheet or with several plain sheets appropriately arranged.

Fig. 1-20.

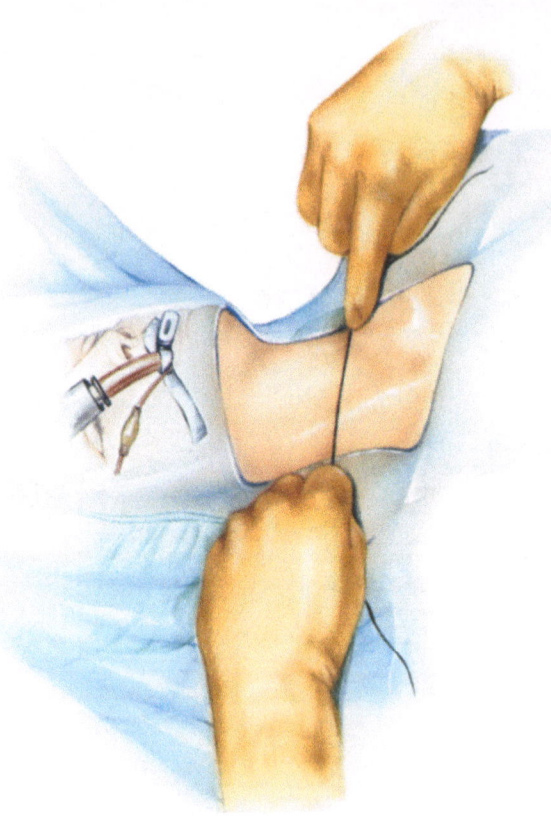

Fig. 1-21. **Incision.** The line of incision is imprinted on the skin by pressure with a fine thread. This follows a horizontal line, which is approximately two fingerbreadths above the sternal notch at midpoint. The skin and subcutaneous tissue are incised down to the platysma.

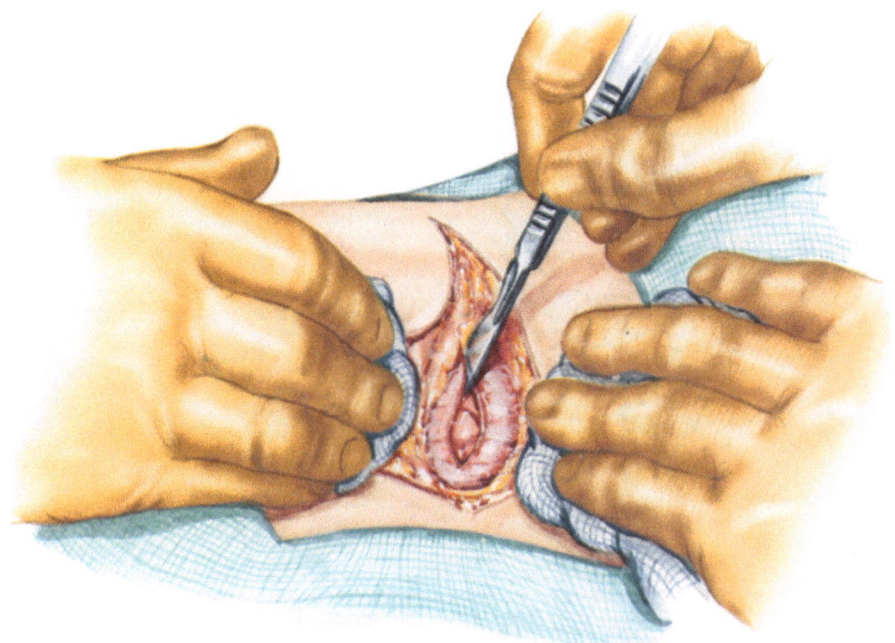

Bleeding from the skin edges is controlled by firm traction on both sides of the incision, and the platysma is divided in the line of the incision to expose the underlying deep investing fascia of the neck and anterior jugular veins.

Fig. 1-22.

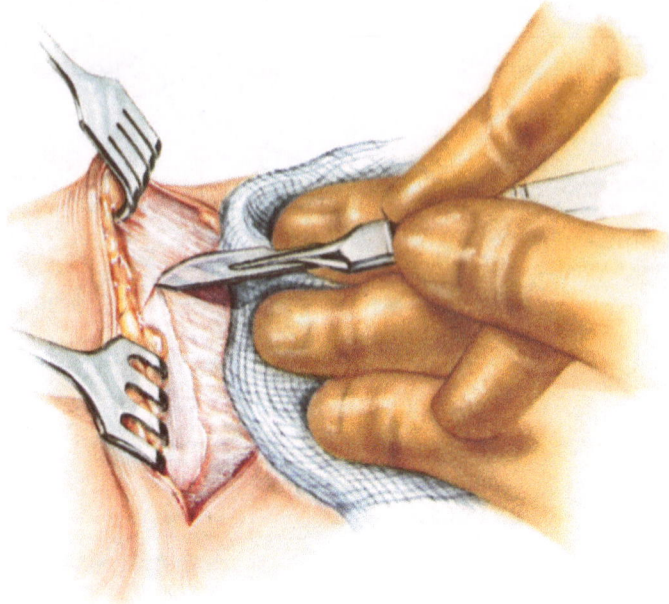

A

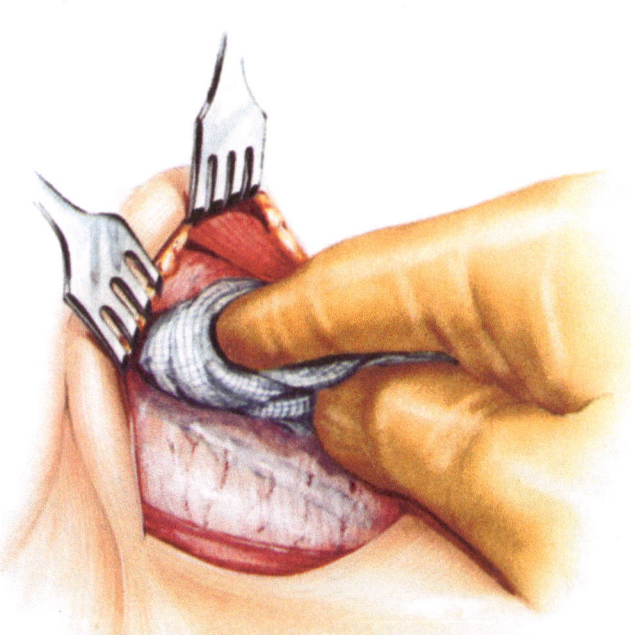

B

Fig. 1-23.   Elevation of the skin flaps. The upper edge of the incision is raised as a flap
up to the notch of the thyroid cartilage using a combination of sharp **(A)** and
then blunt **(B)** dissection. The plane of dissection is the areolar layer immediately subjacent to the platysma. This plane is brought into sharp relief by firm
upward traction of the skin and countertraction below on the midline tissues of
the neck. The lower skin edge is freed in a similar manner to expose the suprasternal notch.

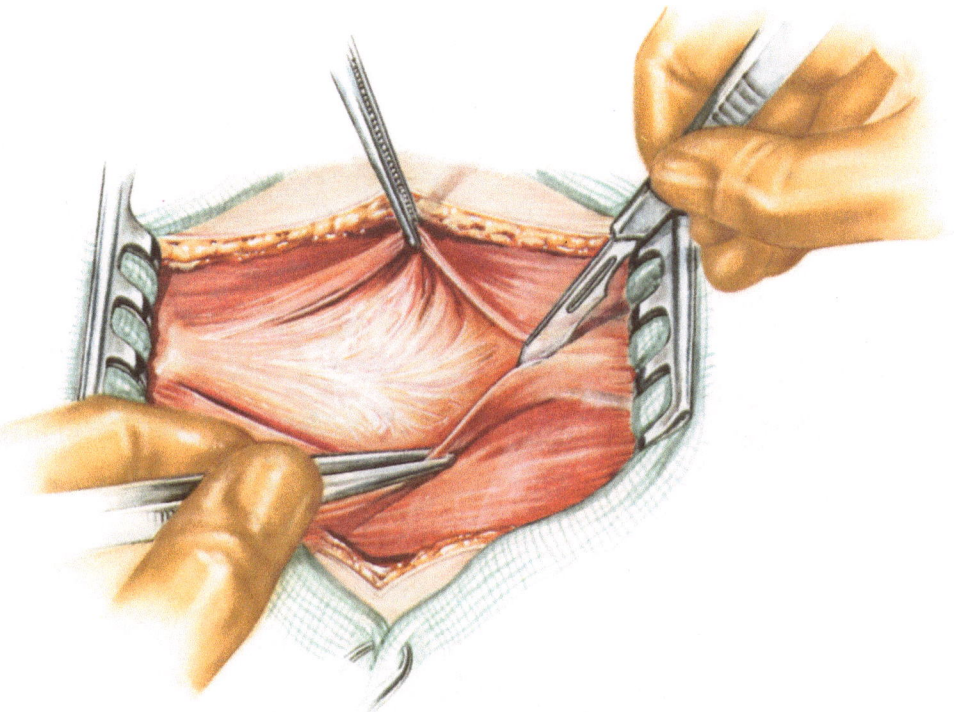

A

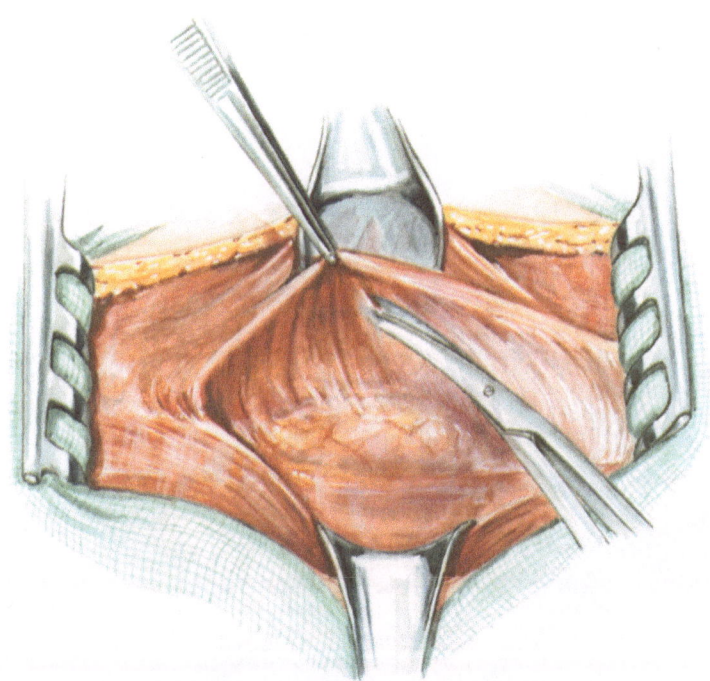

B

Exposure of the thyroid gland. A self-retaining retractor spreads the incision. **A.** The investing fascia of the neck is incised in the midline, from the thyroid cartilage to the sternal notch. The sternohyoid muscles are now retracted away from the midline to expose the underlying thyroid gland, which is partially overlapped by the membranous sternothyroid strap muscles. **B.** These muscles are freed from the thyroid by dissection of their medial areolar attachments to the capsule of the gland.

Fig. 1-24.

Fig. 1-25.

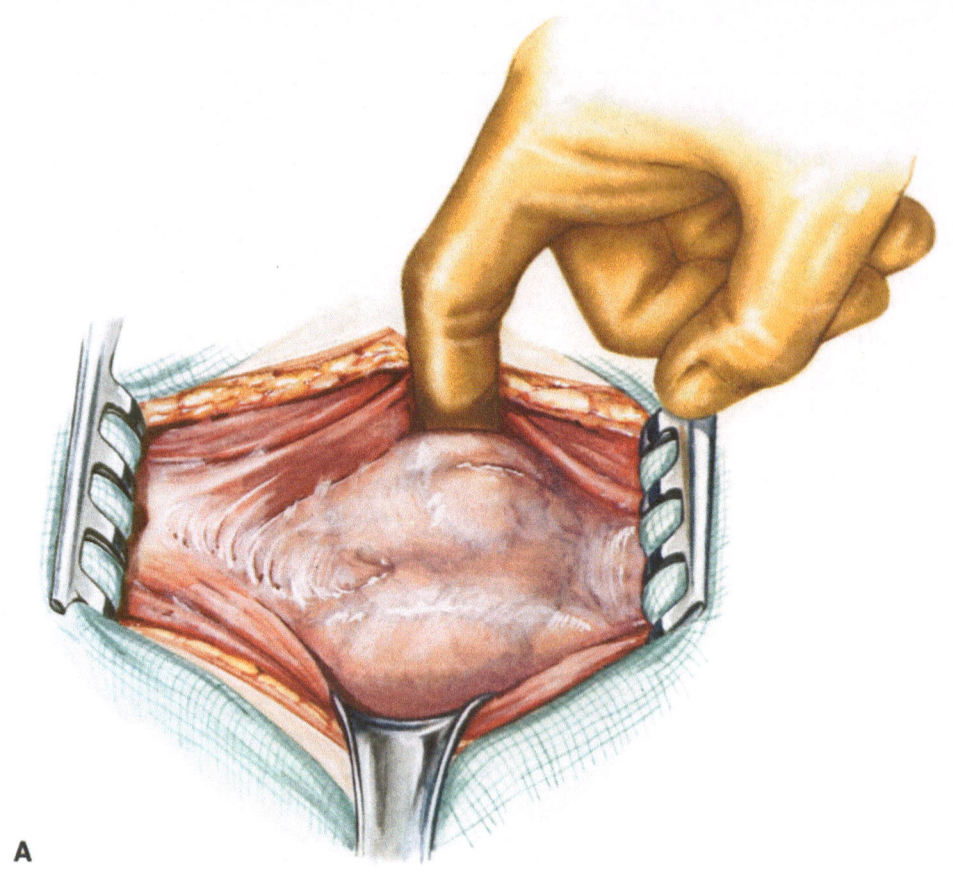

A

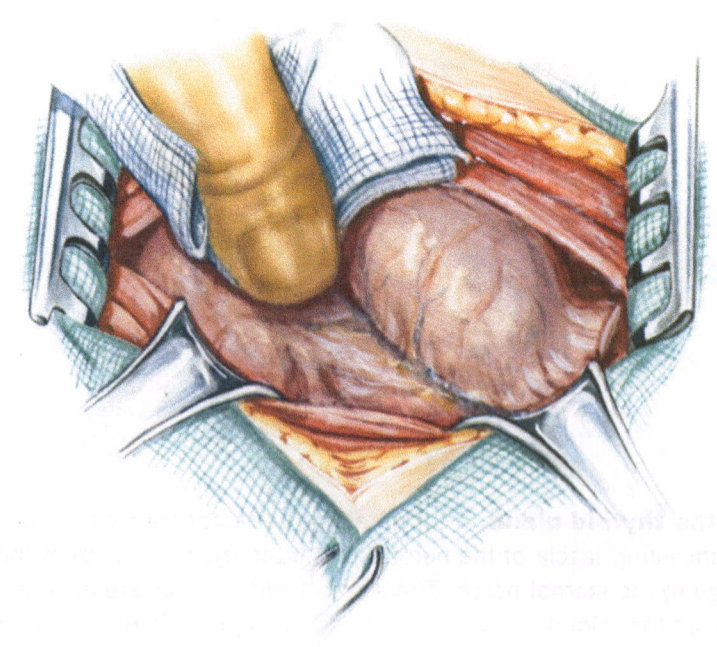

B

Fig. 1-26.

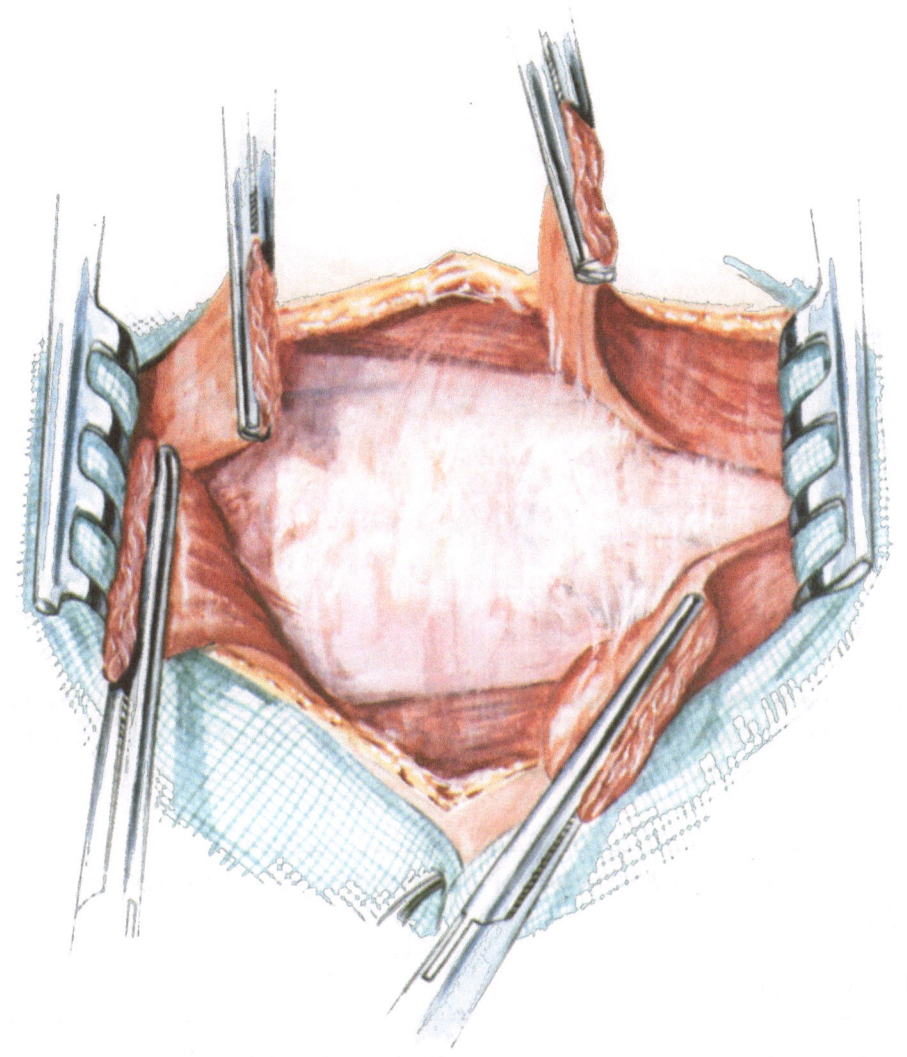

Mobilization of the thyroid for exposure of the parathyroids. **A.** The index finger is insinuated between the thyroid gland and the overlying strap muscles on the left. A sweeping movement frees the thyroid lobe from its lateral areolar attachments. The maneuver is repeated on the right. **B.** The strap muscles are retracted laterally and the right lobe of the thyroid is dislocated forward and medially to bring the lateral aspect of the gland into view. The middle thyroid vein is divided between clips. The surgeon controls the exposure by retracting the thyroid with the left thumb over a gauze sponge.

Fig. 1-25.

Division of the strap muscles: Alternative method of exposure. If the exposure afforded by retraction of the strap muscles is not satisfactory, they may be clamped and divided on each side of the neck at the cricoid level (thereby saving their innervation), as shown. Usually, the authors prefer not to divide the straps. The traction and countertraction possible when the muscles are intact greatly facilitate dissection of the areolar planes of the neck.

Fig. 1-26.

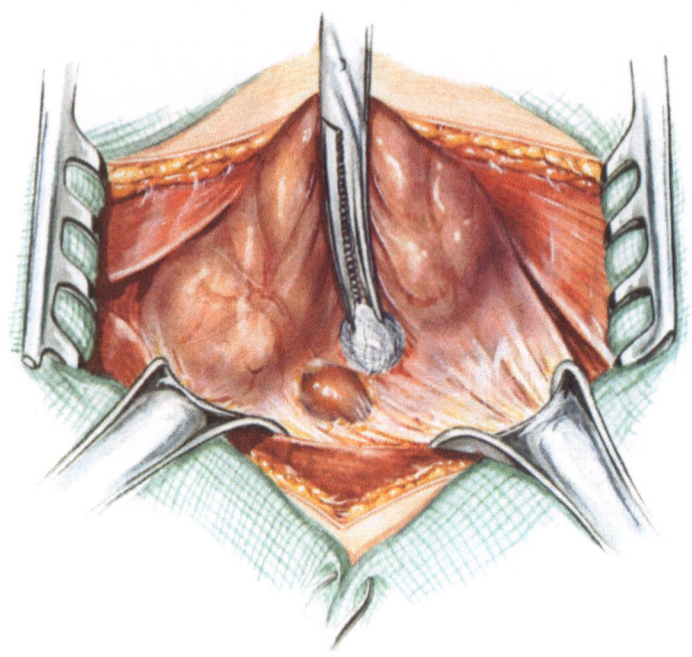

Fig. 1-27. **Adenoma of the right superior parathyroid.** It has a smooth glistening capsule and is not adherent to the surrounding tissues, making it possible for the surgeon to shell it out with relative ease.

CERVICAL EXPLORATION WITH REMOVAL OF A PARATHYROID ADENOMA

"EASY" CASE

On occasion an adenoma is seen as soon as the right lobe of the thyroid gland is reflected forward (Figs. 1-27 and 1-28). The adenoma is removed as shown in Figure 1-29. A biopsy may be used to confirm the identity of a normal-sized parathyroid (Fig. 1-30).

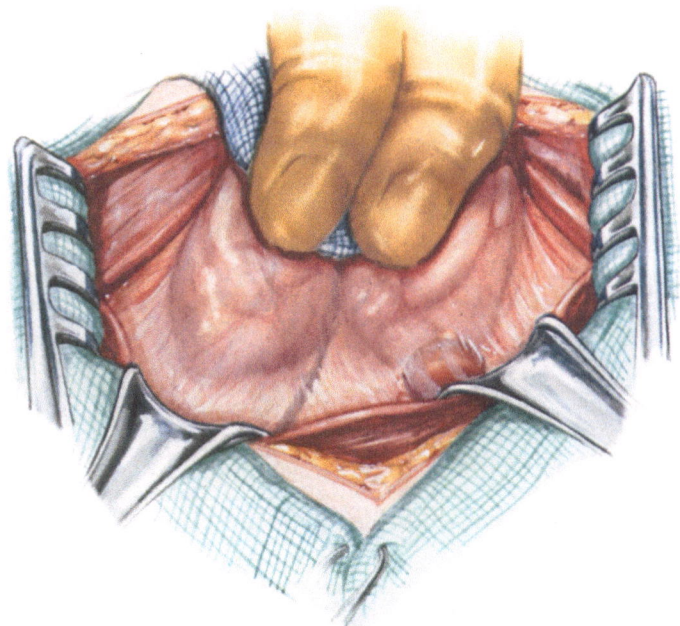

Adenoma of the left superior parathyroid. If an adenoma is not readily   **Fig. 1-28.**
seen or felt on the right side of the neck, attention is directed to the left before
detailed dissection is contemplated. If the surgeon prefers to remain on the
right side of the patient, the thyroid gland is retracted with the fingers of the left
hand, as shown here (viewing the operative field from the patient's left).

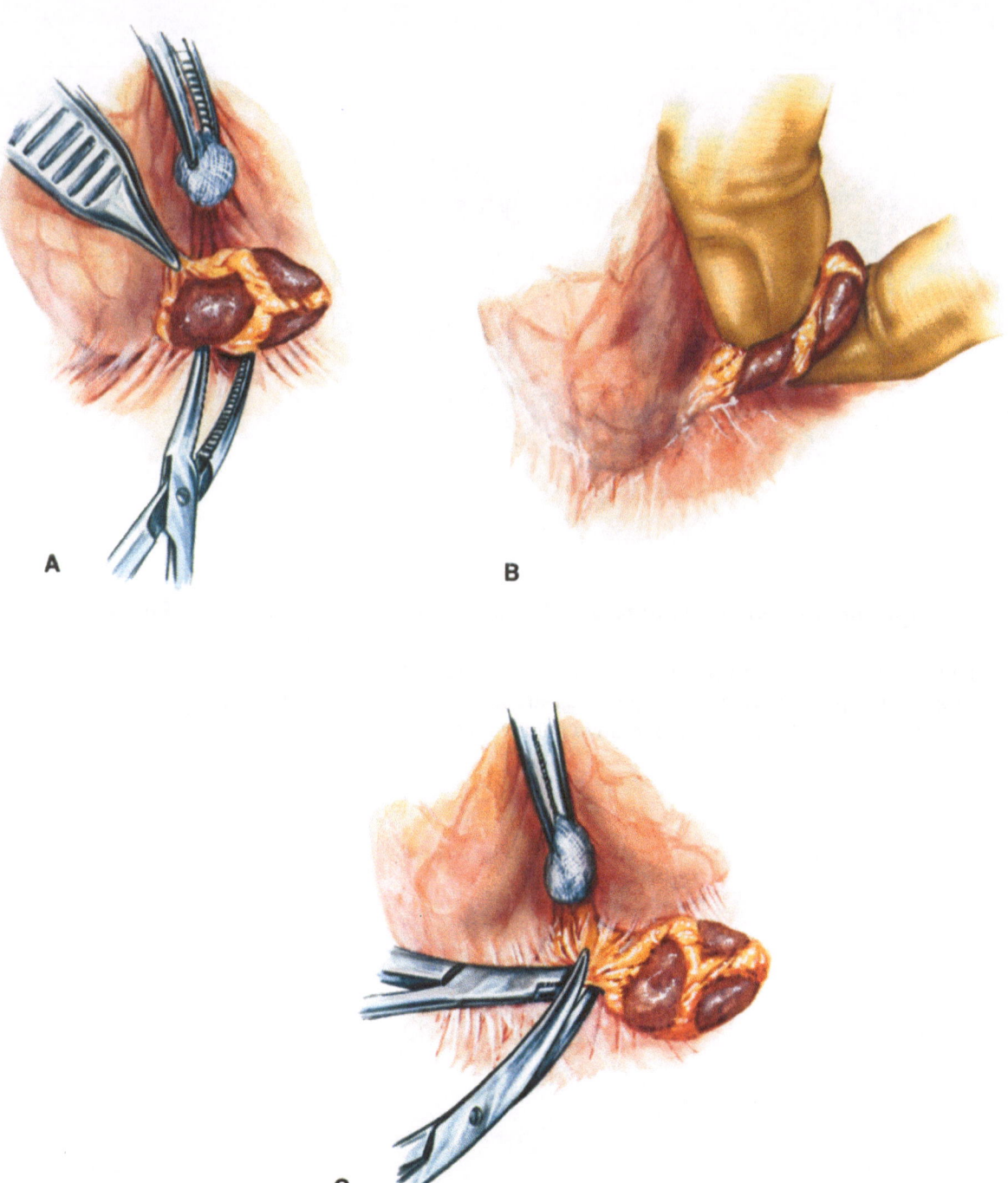

Fig. 1-29. Removal of an adenoma. A and B. Sharp and blunt dissection are carefully used to free the tumor from the surrounding tissues.   **C.** The vascular pedicle is clamped and divided, and the adenoma is removed.

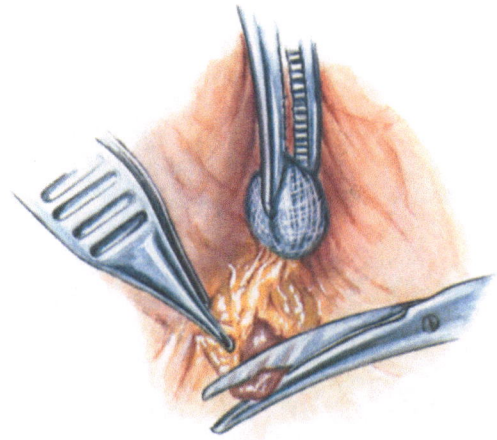

Biopsy of a normal parathyroid gland. Identification of parathyroid glands should be confirmed by biopsy and histologic examination. An *immediate* frozen section examination is necessary if the surgeon is uncertain about the nature of the biopsied tissue. It is possible to mistake lobules of blood-stained fat, protuberant thyroid nodules, small lymph nodes, thymic remnants, and even the bulging hypopharyngeal muscle for parathyroid tissue. Here a biopsy is being taken from a normal parathyroid gland. The normal gland is small, usually weighs about 35–40 mg, and has a tonguelike shape. It is yellow-brown to tan in color and is often concealed by, or closely associated with, a halo of fat. Great care is taken not to disturb its fragile blood supply. The surrounding fat is held to steady the gland and the biopsy is taken from the antihilar tip of the gland. A pair of fine dissecting scissors is used and a small piece of tissue is removed with a single, deliberate snip. Characteristically, blood oozes from the entire cut surface of the remnant.

Fig. 1-30.

Fig. 1-31.

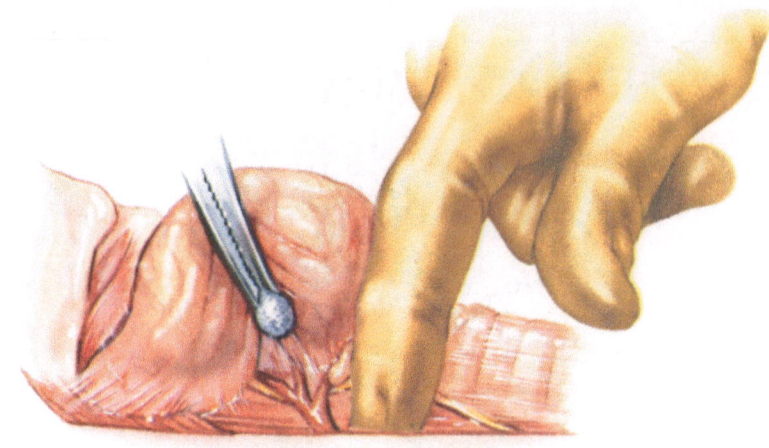

Fig. 1-32.

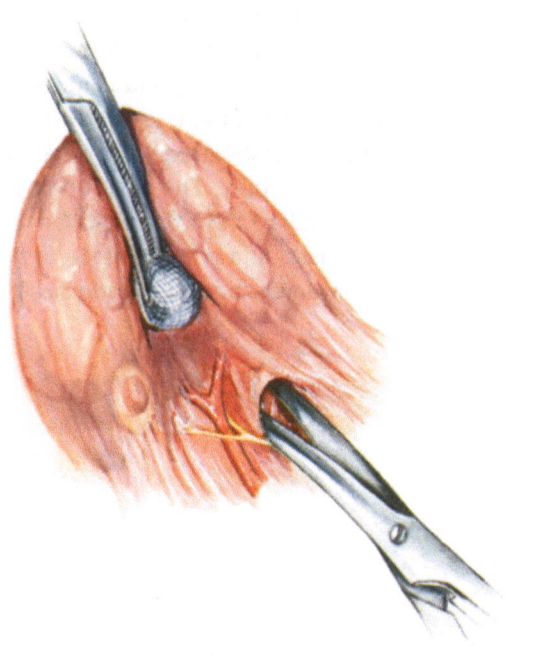

"ROUTINE" CASE

In the usual cervical exploration for primary HPT the adenoma is not immediately evident, and it is necessary to carry out a methodical dissection on both sides of the neck (Figs. 1-31 to 1-33). The recurrent laryngeal nerves are routinely exposed in these cases. Once seen, they are less likely to be damaged. The inferior thyroid artery is usually *not* ligated.

Fig. 1·33.

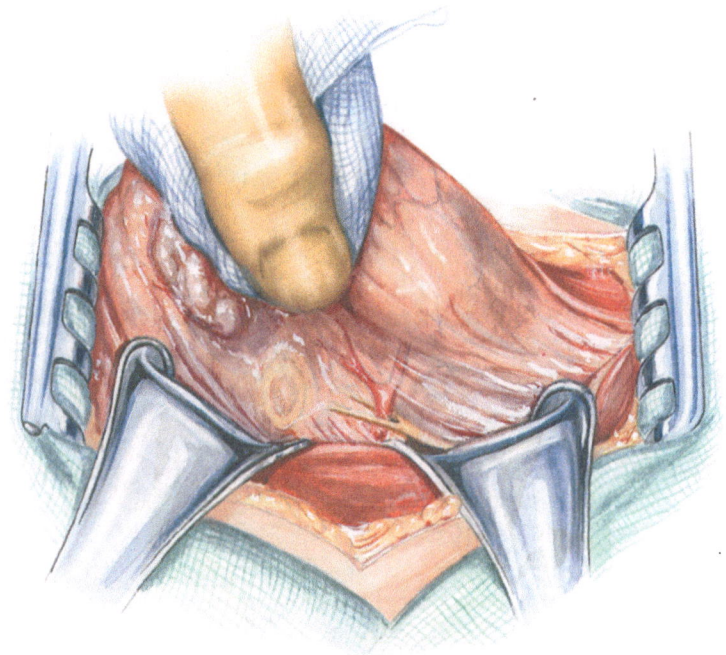

Palpation of the recurrent laryngeal nerve. The nerve often can be palpated before it is actually visualized. It is felt as a cordlike structure that can be
gently "popped" against the lateral aspect of the trachea.

Fig. 1·31.

Dissection technique. Dissection of fatty and areolar tissue surrounding the
recurrent laryngeal nerve must be careful and precise to avoid damage to the
nerve and any unnecessary bleeding. This process is facilitated by "air dissection" of the tissues: traction on the thyroid with countertraction of the strap
muscles sucks air into the connective tissue, or areolar planes, lateral and posterior to the thyroid, thus throwing into sharp relief the vessels, nerve, and
parathyroids. The teasing action of fine thumb forceps or a small pair of dissecting scissors enables gentle and meticulous separation of tissue planes.

Fig. 1·32.

Adenoma of the right inferior parathyroid. Its "classic" location is below
the point of intersection of the recurrent laryngeal nerve with the inferior thyroid
artery, on the lateral or posterior aspect of the lower pole of the thyroid lobe. It
has been uncovered by gently teasing off the fine, overlying areolar capsule. The
anatomic relationships are clearly seen, and branching of the nerve is evident.
The right superior parathyroid is normal in appearance and surrounded by a
characteristic halo of fat.

Fig. 1·33.

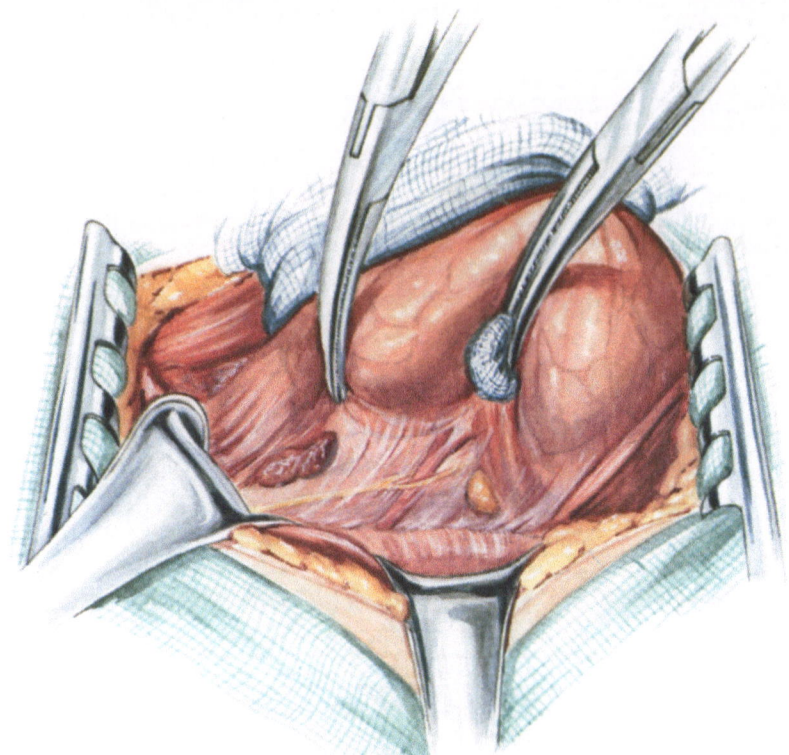

Fig. 1-34. **Adenoma of the left inferior parathyroid.** An adenoma of the left inferior parathyroid has been found by dissecting the areolar tissue below and lateral to the inferior pole of the thyroid (view of the left side of the neck).

"DIFFICULT" CASE

If a parathyroid tumor is not found during the routine dissection of the neck, the missing gland or glands are sought systematically. As a general rule, adenomas arising in a superior gland tend to be displaced inferiorly along the tracheoesophageal groove into the posterior superior mediastinum. Those originating in an inferior gland are often located at the root of the neck (Fig. 1-34) or in the anterior superior mediastinum, where they are intimately associated with the thymus gland (Fig. 1-35). Very rarely, they are found high in the neck (so-called undescended parathymus glands).

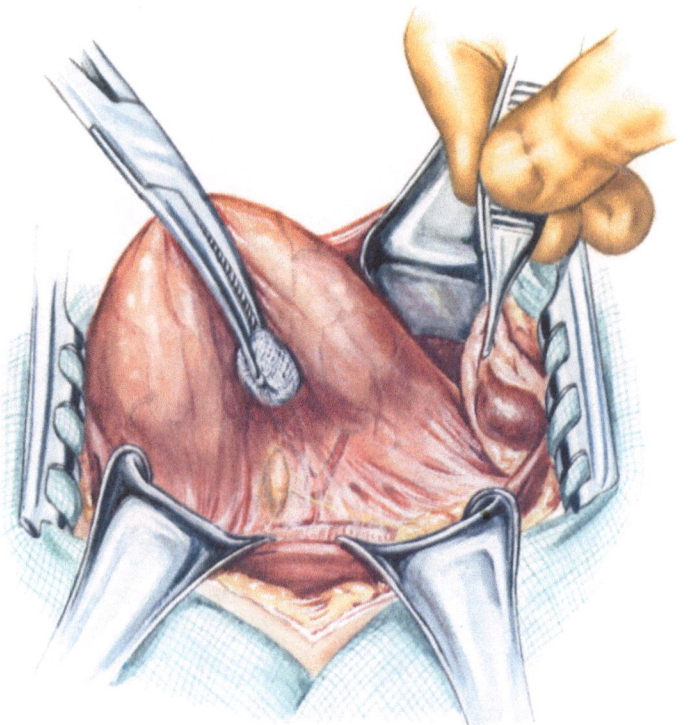

Adenoma of the right inferior parathyroid embedded in the thymus.   **Fig. 1-35.**
Cervical prolongations of the thymus gland are often seen in the root of the
neck and, not uncommonly, an inferior parathyroid tumor is found·partially embedded in the substance of the thymus, as depicted here. If the parathyroid tumor is not visible in the root of the neck, that portion of the thymus can be removed and sectioned grossly to look for intrathymic parathyroid tissue.

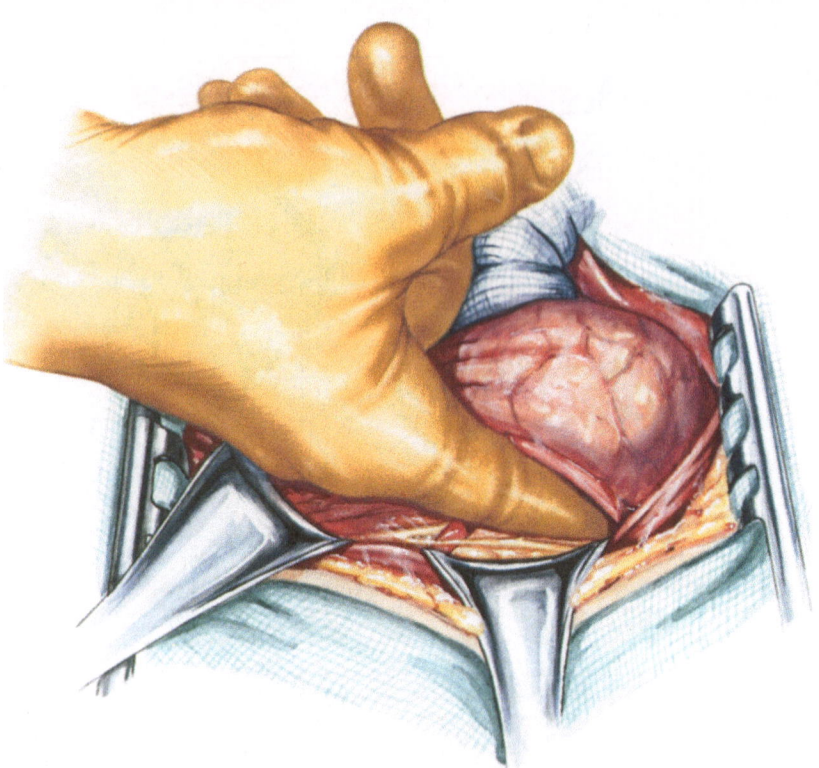

Fig. 1-36. **Examination of the retropharyngeal area.** A missing superior parathyroid gland may be found in the prevertebral space directly behind the esophagus and pharynx. Here the surgeon is carefully examining the retropharyngeal recess close to the upper pole of the thyroid.

If a superior gland cannot be found in its usual location, the tracheoesophageal groove should be explored from the superior pole of the thyroid down into the posterior superior mediastinum, with all fatty and areolar tissue being removed for careful study (Fig. 1-36). The dissection is extended as far as possible under direct vision; care is taken to avoid injury to the recurrent laryngeal nerve.

Although 10% to 20% of all parathyroid adenomas are found in the mediastinum, almost all can be removed via a cervical approach. A formal exploration of the mediastinum through a median sternotomy incision is necessary in less than 1–2% of all cases of primary HPT. It is said that adenomas displaced into the chest often have a prominent vascular pedicle derived from the inferior thyroid artery and that this pedicle guides the surgeon to the tumor. However, the authors have not found this information to be of much practical value. The carotid sheath is opened on the side of the missing gland if other efforts have failed to disclose a tumor.

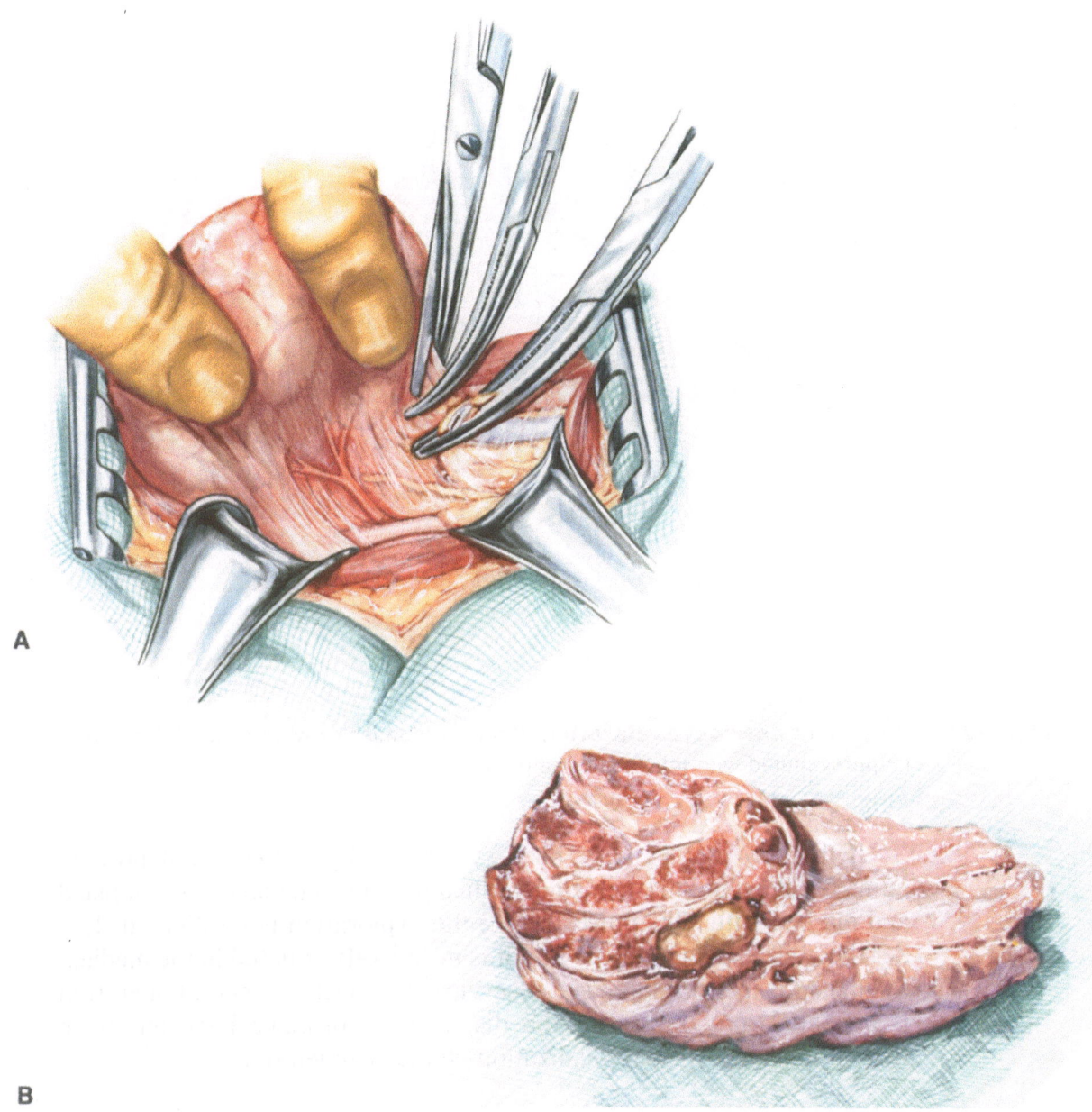

A

B

Thyroid lobectomy. **A.** The thyroid lobe on the side of the missing gland is removed; the recurrent laryngeal nerve is preserved. **B.** The resected specimen has been sectioned to reveal a small parathyroid tumor in the substance of the gland.

Fig. 1-37.

Finally, if no adenoma has been found, subtotal thyroid lobectomy should be performed on the side of the missing parathyroid (Fig. 1-37). It is a rare situation, but the thyroid gland may harbor a parathyroid adenoma; usually, such tumors are not palpable in the substance of the gland.

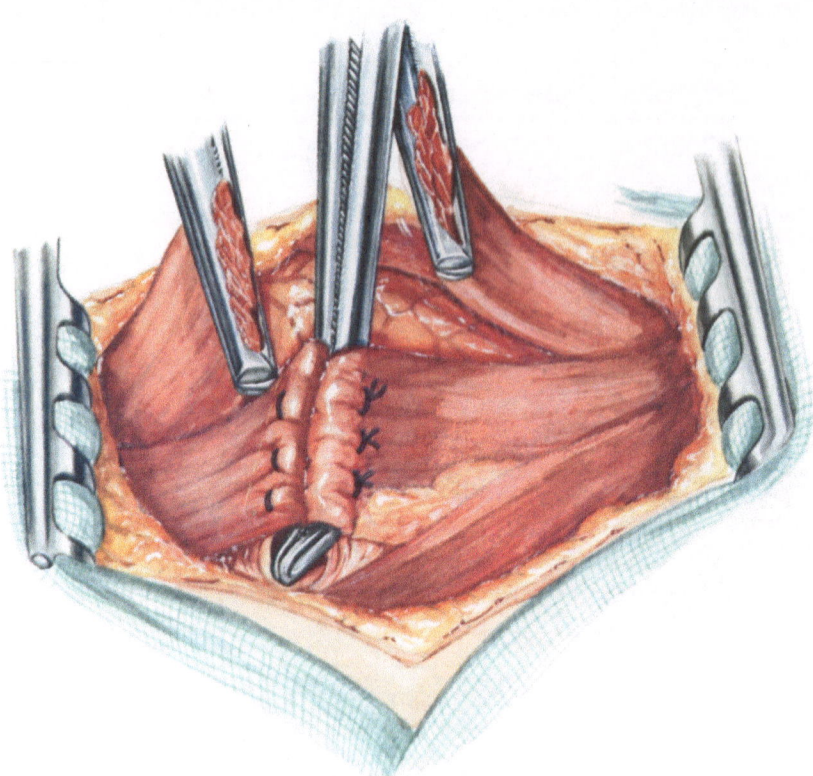

Fig. 1-38. **Closure of cervical exploration.** If the strap muscles were divided, they are reapproximated with interrupted catgut mattress sutures.

If the above steps have been systematically followed but no adenoma has been found, then all identified parathyroid glands are biopsied and marked with silk sutures before the exploration is terminated. Under these circumstances, the tumor is most likely situated in the mediastinum and is inaccessible via the cervical approach. A second operation is indicated, *but* only after the diagnosis of primary HPT has been reconfirmed and special localization studies carried out.

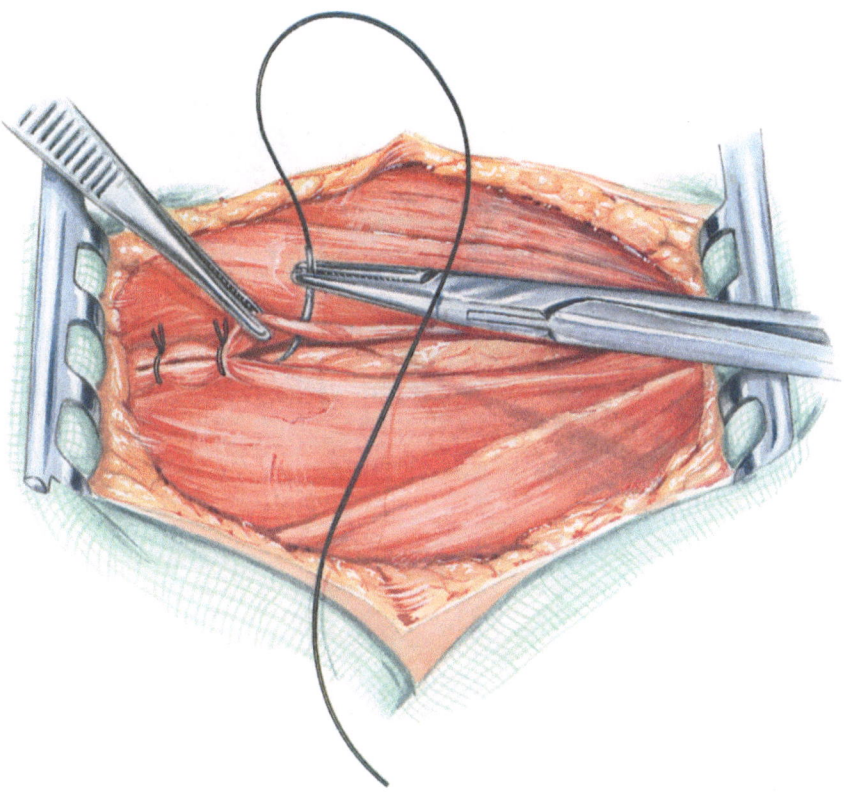

The midline cervical fascia is approximated with interrupted catgut sutures. The **Fig. 1-39.**
platysma and subcutaneous tissue layers are closed with interrupted catgut.

CLOSURE

The tissues of the neck are irrigated with saline and residual bleeding
points are ligated (Figs. 1-38 through 1-41).

Fig. 1-40.

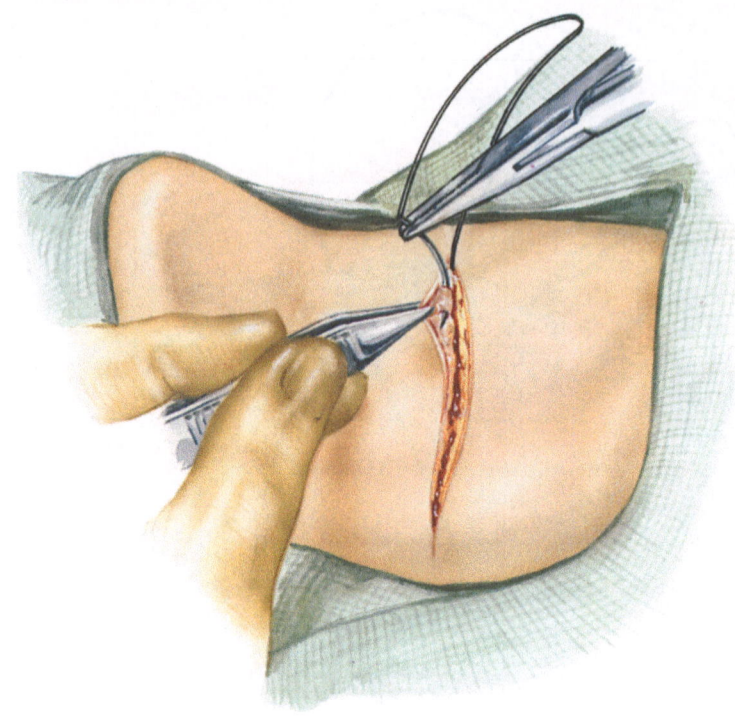

Fig. 1-41.

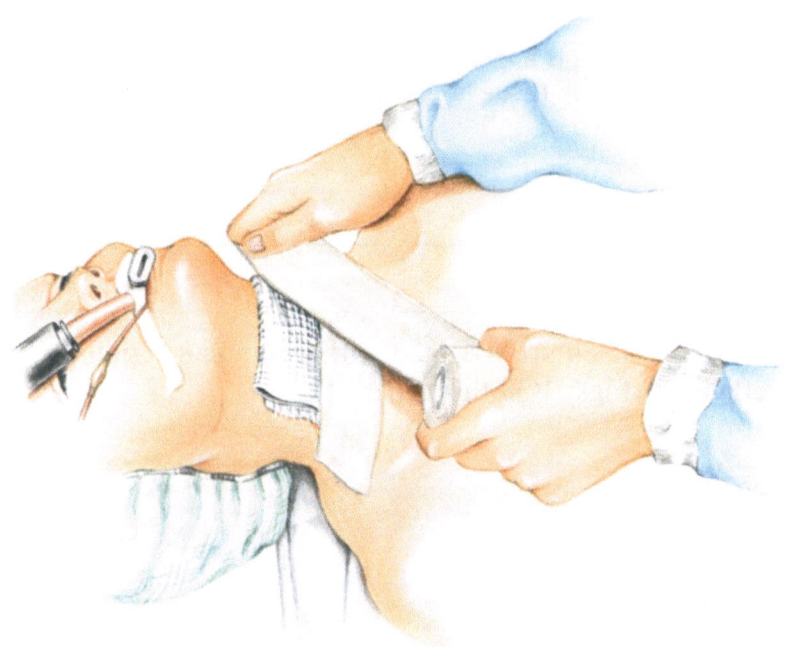

Fig. 1-40. The skin is sutured with a running subcuticular stitch of fine absorbable material.

Fig. 1-41. A loose dressing is applied.

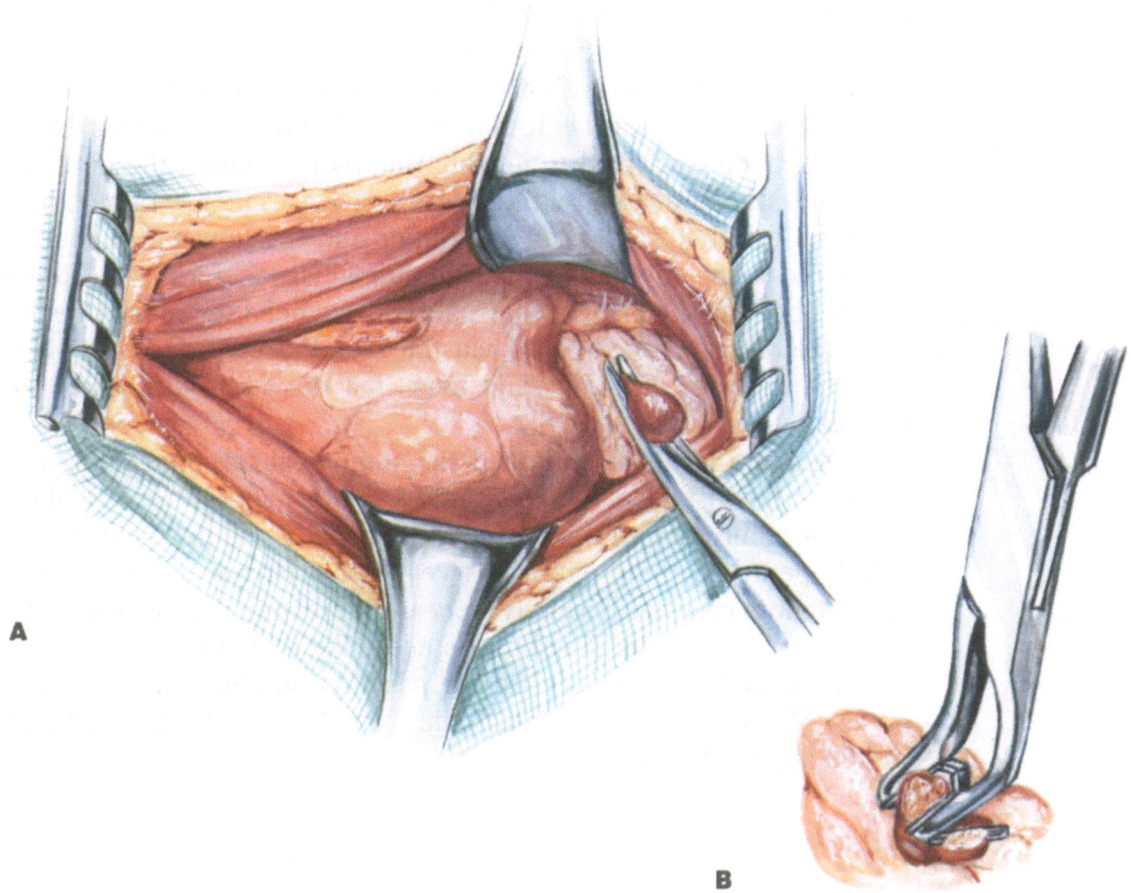

Subtotal parathyroidectomy. **A.** A portion of the left inferior parathyroid is being removed to prepare a small viable remnant. The technique is similar to that of biopsying normal parathyroid gland (see Fig. 1-30). **B.** Several small metal clips are used to control bleeding from the remnant; they also will facilitate its identification should a subsequent operation be required.   **Fig. 1-42.**

SUBTOTAL PARATHYROIDECTOMY FOR HYPERPLASIA

Subtotal parathyroidectomy involves removing three glands and often a portion of the fourth in order to leave a viable remnant (Fig. 1-42), which is the approximate size of a normal gland (30–50 mg). A well-vascularized remnant should be secured before any one of the glands is removed completely. Thus the surgeon will have four opportunities instead of one to obtain a viable functioning remnant.

PARATHYROIDECTOMY FOR CARCINOMA

Parathyroid carcinoma is a very rare entity, accounting for less than 1% of all cases of HPT. The tumor grows slowly and spreads by local invasion, becoming fixed to neighboring tissues. Often the first indications that one is dealing with a parathyroid carcinoma rather than an adenoma are the firmness of the tumor and the unusual difficulty encountered in separating it from surrounding tissues (Fig. 1-43). Regional lymph node involvement is unusual, and the need for radical neck dissection is uncommon. Spread via the blood stream does occur, with a predilection for the lungs and liver, but this is usually a late manifestation.

When the lesion is removed the tumor capsule must not be disrupted, otherwise local implantation of viable malignant cells will result in tumor recurrence. If the tumor recurs locally within 2 years after the initial operation, the prognosis is very poor. However, since some of these tumors grow fairly slowly, repeated resection is worthwhile. Likewise, resection of functional metastases may be beneficial.

The overall 5-year survival for parathyroid carcinoma is approximately 35% (30). Patients usually die from the complications of uncontrolled hypercalcemia.

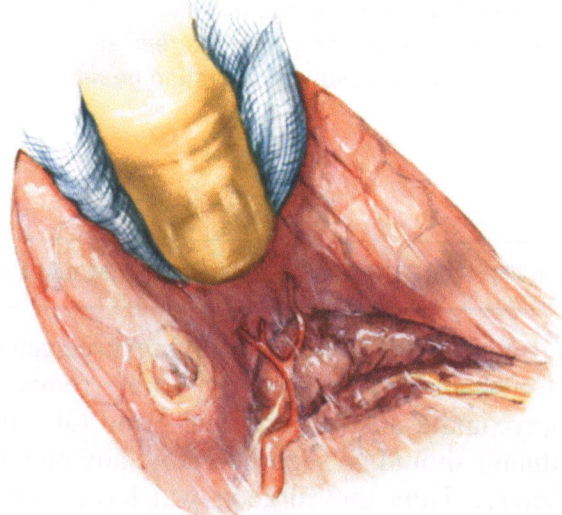

Fig. 1-43.   Resection of parathyroid carcinoma. The adhesive reaction surrounding a parathyroid cancer involves the recurrent laryngeal nerve in this instance. Treatment of this particular lesion, therefore, will involve excision of the tumor along with the ipsilateral thyroid lobe and a segment of the recurrent nerve enbloc.

MEDIASTINAL EXPLORATION FOR PARATHYROID TUMOR

Patients with HPT that persists or recurs after exploration of the neck should undergo studies to localize the hyperfunctioning parathyroid tissue before further surgery is undertaken (see section, Preoperative Localization Studies). If the localizing studies define a mediastinal lesion, formal exploration of the mediastinum via a sternum-splitting incision is indicated (Figs. 1-44 to 1-48). This is an uncommon surgical procedure; in 98%–99% of cases, the lesion or lesions causing HPT can be removed via a cervical incision.

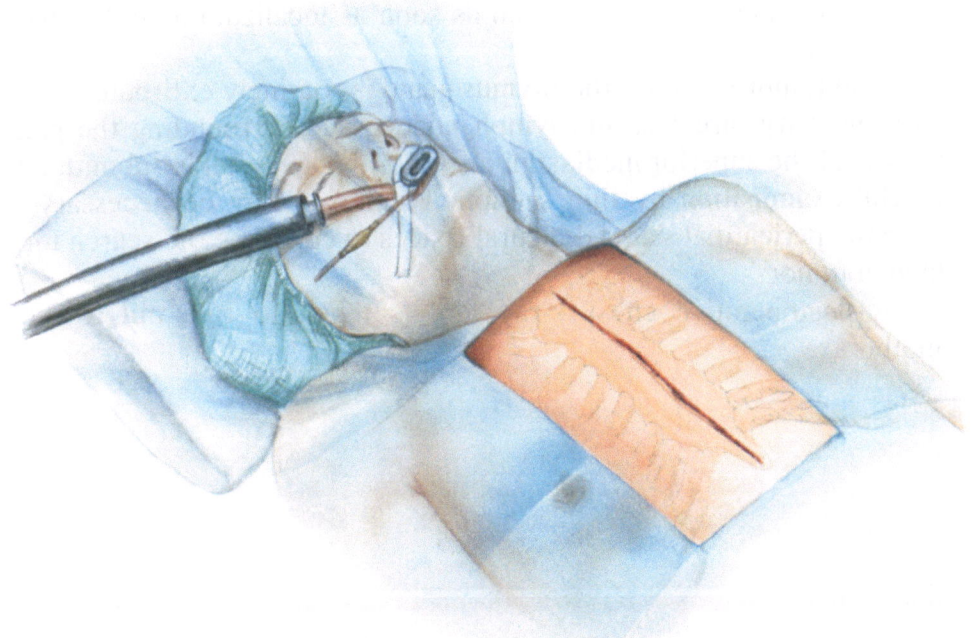

A

Mediastinal Exploration Incision. **A.** With the patient supine, a midline incision is made either part way or entirely from the suprasternal notch to the xiphoid. **B.** The electrocautery is used to carry the incision down to the periosteum.

Fig. 1-44.

Fig. 1-44.

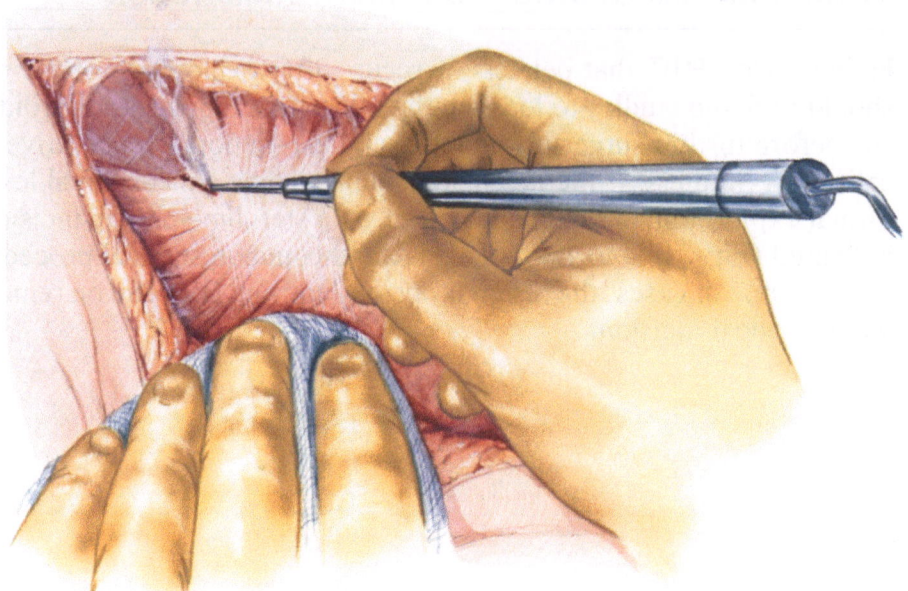

B

If prompt re-exploration is not possible, there is probably some advantage to be gained by delaying the operation 2–3 months so as to allow tissue reaction from the prior cervical and upper mediastinal dissection to resolve. When the hyperparathyroid state is severe, however, reoperation should be undertaken as soon as localization studies have been completed.

If no tumor is found, the thymus gland is routinely extirpated along with the fatty, areolar, and lymph node tissue surrounding the great vessels of the superior mediastinum. All of this material is submitted to careful examination by thin section. Finally, it may be necessary to open the pericardial sac and pleural spaces to complete the search for a hidden tumor.

A postoperative chest x-ray film is taken to rule out a pneumothorax.

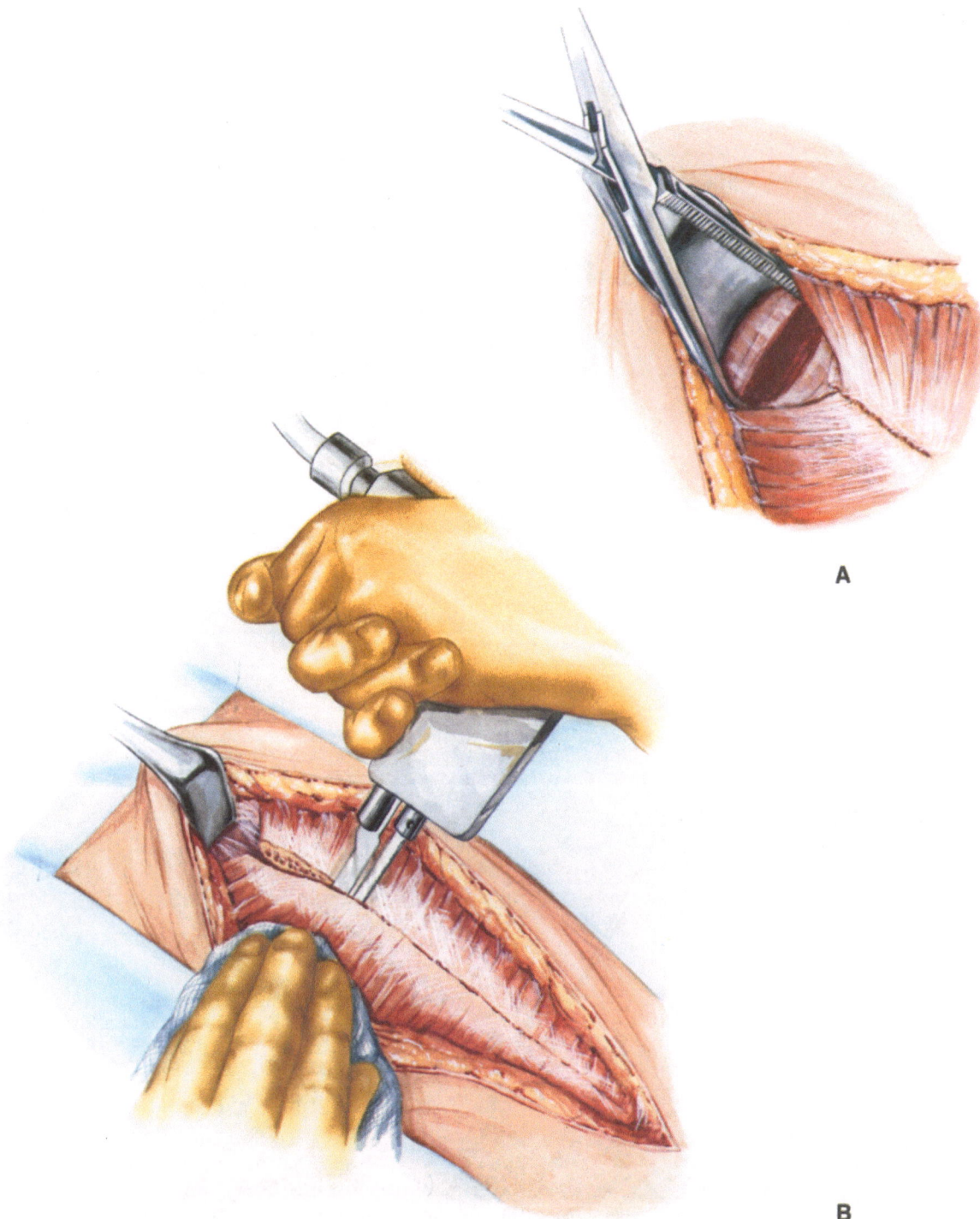

A

B

Splitting the sternum. **A.** The dense fascia immediately above and behind
the suprasternal notch is spread apart to open up a space between the sternum
and underlying great vessels. **B.** An oscillating electric saw is used to divide
the entire sternum in the midline. Bleeding is controlled by electrocoagulation
of the periosteal vessels and impregnation of the marrow with bone wax.

Fig. 1-45.

Fig. 1-46.

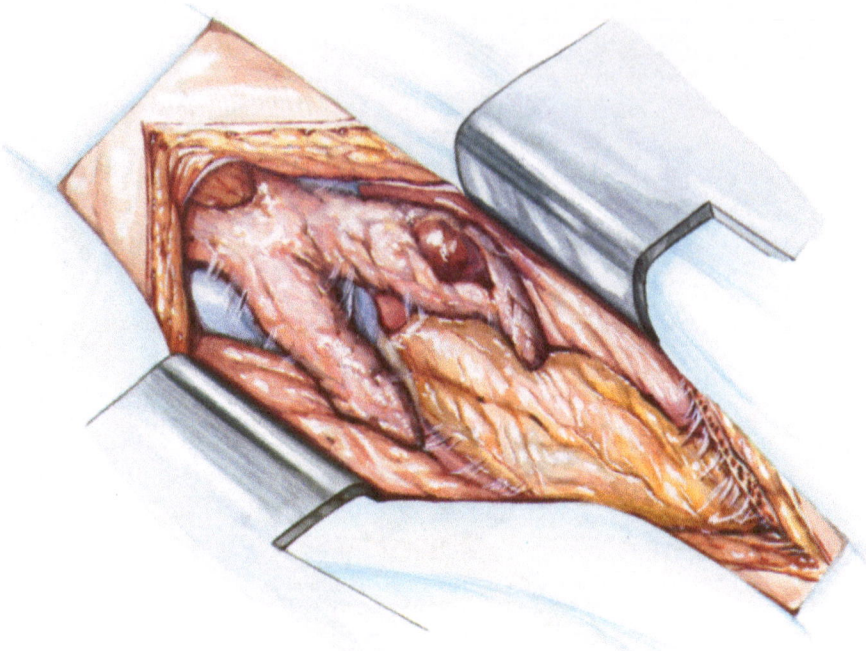

Fig. 1-47.

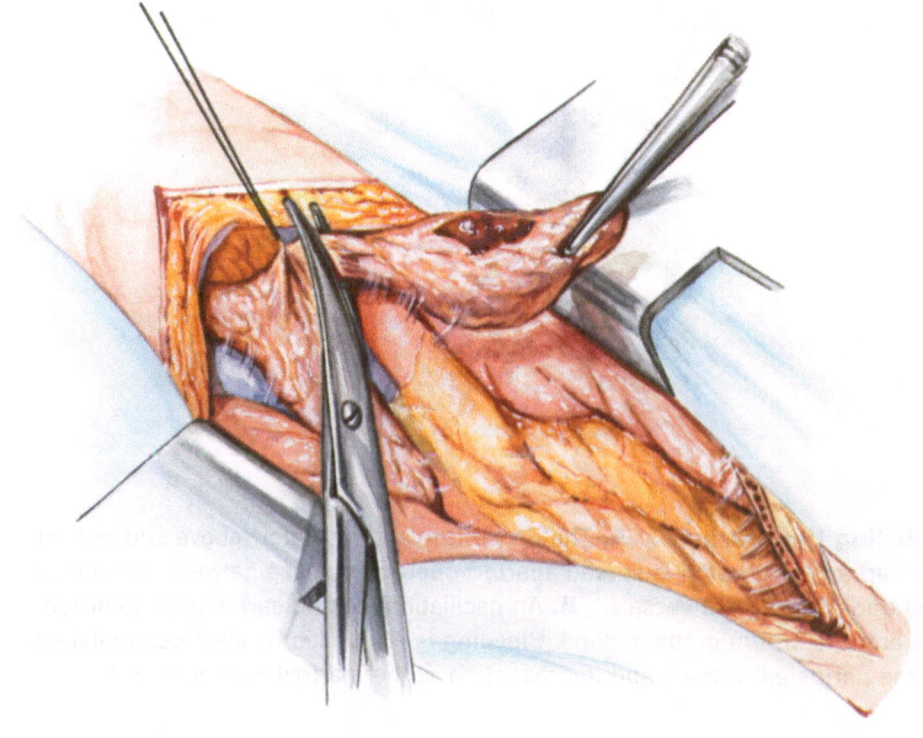

Fig. 1-48.

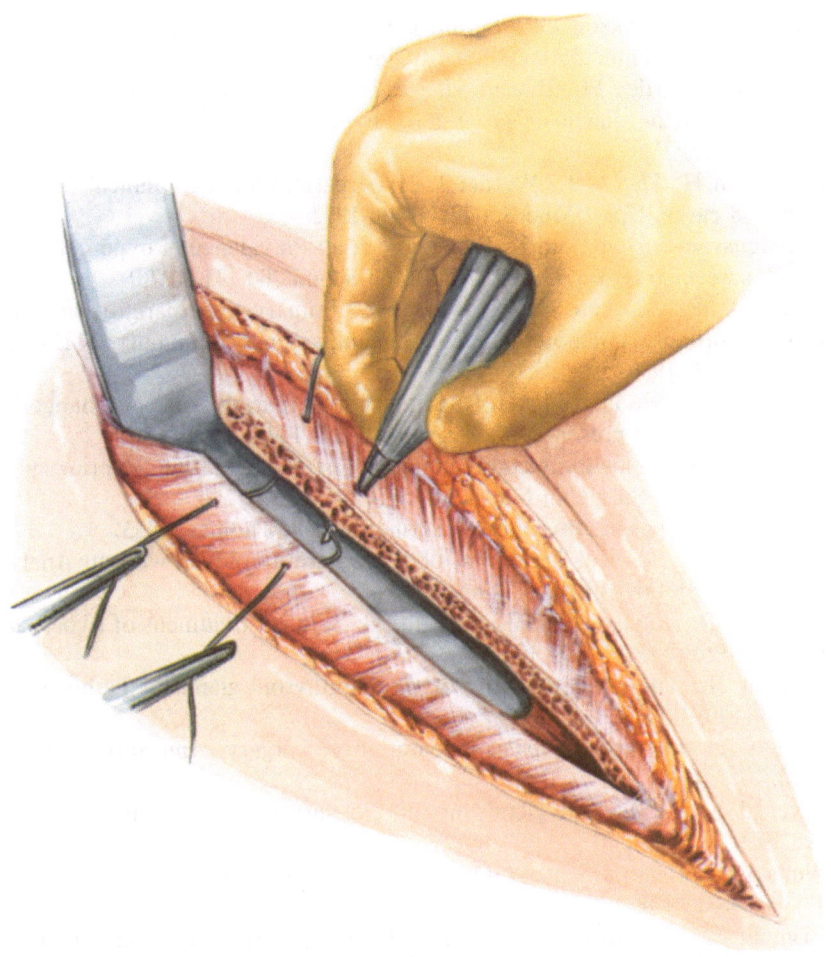

Exposure of the mediastinum. A self-retaining retractor is used to spread the divided sternum. The parietal pleura is freed and pushed away on both sides to fully expose the contents of the superior mediastinum.

Fig. 1-46.

Removal of the left lobe of thymus containing a parathyroid tumor. In this particular case, the parathyroid adenoma was visible immediately upon entering the chest. It was partially embedded in the left lobe of the thymus gland. Here, that portion of the thymus containing the parathyroid tumor is being amputated.

Fig. 1-47.

Closure. The sternum is reapproximated by means of multiple wire sutures inserted through the bone with an awl. The wires are twisted and the exposed tips are buried. Although not shown, a suction catheter is left retrosternally and brought out through the skin to one side of the xiphoid. Fascia and subcutaneous tissues are closed with interrupted sutures and the skin is closed with a running subcuticular stitch.

Fig. 1-48.

References

1. Boonstra CE, Jackson CE: Serum calcium: survey for hyperparathyroidism: result in 50,000 clinic patients. Am J Clin Pathol 55:523–526, 1971.
2. Aitken RE, Bartley PC, Bryant SJ, et al: The effect of multiphasic biochemical screening on the diagnosis of primary hyperparathyroidism. Aust NZ J Med 5:224–226, 1975.
3. Johansson H, Thorén L, Werner I: Hyperparathyroidism: clinical experiences from 208 cases. Ups J Med Sci 77:41–46, 1972.
4. Christensson T, Hellström K, Wengle B, et al: Prevalence of hypercalcemia in a health screening in Stockholm. Acta Med Scand 200:131, 1976.
5. Heath H III, Hodgson SF, Kennedy MA: Primary hyperparathyroidism: incidence, morbidity, and potential economic impact in a community. N Engl J Med 302:189–193, 1980.
6. Mundy GR, Cove DH, Fisken R: Primary hyperparathyroidism: changes in the pattern of clinical presentation. Lancet 1:1317–1320, 1980.
7. Edis AJ: Surgical anatomy and technique of neck exploration for primary hyperparathyroidism. Surg Clin North Am 57:495–504, 1977.
8. Black BM: Hyperparathyroidism. Springfield, Ill, Thomas, 1953.
9. Bruining HA: Surgical Treatment of Hyperparathyroidism with an Analysis of 267 Cases. Springfield, Ill, Thomas, 1971.
10. Romanus R, Heimann P, Nilsson O, et al: Surgical treatment of hyperparathyroidism. Prog Surg 12:22, 1973.
11. Gilmour JR: The gross anatomy of the parathyroid glands. J Pathol Bacteriol 46:133–149, 1938.
12. Wang CA: The anatomic basis of parathyroid surgery. Ann Surg 183:271–275, 1976.
13. Alveryd A: Parathyroid glands in thyroid surgery. Acta Chir Scand [Suppl] 398:1968.
14. Wells SA Jr, Leight GS, Ross AJ: Primary hyperparathyroidism. Curr Probl Surg 17:398–463, 1980.
15. Grimelius L, Åkerström G, Johansson H: The parathyroids: location and histopathological diagnosis. Centraltryckeriet AB Upsala, 1981.
16. Norris EH: The parathyroid glands and the lateral thyroid in man: their morphogenesis, topographic anatomy and prenatal growth. Contrib Embryol 26:247, 1937.
17. Boyd JD: Development of the thyroid and parathyroid glands and the thymus. Ann R Coll Surg Engl 7:455, 1950.
18. Gilmour JR: The normal histology of the parathyroid glands. J Pathol Bacteriol 48:187–222, 1939.
19. Edis AJ, Purnell DC, van Heerden JA: The undescended 'parathymus': an occasional cause of failed neck exploration for hyperparathyroidism. Ann Surg 190:64–68, 1979.
20. Cope O: Surgery of hyperparathyroidism: the occurrence of parathyroids in the anterior mediastinum and the division of the operation into two stages. Ann Surg 114:706–731, 1941.
21. Russell CF, Edis AJ, Scholz DA, et al: Mediastinal parathyroid tumors—experience with 38 tumors requiring mediastinotomy for removal. Ann Surg 193:805–809, 1981.
22. Weller CL Jr: Development of the thyroid, parathyroid and thymus glands in man. Contrib Embryol 24:93–139, 1933.
23. Arnaud CD, Brewer HB Jr: Parathyroid hormone: structure and immuno-heterogeneity. *In* Kuhlencordt F, Kruse HP (eds): Calcium Metabolism, Bone and Metabolic Bone Diseases. New York, Springer-Verlag, 1975, pp 295–315.
24. Martin KJ, Hruska KA, Freitag JJ, et al: The peripheral metabolism of parathyroid hormone. N Engl J Med 301:1092–1098, 1979.

25. Austin LA, Heath H III: Calcitonin physiology and pathophysiology. N Engl J Med 304:269, 1981.
26. DeLuca HF: Vitamin D endocrinology. Ann Intern Med 85:367–377, 1976.
27. Verdonk CA, Edis AJ: Parathyroid "double adenomas": fact or fiction? Surgery 90:523, 1981.
28. Ejerblad S, Grimelius L, Johansson H, et al: Studies on the non-adenomatous glands in patients with a solitary parathyroid adenoma. Ups J Med Sci 81:31, 1976.
29. Weiland LH, Garrison RC, ReMine WH, et al: Lipoadenoma of the parathyroid gland. Am J Surg Pathol 2:3, 1978.
30. van Heerden JA, Weiland LH, ReMind WH, et al: Cancer of the parathyroid glands. Arch Surg 114:475, 1979.
31. Schantz A, Castleman B: Parathyroid carcinoma: a study of 70 cases. Cancer 31:600, 1973.
32. Edis AJ, Beahrs OH, van Heerden JA, et al: "Conservative" versus "liberal" approach to parathyroid neck exploration. Surgery 82:466, 1977.
33. Roth SI: Recent advances in parathyroid pathology. Am J Med 50:612, 1971.
34. Black WC III, Utley JR: The differential diagnosis of parathyroid adenoma and chief cell hyperplasia. Am J Clin Pathol 49:761, 1968.
35. Esselstyn CB Jr: Parathyroid pathology: its relation to choice of operation for primary hyperparathyroidism. World J Surg 1:701, 1977.
36. Grimelius L, Åkerström G, Johansson H, et al: Estimation of parenchymal cell content of human parathyroid glands using the image analyzing computer technique. Am J Pathol 93:793, 1978.
37. Wang CA, Rieder SV: A density test for the intraoperative differentiation of parathyroid hyperplasia from neoplasia. Ann Surg 187:63, 1978.
38. Irvin GL, Bagwell CB: Identification of histologically undetectable parathyroid hyperplasia by flow cytometry. Am J Surg 138:567, 1979.
39. Woltering EA, Emmott RC, Javadpour N, et al: ABO (H) cell surface antigens in parathyroid adenoma and hyperplasia. Surgery 90:1–9, 1981.
40. Roth SI, Gallagher MJ: The rapid identification of "normal" parathyroid glands by the presence of intracellular fat. Am J Pathol 84:521, 1976.
41. Russell C, Edis AJ: Surgical treatment of presumptive primary hyperparathyroidism: results in 500 consecutive cases with an evaluation of the role of surgery in the asymptomatic patient. Br J Surg. 69:244, 1982.
42. Keating RF Jr: Diagnosis of primary hyperparathyroidism. JAMA 178:547, 1961.
43. Purnell DC, Scholz DA, Smith LH: Diagnosis of primary hyperparathyroidism. Surg Clin North Am 57:543, 1977.
44. Jackson CE, Frame B: Diagnosis and management of parathyroid disorders. Orthop Clin North AM 3:699, 1972.
45. Pyrah LN, Hodgkinson A, Anderson CK: Primary hyperparathyroidism. Br J Surg 53:245, 1966.
46. Purnell DC, Smith LH, Scholz DA, et al: Primary hyperparathyroidism: a prospective clinical study. Am J Med 50:670, 1971.
47. Yendt ER, Gagne RJA: Detection of primary hyperparathyroidism, with special reference to its occurrence in hypercalciuric females with "normal" or borderline calcium. Can Med Assoc J 98:331, 1968.
48. Sherwood LM: The multiple causes of hypercalcemia in malignant disease. N Engl J Med 303:1412, 1980.
49. Aurbach GD, Mallette LE, Patten BM, et al: Hyperparathyroidism: recent studies. Ann Intern Med 79:566, 1973.
50. Alveryd A, Bostrom H, Wengle B, et al: Indications for surgery in the elderly patient with primary hyperparathyroidism. Acta Chir Scand 142:491, 1976.
51. Wang CA, Guyton SW: Hyperparathyroid crisis: clinical and pathologic studies of 14 patients. Ann Surg 190:782, 1979.

52. Schweitzer VG, Thompson NW, Harness JK, et al: Management of severe hypercalcemia caused by primary hyperparathyroidism. Arch Surg 113:373, 1978.

53. Casey JH: Endocrine emergencies. Med J Aust 2:304, 1980.

54. Cope O: Hyperparathyroidism: diagnosis and management. Am J Surg 99:394, 1960.

55. Linos DA, van Heerden JA, Abboud CF, et al: Primary hyperparathyroidism and peptic ulcer disease. Arch Surg 113:384, 1978.

56. Barreras RF, Donaldson RM Jr: Effects of induced hypercalcemia on human gastric secretion. Gastroenterology 52:670, 1967.

57. Wilson SD, Singh RB, Kalkhoff RK, et al: Does hyperparathyroidism cause hypergastrinemia? Surgery 80:231, 1976.

58. Bess MA, Edis AJ, van Heerden JA: Hyperparathyroidism and pancreatitis: chance or a causal association? JAMA 243:246, 1980.

59. Rosin RD: Pancreatitis and hyperparathyroidism. Postgrad Med J 52:95, 1976.

60. Scholz DA: Hypertension and hyperparathyrodism. Arch Intern Med 137:1123, 1977.

61. Christensson T, Einarsson K: Cholelithiasis in subjects with hypercalcemia and primary hyperparathyroidism detected in a health screening. Gut 18:543, 1977.

62. Berkson J: Limitations of the application of fourfold table analysis to hospital data. Biomet Bull 2:47, 1946.

63. Christensson T: Hyperparathyroidism and radiation therapy. Ann Intern Med 89:216, 1978.

64. Rao SD, Frame B, Miller MJ, et al: Hyperparathyroidism following head and neck irradiation. Arch Intern Med 140:205, 1980.

65. Purnell DC, Scholz DA, Smith LH: Diagnosis of primary hyperparathyroidism. Surg Clin North Am 57:543, 1977.

66. Keating FR: Diagnosis of primary hyperparathyroidism. JAMA 178:547, 1961.

67. Broadus AE, Horst RL, Littledike ET, et al: Primary hyperparathyroidism with intermittent hypercalcemia: serial observations and simple diagnosis by means of oral calcium tolerance test. Clin Endocrinol 12:225, 1980.

68. Benson RC Jr, Riggs BL, Pickard BM, et al: Radioimmunoassay of parathyroid hormone in hypercalcemic patients with malignant disease. Am J Med 56:821, 1974.

69. Foley TP Jr, Harrison HC, Arnaud CD, et al: Familial benign hypercalcemia. J Pediatr 81:1060, 1972.

70. Marx SJ: Familial hypocalciuric hypercalcemia. N Engl J Med 303:810, 1980.

71. Arnaud CD, Tsao HS, Littledike EF: Radioimmunoassay of human PTH in serum. J Clin Invest 50:21, 1971.

72. Palmer FJ, Nelson JC, Bacchus H: The chloride–phosphate ratio in hypercalcemia. Ann Intern Med 80:200, 1974.

73. Monchik JM, Martin HF: Ionized calcium in the diagnosis of primary hyperparathyroidism. Surgery 88:185, 1980.

74. Broadus AE, Mahattey JE, Barker FC, et al: Nephrogenous cyclic adenosine monophosphate as a parathyroid function test. J Clin Invest 60:771, 1977.

75. Clark OH: Methods for diagnosing the cause of hypercalcemia. In Najarian JS, Delaney JP (eds): Endocrine Surgery. Miami, Symposia Specialists, 1981, pp 201–209.

76. Brennan MF, Krudy AG, Doppman JL: Localization of functionally abnormal parathyroid tissue. In Najarian JS, Delaney JP (eds): Endocrine Surgery. Miami, Symposia Specialists, 1981, pp 211–225.

77. Bradley EL III, McGarity WC: Surgical evaluation of parathyroid arteriography. Am J Surg 126:67, 1973.

78. Krementz ET, Yeager R, Hawley W, et al: The first 100 cases of parathyroid tumor from Charity Hospital of Louisiana. Ann Surg 173:872, 1971.

79. Mishkin MM, Baum S, DiChiro G: Emergency treatment of angiography-induced

paraplegia and tetraplegia. N Engl J Med 288:1184, 1973.

80. Seldinger SI: Localization of parathyroid adenoma by arteriography. Acta Radiol 42:353, 1954.

81. Edis AJ, Sheedy PF II, Beahrs OH, et al: Results of reoperation for hyperparathyroidism with evaluation of preoperative localization studies. Surgery 84:384, 1978.

82. Rothmund M, Diethelm L, Brünner H, et al: Diagnosis and surgical treatment of mediastinal parathyroid tumors. Ann Surg 183:139, 1976.

83. Eisenberg H, Pallotta J, Sherwood LM: Selective arteriography, venography and venous hormone assay in diagnosis and localization of parathyroid lesions. Am J Med 56:810, 1974.

84. Brennan MF, Doppman JL, Marx SJ, et al: Reoperative parathyroid surgery for persistent hyperparathyroidism. Surgery 83:669, 1978.

85. Grant CS, Edis AJ, James EM, et al: Parathyroid ultrasound and computed tomography. *In* Rothmund M, Kümmerle F (eds): Fortschritte der endokrinologischen Chirurgie. Stuttgart, New York, Georg Thieme Verlag, 1981, p 109–114.

86. Edis AJ, Evans TC Jr: High-resolution, real-time ultrasonography in the preoperative location of parathyroid tumors. N Engl J Med 301:532, 1979.

87. Reading CC, Charboneau JW, James EM, et al: High resolution parathyroid sonography. AJR 139:539–546, 1982.

88. Sherwood JK, Ackroyd FW, Garcia M: Cimetidine in hyperparathyroidism. Lancet 1:1298, 1980.

89. Caro JF, Castro JH, Glennon JA: Effect of long-term propranolol administration on parathyroid hormone and calcium concentration in primary hyperparathyroidism. Ann Intern Med 91:740, 1979.

90. Aurbach GD, Mallette LE, Patten BM, et al: Hyperparathyroidism: recent studies. Ann Intern Med 79:566, 1973.

91. Heath DA, Wright AD, Barnes AD, et al: Surgical treatment of primary hyperparathyroidism in the elderly. Br Med J June 14th, p 1406, 1980.

92. Scholz DA, Purnell DC: Asymptomatic primary hyperparathyroidism 10-year prospective study. Mayo Clin Proc 56:473, 1981.

93. Hodgson SF, Heath H III: Asymptomatic primary hyperparathyroidism: treat or follow? Mayo Clin Proc 56:521, 1981.

94. Graham JJ, Harding PE, Hoare LL, et al: Asymptomatic hyperparathyroidism: an assessment of operative intervention. Br J Surg 67:115, 1980.

95. Bruining HA, van Houten H, Juttman JR, et al: Results of operative treatment of 615 patients with primary hyperparathyroidism. World J Surg 5:85, 1981.

96. Satava RM, Beahrs OH, Scholz DA: Success rate of cervical exploration for hyperparathyroidism. Arch Surg 110:625, 1975.

97. Coe FL, Favus MJ: Does mild, asymptomatic hyperparathyroidism require surgery? N Engl J Med 302:224, 1980.

98. Kaplan RA, Snyder WH, Stewart A, et al: Metabolic effects of parathyroidectomy in asymptomatic primary hyperparathyroidism. J Clin Endocrinol Metab 42:415, 1976.

99. Tougaard L, Han C, Rodbrop P, et al: Bone mineralization and bone mineral content in primary hyperparathyroidism. Act Endocrinol 84:314, 1977.

100. Edis AJ, van Heerden JA, Scholz DA: Results of subtotal parathyroidectomy for primary chief cell hyperplasia. Surgery 86:462, 1979.

101. Block MA, Frame B, Jackson CE: The efficacy of subtotal parathyroidectomy for primary hyperparathyroidism due to multiple gland involvement. Surgery 147:1, 1978.

102. Clark OH, Way LW, Hunt TK: Recurrent hyperparathyroidism. Ann Surg 184:391, 1976.

103. Wells SA Jr, Farndon JR, Dale JK, et al: Long-term evaluation of patients with primary parathyroid hyperplasia managed by total parathyroidectomy and

heterotopic autotransplantation. Ann Surg 192:451, 1980.

104. Roth SI, Wang CA, Potts JT Jr: The team approach to primary hyperparathyroidism. Human Pathol 6:645, 1975.

105. Edis AJ, Sheedy PF II, Beahrs OH, et al: Results of reoperation for hyperparathyroidism, with evaluation of preoperative localization studies. Surgery 84:384, 1978.

106. Brennan MF, Doppman JL, Marx SJ, et al: Reoperative parathyroid surgery for persistent hyperparathyroidism. Surgery 83:669, 1978.

107. van Vroonhoven TJ, Muller H: Causes of failure in the surgical treatment of primary hyperparathyroidism. Br J Surg 65:297, 1978.

108. Wang CA: Parathyroid reexploration. A clinical and pathological study of 112 cases. Ann Surg 186:140, 1977.

109. Wang CA, Mahaffey JE, Axelrod L, et al: Hyperfunctioning supernumerary parathyroid glands. Surg Gynecol Obstet 148:711, 1979.

110. Palmer JA, Sutton FR: Importance of a fifth parathyroid gland in the surgical treatment of hyperparathyroidism. Can J Surg 21:350, 1978.

111. Russell CF, Edis AJ, Scholz DA, et al: Mediastinal parathyroid tumors—experience with 38 tumors requiring mediastinotomy for removal. Ann Surg 193:805, 1981.

112. Saxe AW, Brennan MF: Strategy and technique of reoperative parathyroid surgery. Surgery 89:417, 1981.

113. Edis AJ, Beahrs OH, Sheedy PF II: Reoperation for hyperparathyroidism. World J Surg 1:731, 1977.

114. Hellström J: The causes of unsuccessful or inadequate parathyroidectomy in hyperparathyroidism. Acta Chir Scand 112:79, 1957.

115. Edis AJ, Beart RW Jr: Parathyroid autotransplantation: an innovative approach. Hosp Pract Jan 1979, pp 78–84.

116. Brennan MF, Brown EM: Prediction of in vivo function of human parathyroid tissue autografts by in vitro testing. World J Surg 4:747, 1980.

117. Saxe AW, Brennan MF: Reoperative parathyroid surgery for primary hyperparathyroidism caused by multiple-gland disease: total parathyroidectomy and autotransplantation with cryopreserved tissue. Surgery 91:616, 1982.

118. Hanley DA, Sherwood LM: Secondary hyperparathyroidism in chronic renal failure. Pathophysiology and treatment. Med Clin North Am 62:1319, 1978.

119. Arnaud CD: Hyperparathyroidism and renal failure. Kidney Int 4:89, 1973.

120. Johnson WJ, Goldsmith RS, Beabout JW, et al: Prevention and reversal of progressive secondary hyperparathyroidism in patients maintained by hemodialysis. Am J Med 56:827, 1974.

121. Clark OH: Secondary and tertiary hyperparathyroidism. In Najarian JS, Delaney JP (eds): Endocrine Surgery. Miami, Symposia Specialists, 1981, pp 239–247.

122. Cordell LJ, Maxwell JG, Warden GD: Parathyroidectomy in chronic renal failure. Am J Surg 138:951, 1979.

123. Gordon HE, Coburn JW, Passaro E Jr: Surgical management of secondary hyperparathyroidism. Arch Surg 104:520, 1972.

124. Sivula A, Kuhlback, B, Kock B, et al: Parathyroidectomy in chronic renal failure. Acta Chir Scand 145:19, 1979.

125. Bigos ST, Neer RM, St Goar WJ: Hypercalcemia of seven years' duration after kidney transplantation. Am J Surg 132:83, 1976.

126. Gittes RF, Radde IC: Experimental model for hyperparathyroidism: effect of excessive numbers of transplanted isologous parathyroid glands. J Urol 95:595, 1966.

127. David DS, Sakai S, Brennan BL, et al: Hypercalcemia after renal transplantation. Long-term follow-up data. N Engl J Med 289:398, 1973.

Surgery of the Thyroid

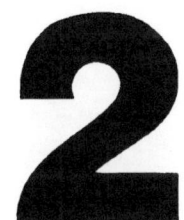

In the early half of this century, thyroidectomy was used to treat practically all diseases of the thyroid except deficiency states. Today, however, it is limited principally to the management of solitary nodules and cancer of the thyroid. Other, less frequent indications for thyroidectomy include the control of hyperthyroidism in patients with hyperfunctioning adenomatous goiter and selected patients with Graves' disease, and the alleviation of symptoms due to thoracic inlet compression by large, nodular goiters. Classic endemic colloid goiter has virtually been eliminated by the supplementation of foodstuffs with iodides, and effective nonoperative therapies have been developed for Graves' disease, thyroiditis, and many cases of nontoxic adenomatous goiter.

The antithyroid drugs, introduced by Astwood in 1943 (1), posed the first serious challenge to operative treatment of hyperthyroidism. Radioiodine became available 3 years later and gained immediate popularity. In the ensuing years, radioiodine has almost totally supplanted thyroidectomy as the treatment of choice for Graves' disease in the United States. Greer and Astwood (2) were responsible for promoting the medical treatment of nontoxic goiter with thyroid hormone.

With a decrease in the total number of goiters and in the number of patients with thyroid disease coming to surgery, there has been less and less opportunity for surgical residents to become proficient in removing the thyroid gland. Black (3) has been prompted to write that "the quality of surgery of the thyroid will undoubtedly decline in time, if it has not done so already, making nonsurgical methods of treatment comparably even more attractive." Nonetheless, surgeons should be thoroughly familiar with the operative technique. According to the American Cancer Society, there are more than 9000 new cases of thyroid cancer in the United States each year and surgery remains the first and, in some cases, the only therapy for this condition. Until recently, thyroidectomy was the only definitive way to exclude malignancy in a thyroid nodule; however, it is to be hoped that the increasing use of fine-needle aspiration cytology in the diagnostic evaluation of thyroid nodules will help limit the number of operations on benign lesions in the future.

**General
Introduction**

SURGICAL ANATOMY

ORIENTATION

The thyroid gland has a bipartite origin from the primitive pharynx and the neural crest (Fig. 2-1). The normal adult thyroid weighs about 15 g and is composed of two lateral lobes, a midline isthmus, and, in about 30% of patients, a pyramidal lobe that extends upward for a variable distance from the left side of the isthmus. The gland is wrapped around the anterolateral portions of the trachea and larynx, each lobe occupying a bed between the trachea and esophagus medially and the carotid sheath and sternocleidomastoid muscle laterally.

A delicate, adherent connective tissue capsule (the true capsule) invests the gland and sends septa into its substance, breaking it up into a number of anatomic lobes and lobules. A richly anastomosing network of vessels courses in the true capsule of the thyroid and it is this unique arrangement of the vessels that allows easy clamping and control of bleeding during subtotal thyroidectomy.

Each lobe is composed of many tightly packed macroscopic discs or lobules, and each lobule, in turn, is made up of clusters of 20–40 follicles bound together by a fine connective tissue sheath. The lobule, serviced by its own individual artery and vein, constitutes the basic structural and functional unit of the thyroid gland.

On histologic section, the follicles vary widely in size (30–500 μm in diameter) because they are cut in different planes (Fig. 2-2). They are lined with cuboidal epithelial cells and are filled with colloidal material (thyroglobulin), which is the storage form of thyroid hormone. The parafollicular or C cells are difficult to identify in the usual hematoxylin and eosin sections of normal human thyroid but may be demonstrated with the use of special immunocytochemical techniques.

Also surrounding the gland is a covering of pretracheal fascia known as the surgical capsule. Anteriorly and laterally, this sheath is thin, transparent, and easy to separate; medially and posteriorly, however, it condenses to attach the lobes of the thyroid firmly to the cricoid cartilage and the upper two tracheal rings. This is the so-called adherent zone of the surgical capsule, or suspensory ligament of Berry.

Thyroid physiology and metabolism. The thyroid follicle produces two physiologically active hormones: thyroxine (T4) and 3,5,3'-triiodothyronine (T3). Since T3 is four times more metabolically active than T4 on a milligram-to-milligram basis, and because T3 is the principal intracellular form of thyroid hormone, it is now generally agreed that T4 is a prohormone and T3 is the active hormone.

The hormone calcitonin is secreted by the parafollicular or C cells of the thyroid. Its putative physiologic functions relate to plasma calcium homeostasis; however, thyroidectomized persons with no detectable calcitonin in the blood do not appear to have any significant disturbance of calcium metabolism.

Iodide is extracted from the blood, oxidized, and coupled intramolecularly with tyrosine radicals to form thyroglobulin. Thyroglobulin, which is a mixture

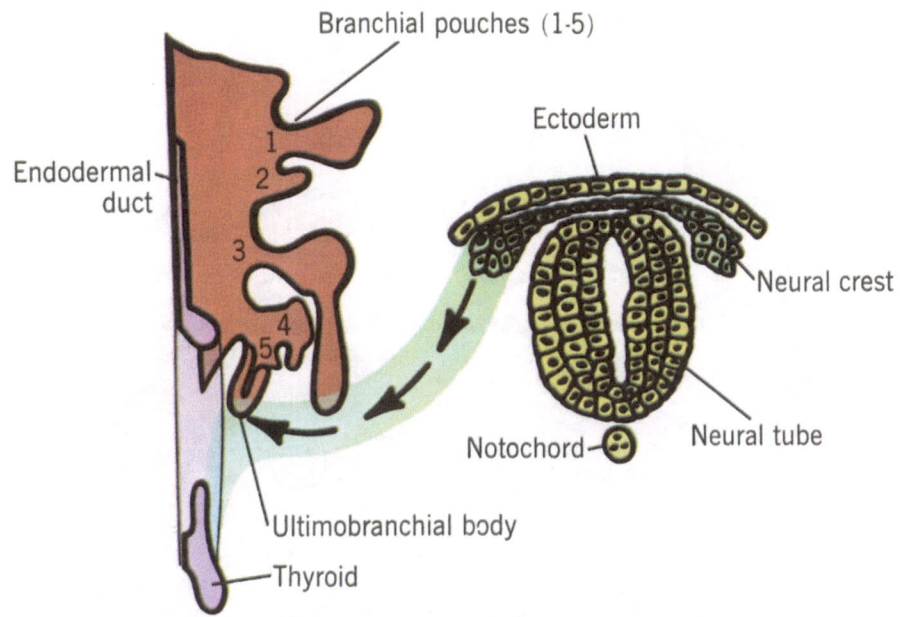

Branchial pouches (1-5)

Ectoderm

Endodermal duct

1
2
3
4
5

Neural crest

Notochord

Neural tube

Ultimobranchial body

Thyroid

Development of the thyroid. The main body of the thyroid gland is derived from the endoderm of the primitive foregut. It descends in the midline of the neck from the pharyngeal floor and develops as a bilateral encapsulated structure. The foramen cecum of the tongue, lingual, and other midline thyroid ectopia, thyroglossal duct cysts, and the pyramidal lobe are all part of this embryologic ontogeny. The parafollicular or "C" (for calcitonin-producing) cells found scattered throughout the thyroid gland are derived from the neural crest. These cells migrate from the neural crest to the ultimobranchial bodies of the 4th and 5th branchial pouches and eventually populate the thyroid by way of its lateral anlagen (4). These cells belong to a larger system of cells comprising what is known as the APUD system (so named because most of these cells share the capacity for amine precursor uptake and decarboxylation) or neuroendocrine series (5,6). They are all believed to come from the neural ectoderm or neuroendocrine-programed ectoblast of the developing embryo. Together they make up the central and peripheral components of the neuroendocrine system (see section in Chapter 1, Common Denominators in Endocrine Neoplasia).

Fig. 2-1.

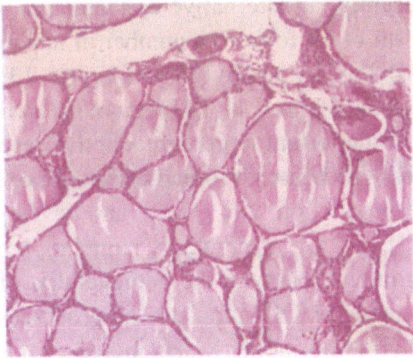

Histologic specimen of normal thyroid. The normal thyroid follicle consists of a single layer of cuboidal epithelial cells resting on a basement membrane and surrounding a central colloid mass.

Fig. 2-2.

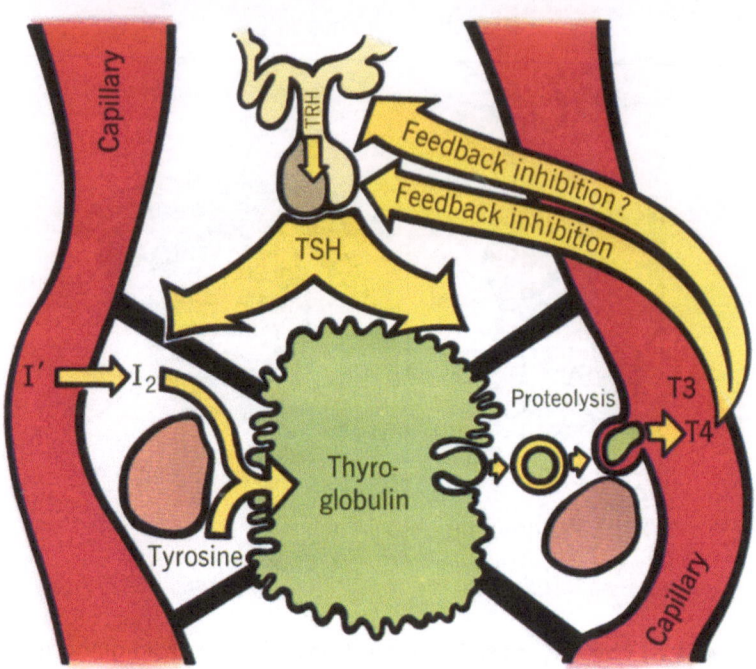

Fig. 2-3. **Thyroid physiology and metabolism.** Through the action of TRH from the hypothalamus, TSH is released from the anterior pituitary. TSH stimulates all processes leading to the synthesis and release of thyroid hormone. Following extraction from the blood, iodide is oxidized and coupled with tyrosine to form thyroglobulin. Release of T3 and T4 into the bloodstream occurs by reverse pinocytosis. These hormones cause a negative feedback on TSH, a "servo" control mechanism which is characteristic of endocrine systems.

of iodotyrosines, T3, and T4, is stored as colloid in the lumen of the follicle. Release of active hormones into the circulation involves reverse pinocytosis of intrafollicular colloid and intracellular proteolysis (Fig. 2-3).

In plasma, T3 and T4 are bound to globulin and albumin. T4 undergoes monodeiodination to form the more active T3 in the periphery (principally in the liver and kidney); more recently, an alternative de-iodinative pathway has been described for the metabolism of T4 to form a number of apparently biologically inactive products, such as 3,3′,5′-triiodothyronine (reverse T3; rT3). This alternative pathway, which permits shunting of T4 metabolism away from active T3, toward inactive rT3, may be important in certain adaptive responses to starvation and nonthyroidal illness. T3 has widespread effects on cellular metabolism, oxygen consumption, heat production, and growth and development. The evidence suggests that these effects are mediated by stimulation of gene transcription of the nucleus and by interaction with the mitochondria of target cells (7).

Thyroid-stimulating hormone (TSH) stimulates all processes leading to the synthesis and release of thyroid hormone. It also increases the cellularity and vascularity of the thyroid gland. The secretion of TSH is regulated, in turn, by the concentration of unbound thyroid hormones in the blood via a negative-feedback or "servo" control mechanism exerted mainly at the level of the pituitary

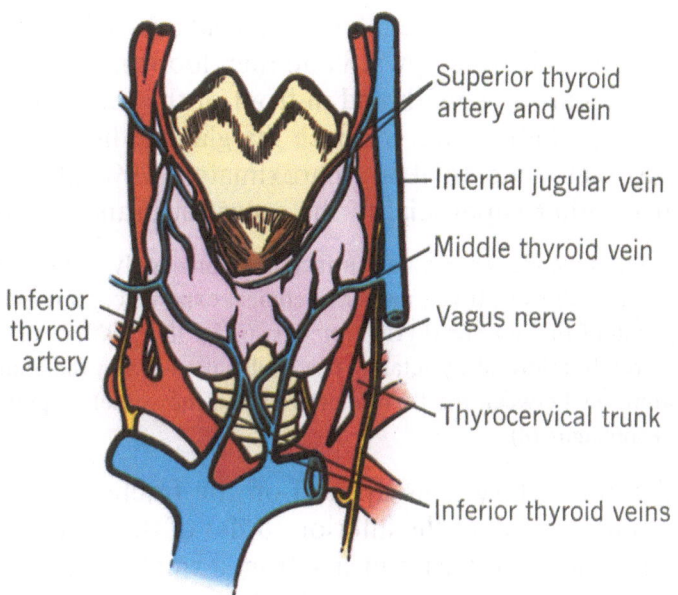

Blood supply of the thyroid.   **Fig. 2-4.**

(Fig. 2-3). It is thought that the hypothalamus simply determines the set-point of the feedback threshold, presumably through the secretion of thyrotropin-releasing hormone (TRH).

The concentration of intrathyroidal iodide exerts an important autoregulatory control over thyroid function. The size of the organic iodide pool inversely influences the iodide transport mechanism (iodide trap) and the thyroid's response to TSH. High concentrations of iodide decrease the rate at which active hormone is formed and released into the bloodstream (the Wolff-Chaikoff effect). This mechanism forms the basis for the preoperative use of Lugol's iodine or SSKI to rapidly control thyrotoxicity and cause involution of the gland in patients with Graves' disease. It should be noted, however, that the effect is usually transient and "escape" from the iodine effect eventually occurs after several weeks.

BLOOD SUPPLY

Arterial Supply. The thyroid gland is supplied by two arteries—the superior and inferior thyroid arteries (Fig. 2-4)—and sometimes an additional midline artery, the thyroidea ima, derived most commonly from the innominate artery. The superior thyroid artery is the first branch of the external carotid. It arises a little above the thyroid cartilage and runs downward on the inferior constrictor of the pharynx, alongside the superior laryngeal nerve and deep to the sternothyroid muscle, to enter the thyroid at its upper pole. Terminal branches anastomose within the gland with those of the ipsilateral thyroid artery and the superior thyroid artery of the opposite side. The inferior thyroid artery is a branch of the thyrocervical trunk. It runs upward and then loops medially and downward behind the carotid sheath and in front of the longissimus cervicis muscle and sympathetic trunk to reach the gland. The recurrent laryngeal nerve crosses deep to it in approximately 70% of cases; in the remainder it is either superficial to the artery or branches around it.

> The parathyroid glands receive their principal blood supply from the inferior thyroid artery on each side. It is a matter of clinical experience, however, that bilateral ligation of the inferior thyroid arteries, or for that matter, all four thyroid arteries, is rarely followed by tetany. The explanation lies in the abundant collateral anastomoses between the thyroid arteries and the vessels supplying the trachea and esophagus (8).

The thyroidea ima artery runs upward on the trachea from the aortic arch or innominate trunk to the inferior border of the thyroid gland. It is not always present and it varies in size from a small arteriole to a vessel rarely as large as the inferior thyroid artery, which it sometimes replaces.

Venous Drainage. Large, thin-walled veins anastomose freely in the capsule of the thyroid gland to form a characteristic surface network. Their tributaries, which drain the substance of the gland, are of small caliber. Therefore, provided the capsular vessels are clamped, partial excision of the thyroid is usually a relatively bloodless procedure. The capsular plexus is drained by the superior thyroid veins above (either directly or indirectly into the internal jugular vein), by the middle thyroid vein from the midportion of the gland (directly into the internal jugular vein), and by the inferior thyroid veins from the lower pole (into the innominate vein or internal jugular).

LYMPHATIC DRAINAGE

Dye injected into the isthmus of the thyroid drains down into the mediastinal nodes and upward into the prelaryngeal (or so-called Delphian) nodes immediately above the isthmus. Dye injected into the central or lower parts of the lateral lobes drains into the tracheoesophageal lymph nodes which lie behind the thyroid and along the course of the recurrent laryngeal nerves. Only when dye is injected into the superior pole of the thyroid does it appear to drain directly into the nodes of the lateral neck along the lymphatics of the superior thyroid vessels (9).

It would appear from these observations that the nodes of the lateral cervical region (jugular chain, posterior triangle) are not primary but secondary zones of lymphatic drainage for the thyroid (Fig. 2-5). Thus, in thyroid cancer, it is the nodes of the middle, or visceral, compartment

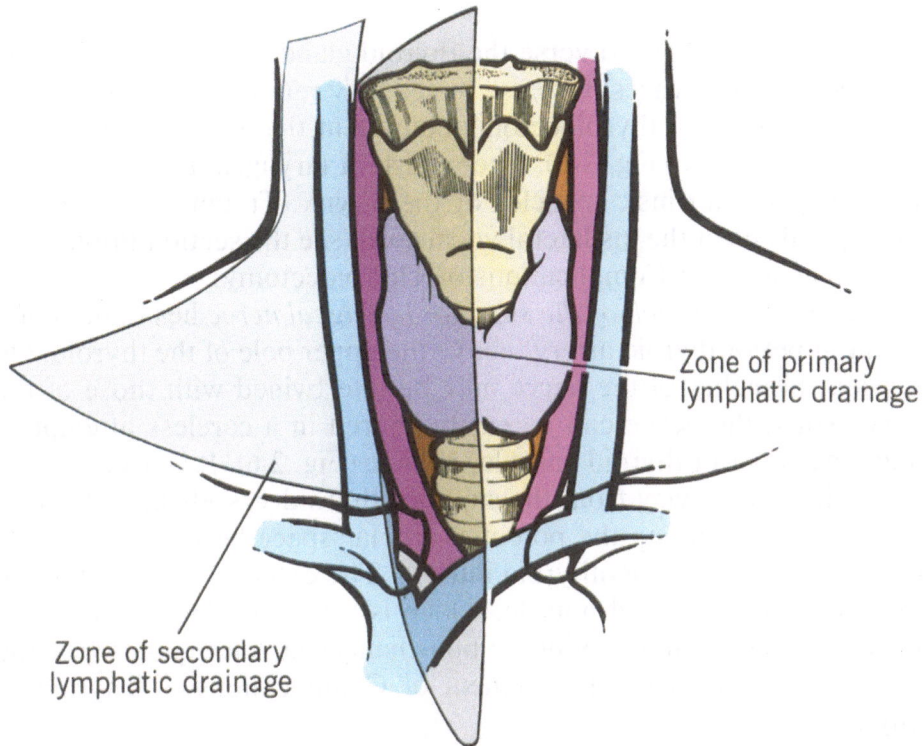

Zone of primary
lymphatic drainage

Zone of secondary
lymphatic drainage

Lymphatic drainage of the thyroid. The primary zone of lymphatic drainage
is to the midline pretracheal, prelaryngeal (Delphian), tracheoesophageal, and
superior mediastinal nodes. The nodes of the lateral neck (internal jugular, posterior triangle) constitute a zone of secondary drainage.

Fig. 2-5.

of the neck that are usually the first site of metastasis; the nodes of the
lateral neck become involved with tumor spread later in the course of
the disease.

IMPORTANT RELATIONS

The relationships to the thyroid of the recurrent and superior laryngeal
nerves, the cervical sympathetic trunk, and the parathyroid glands are
of great importance in thyroidectomy.

The *recurrent laryngeal nerve* ascends on each side either in the
tracheoesophageal sulcus or just lateral to it, to reach the junction of the
lower and middle thirds of the thyroid gland. Here, the nerve assumes a
variable relationship with the inferior thyroid artery, frequently dividing
into several branches before it courses through the adherent zone of the
surgical capsule. It finally enters the larynx deep to the cricopharyngeus
muscle and posterior to the cricothyroid articulation and the inferior
horn of the thyroid cartilage (see Fig. 2-31). In about 10% of patients,

the nerve may actually traverse the thyroid gland itself before entering the larynx. In such cases it is easy to see how retraction on the thyroid lobe in the course of thyroidectomy could tent the nerve up, making it vulnerable to injury (Fig. 2-6). The recurrent laryngeal nerves on each side supply the intrinsic muscles of the larynx. Trauma to the nerve causes paralysis of the ipsilateral vocal cord (see the section Prevention and Management of Complications of Thyroidectomy).

The *external branch of the superior laryngeal nerve* lies right alongside the superior thyroid artery, above the upper pole of the thyroid. On occasion, branches of the nerve may be intertwined with those of the artery. Thus, the nerve can be easily injured in a careless attempt to secure the superior thyroid vascular pedicle (Fig. 2-6). It is necessary to dissect the nerve away from the superior thyroid vessels prior to their ligation, by opening up the potential areolar space between the upper lobe vessels and the cricothyroid muscle. The external laryngeal nerve supplies the cricothyroid muscle, which is a tensor of the vocal cord. Injury to the nerve may produce subtle changes in voice quality (see the section Prevention and Management of Complications of Thyroidectomy).

The *cervical sympathetic chain* lies in close proximity to the inferior thyroid artery where the latter arches medially toward the thyroid gland. It is therefore vulnerable if one attempts to dissect out and ligate the inferior thyroid artery too far laterally (Fig. 2-6). The resulting miosis and ptosis usually persist for long periods and are often permanent. For some unknown reason, cutaneous vascular dilatation, which is usually part of Horner's syndrome, is absent or transient in these patients (10).

The *parathyroid glands* are situated in close relationship to the posterior and lateral aspects of the thyroid. Their detailed anatomy is discussed in Chapter 1 (see Fig. 1-1). The parathyroids may be injured, devascularized, or inadvertently removed during thyroidectomy. Every effort should be made to preserve these glands and to keep their blood supply intact. In those few instances in which a parathyroid gland is devascularized in the course of thyroidectomy, it should be diced up into 1–2 mm pieces and transplanted into separate pockets in the sternocleidomastoid muscle. Such autotransplanted tissue can be expected to survive and function (see Chapter 1 section, Strategy and Technique of Reoperative Parathyroid Surgery for Persistent or Recurrent HPT). With due caution and meticulous technique in preserving the parathyroid blood supply, and with resort to parathyroid autotransplantation when necessary, the incidence of permanent hypoparathyroidism after subtotal thyroidectomy should be almost zero, and after total thyroidectomy, less than 1% (see the section Prevention and Management of Complications of Thyroidectomy).

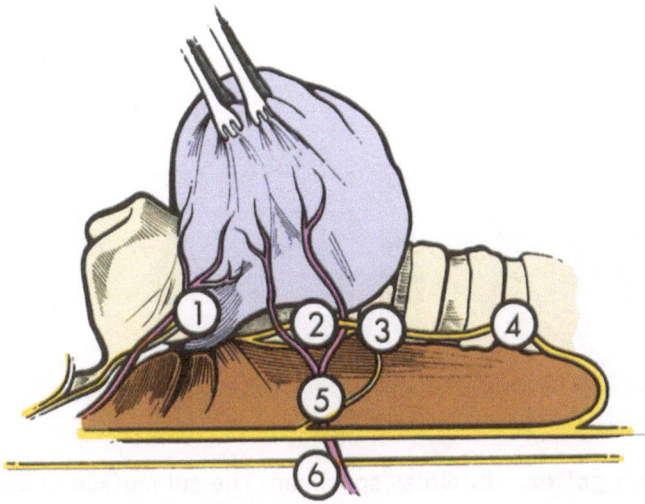

Sites of possible nerve injury in thyroidectomy. *1:* External laryngeal nerve during ligation of the superior thyroid vascular pedicle. *2:* Recurrent laryngeal nerve as it traverses the ligament of Berry during lobectomy. *3:* Recurrent laryngeal nerve during ligation of the inferior thyroid artery. *4:* Recurrent laryngeal nerve during ligation of the inferior thyroid veins. Note that in a small proportion of cases the nerve may be sufficiently anterolateral to the trachea such that it could be caught up and injured during ligation of the veins. *5:* Nonrecurrent nerve during ligation of the inferior thyroid artery. A nonrecurrent nerve may be mistaken for the inferior thyroid artery and ligated because it takes a parallel horizontal course from the cervical vagus to the larynx. Fortunately, this anatomic variant is rare (about 1 in 400 cases), and with routine exposure of the nerve prior to ligation of the artery, injury to the nerve should be avoided. *6:* Cervical sympathetic trunk during ligation of the inferior thyroid artery.

Fig. 2-6.

The principal indication for thyroidectomy today is to rule out malignancy in a discrete or dominant thyroid nodule. Other goiters may be removed for cosmetic reasons or because they have enlarged sufficiently to cause symptoms due to compression of the trachea, esophagus, or major vessels at the thoracic inlet, or because they are causing hyperthyroidism.

Nodular Goiter and Thyroid Carcinoma

PATHOLOGY

Thyroid nodules are palpable in approximately 5% of the U.S. population, with regional variation from 2% to 10% (11–13). The vast majority are dominant "colloid" or "macrofollicular" adenomatous goiters (Fig. 2-7), some are cases of focal thyroiditis (Fig. 2-8), and others are true benign neoplasms or adenomas (Fig. 2-9). Comparatively few (probably less than 5%) (21) are carcinomas. Indiscriminate removal of thyroid nodules is therefore clearly unwarranted.

> **Adenomatous Goiter.** This condition (Fig. 2-7) is believed to be the end product of repeated episodes of focal hyperplasia and involution caused by intermittent

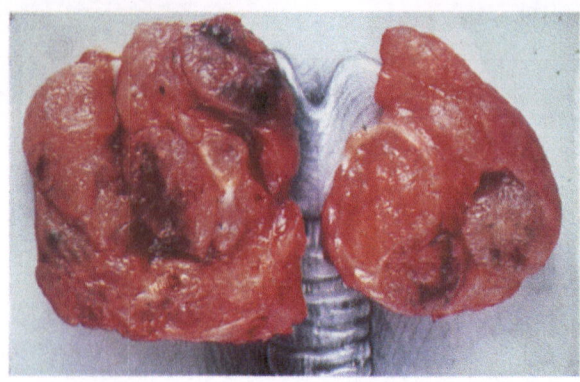
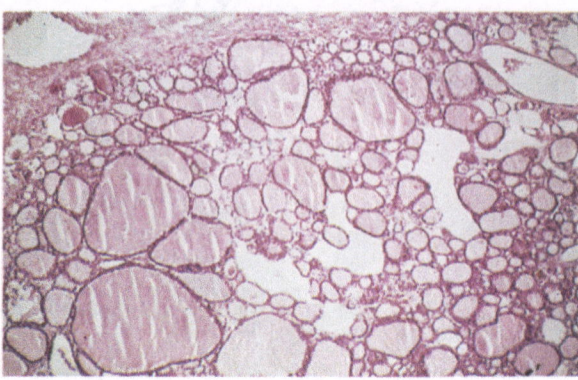

A   B

Fig. 2-7. **Adenomatous goiter.** **A.** Gross specimen. The cut surface of an adenomatous goiter presents a spectrum of pathologic findings: localized colloid nodules, areas of scarring, cystic degeneration, calcification, and hemorrhage. Bleeding into a cyst may produce a sudden increase in the size of the goiter, accompanied by pain and symptoms of thoracic inlet compression. **B.** Histologic specimen. Typical array of micro- and macrofollicles lined with flattened follicular epithelium.

TSH secretion as a compensatory response to impaired thyroid hormone synthesis. Iodine deficiency, dietary goitrogens, autoimmune disease, and inherent biosynthetic defects within the thyroid have all been implicated.

Hashimoto's Thyroiditis (Fig. 2-8A). This is an autoimmune disorder closely related to Graves' disease. Detection of thyroid autoantibodies in the serum and needle biopsy are the most useful diagnostic tests available to the physician. About 25% of patients are hypothyroid when first seen, although transient hyperthyroidism, associated with blocked radioiodine uptake, can also occur (see the section Hashitoxicosis). The condition usually presents in women of middle age, as a moderately enlarged and rubbery firm gland with a bosselated rather than a truly nodular surface. On rare occasions, the disease is focal and may simulate thyroid carcinoma. Sometimes, progressive enlargement of the gland may occur despite treatment with thyroid hormone, leading one to suspect underlying lymphoma. In either case operation may be indicated. If thyroidectomy is performed, thyroid hormone should be given postoperatively and continued indefinitely (15).

Granulomatous (De Quervain's) Thyroiditis. This is a self-limited thyroiditis (Fig. 2-8B), probably caused by an echovirus or enterovirus (16), which presents after a mild flu prodrome, with fever, malaise, and a diffusely enlarged, painful, and tender thyroid. The atypical case may present with focal disease, which is limited to one lobe, and pain and tenderness may be completely absent. Thyroidectomy is advised in such instances to rule out malignancy (15,17). Occasionally, granulomatous thyroiditis causes transient hyperthyroidism associated with blocked uptake of radioiodine (see the section Graves' Disease).

Riedel's Thyroiditis. This is an exceedingly rare and peculiar type of chronic fibrosing inflammation of the thyroid (Fig. 2-8C) indistinguishable clinically from cancer (18). In approximately one-third of cases there is associated retroperitoneal or mediastinal fibrosis (19). The gland is typically very hard, fixed, and usu-

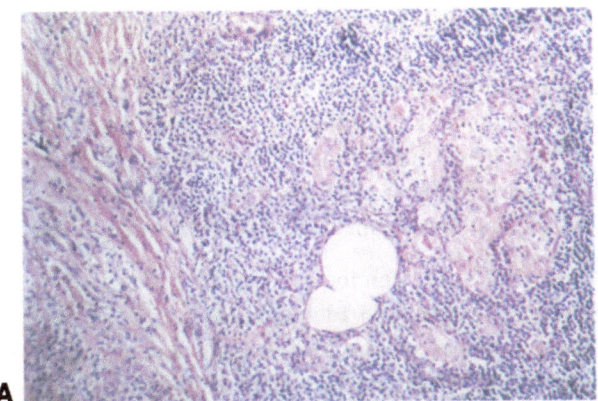

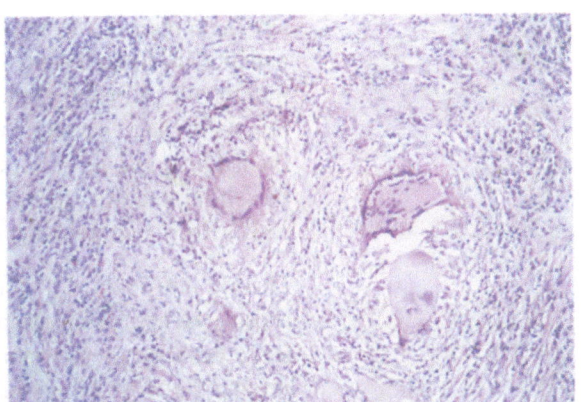

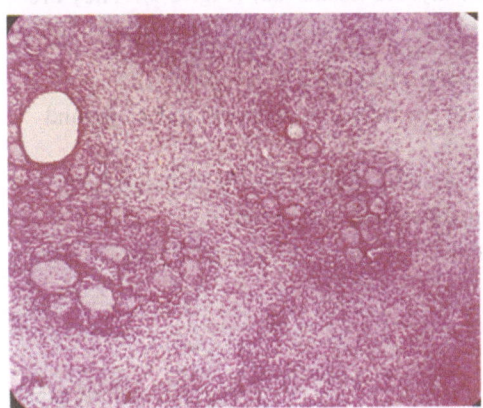

Histologic specimens of thyroiditis. **A.** Hashimoto's thyroiditis. Lympho-   **Fig. 2-8.**
cytic and plasma cell infiltration are seen with oxyphilic epithelium, epithelial
destruction, and fibrosis (14). **B.** Granulomatous (De Quervain's) thyroiditis.
The granulomatous focus of inflammation with foreign body giant cells enclos-
ing fragments of colloid is typical. **C.** Riedel's thyroiditis. There is almost complete destruction of thyroid parenchyma and replacement with fibrotic reaction.
(Used with permission from Woolner LB, McConahey WM, Beahrs OH: Stroma
lymphomatosa (Hashimoto's thyroiditis) and related thyroidal disorders. J Clin
Endocrinol 19:57–81, 1959.)

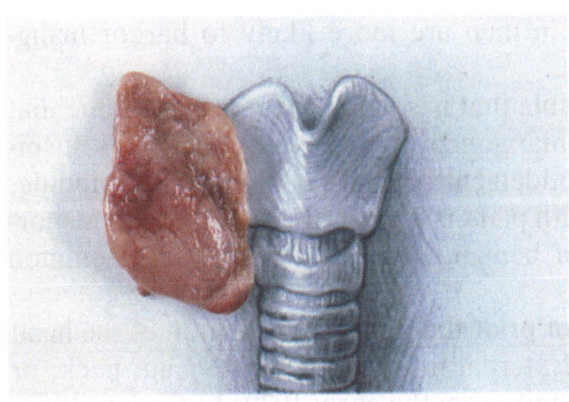

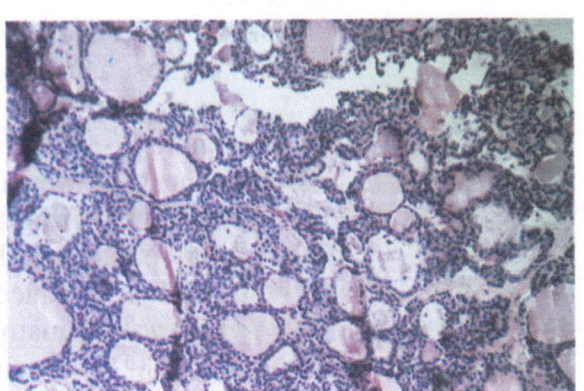

Thyroid adenoma. **A.** Gross specimen of a true follicular adenoma. **B.** His-   **Fig. 2-9.**
tologic specimen of typical microfollicular adenoma.

ally nontender. Obstructive symptoms may be present and up to one-half of the patients are hypothyroid when first seen. All patients require surgical exploration to rule out carcinoma and to free the trachea from the constricting mass of fibrous tissue. The surgical procedure consists essentially of wedge resection of the isthmus and inner aspects of both lobes. Interestingly, the process appears to be self-limited and, in the authors' experience, freeing the trachea has proved a satisfactory guarantee against subsequent development of airway obstruction (15).

Thyroid Adenoma. The term "adenoma" has been loosely applied to focal encapsulated areas of hyperplasia occurring within an adenomatous goiter. We prefer to describe these lesions as adenomatous, colloid, or follicular nodules, reserving the term "adenoma" to describe benign, encapsulated cellular neoplasms loosely surrounded by otherwise normal thyroid tissue (20) (Fig. 2-9). They are classified as follows:

1. Embryonal: composed of cords and strands of cells forming acini.
2. Fetal: composed of small acini with abundant interacinar, loose, ground substance.
3. Follicular: showing mature acinar development and usually comprising a mixture of microfollicles and compact cellular aggregates.
4. Hürthle cell: another variant composed of large, pale acidophilic cells arranged in a trabecular pattern.

DIAGNOSIS

CLINICAL FEATURES: EVALUATION OF THYROID NODULES FOR MALIGNANCY

A selective approach to the management of thyroid nodules involves an assessment of known clinical risk factors, the physical characteristics of the goiter, and certain laboratory studies.

Clinical Risk Factors

1. *Age.* The risk of carcinoma in a dominant thyroid nodule in a child under 14 years of age is approximately 50% (22). The risk in an adult is probably less than 10% overall, with a slightly greater risk after age 60 years.

2. *Sex.* Thyroid nodules in men are more likely to harbor malignancy than those in women.

3. *Growth Pattern.* A nodule that has appeared recently or one that has undergone progressive enlargement over several months is suspicious for cancer. However, sudden enlargement of a preexisting nodule, especially if it is associated with pain, is almost invariably due to hemorrhage into a colloid nodule or benign adenoma. Pain is an uncommon symptom of thyroid cancer.

4. *Irradiation.* A history of prior therapeutic irradiation of the head and neck should be sought. External irradiation of the head, neck, or upper thorax was used commonly from the early 1920s to the late 1950s to treat a variety of benign conditions (such as cervical lymphadenopathy, thymic enlargement, enlarged tonsils or adenoids, acne, heman-

gioma, or keloids). It is now clearly recognized that such exposure, particularly during childhood, results in an increased incidence of various head and neck tumors—including thyroid neoplasia (23), parathyroid adenomas (24), and salivary gland and neurogenic tumors (25,26). The risk of developing thyroid cancer is proportional to the dose of external radiation, but induction of cancer may occur with as little as 7 rads exposure to the thyroid (27). In the absence of any palpable abnormality in the thyroid the risk of cancer is no higher than 7% and is more likely to be in the range of 1% or less (28). The reported risk of thyroid cancer in patients who have palpable thyroid nodules and a history of therapeutic irradiation of the head and neck varies from less than 20% to 50% (23,28,29). The latency period for the development of clinically apparent thyroid cancer following external irradiation may be as long as 25 years (29,30).

5. *Family History*. A family history of thyroid cancer (indeed of any endocrine tumor) must be explored in detail. Medullary thyroid carcinoma (MTC), which accounts for approximately 5% of all thyroid cancers, is familial in 40% of cases; it is transmitted as an autosomal dominant trait. Familial MTC may occur in association with bilateral pheochromocytomas and/or hyperparathyroidism, i.e., multiple endocrine neoplasia type 2 syndrome (MEN-II). Thus, a positive family history has twofold significance: (a) the patient may have associated but as yet undetected endocrine disease as part of MEN-II, and (b) other members of the family may be harboring similar, potentially lethal endocrine tumors.

Physical Characteristics of the Goiter. (See Fig. 2-10 for physical examination of the thyroid gland.)

1. *Single versus multiple*. A dominant or clinically "solitary" nodule is considered much more likely to be cancerous (about 18%–35%) than a multinodular gland (about 5%) (3,31). As implied, most nodules described as solitary on clinical examination are found at operation to be simply the largest nodule in an otherwise multinodular adenomatous goiter.

2. *Consistency*. If the nodule is firm to hard in consistency, cancer is more likely than if the tumor is soft and cystic. However, this criterion is not entirely reliable because some papillary cancers are cystic, and follicular carcinomas can be relatively soft. A rock-hard nodule usually results from extensive calcification in a degenerative colloid nodule.

3. *Fixation*. A lesion that is fixed to surrounding anatomic structures is more suspect as cancerous than a freely mobile one.

4. *Lymph Nodes*. Associated palpable cervical lymphadenopathy points strongly to cancer.

5. *Recurrent Nerve Paralysis*. In the absence of a previous history of neck surgery, a fixed vocal cord in the presence of a thyroid mass is virtually pathognomic of malignancy.

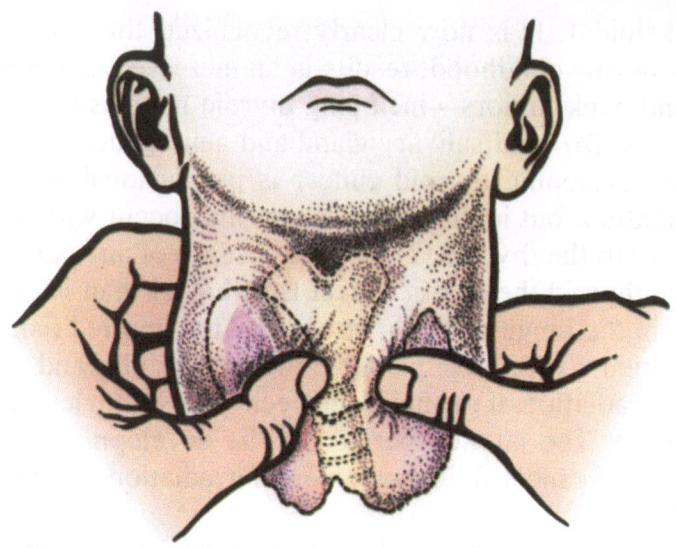

Fig. 2-10. **Examination of the thyroid gland.** The patient stands and faces the examiner. Enlargement or irregularity of the thyroid is often apparent immediately on inspection. Operative scars and trophic skin changes resulting from prior irradiation therapy are noted. The gland is depressed on one side of the trachea to displace the opposite lobe forward, where it can be grasped and palpated between the thumb and fingers. As the patient swallows and the gland moves up and down, nodules, areas of thickening, or fixity of the gland are appreciated quite readily. Substernal extension of the thyroid is suggested when the examiner is unable to palpate the inferior pole. The areas immediately above and below the isthmus and lateral cervical regions are felt for enlarged lymph nodes.

LABORATORY STUDIES

A large number of laboratory tests are available for studying thyroid morphology and function. However, the only tests of specific diagnostic value in the detection of thyroid malignancy are needle biopsy and the serum calcitonin level (for MTC).

There are serious limitations to conventional thyroid function tests and imaging studies in the evaluation of solitary thyroid nodules.

Thyroid Function Tests (see Laboratory Studies in the section, Graves' Disease). Biochemical blood tests, including thyroid hormone levels and thyroid antibody titers, are of limited value in the differential diagnosis of solitary nodules because malignancy may coexist with chronic thyroiditis and Graves' disease. Initially, it was thought that the serum thyroglobulin concentration might serve as a tumor marker for thyroid malignancy; however, thyroglobulin levels have also been shown to be elevated in a number of benign thyroid conditions (32).

Thyroid Imaging Tests. *Thyroid scanning* can be done with isotopes of iodine, which are trapped and organified by the thyroid parenchyma; technetium-99m pertechnetate (^{99m}Tc) is the other commonly used scanning agent, which is trapped but not organified by the thyroid. In general, ^{99m}Tc or ^{123}I are used in the

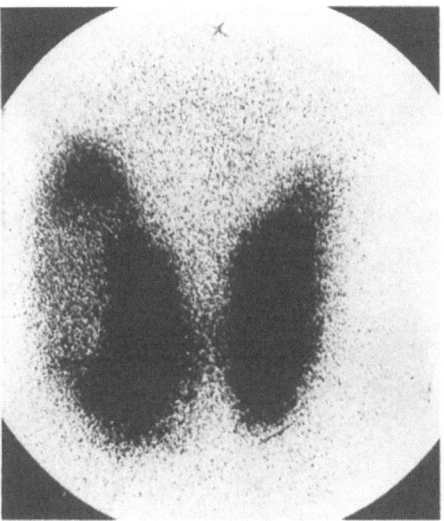

⁹⁹ᵐTc scan of the thyroid. A "cold" nodule is demonstrated in the right lobe of the thyroid. Such scans are of little diagnostic value in discriminating between benign and malignant thyroid nodules.   **Fig. 2-11.**

evaluation of thyroid nodules because both deliver much less radiation to the thyroid than ¹³¹I. If a gamma camera is used with a pinhole collimator, then nodules measuring 8 mm and even less in diameter can be detected. ¹³¹I is still used for the detection of metastatic thyroid cancer after thyroidectomy, in cases of suspected ectopic thyroid tissue (struma ovarii, lingual thyroid), and in cases of retrosternal goiter (because there is less background radioactivity and less attenuation of the emitted radiation by overlying tissues).

A thyroid scan performed on a patient with a clinically solitary nodule may have three possible outcomes (33): it may reveal a single nonfunctioning or "cold" nodule (54%) (Fig. 2-11); it may show a multinodular goiter (36%), with the majority of the nodules being impalpable; or it may show a functioning nodule (10%), which is one that accumulates significantly more tracer than surrounding thyroid tissue and is thus classified as "warm" or "hot." So-called warm nodules should be regarded as nonfunctioning nodules since the apparent tracer uptake is most often due to overlying normal thyroid tissue (34). Hot nodules are almost invariably benign; however, there have been well-documented exceptions (35). Thyroid cancers most commonly appear as hypofunctional or cold nodules on scan, but so do most benign nodules. Thus, unless the area in question is hyperfunctioning, thyroid scanning alone is of relatively little discriminatory value in the identification of thyroid cancer (36,37).

Thyroid ultrasonography (Fig. 2-12) can distinguish cystic from solid nodules with 90% accuracy. However, this information can be obtained expeditiously and at no extra cost at the time of needle aspiration (see below). The wider application of needle biopsy has virtually rendered thyroid ultrasonography obsolete as far as the assessment of solitary nodules is concerned.

In the past it was said that thyroid cysts were rarely malignant. This may be true of cysts less than 4 cm in diameter—less than 2% of cystic thyroid nodules of this size are malignant and can therefore initially be treated conservatively by needle aspiration (39,40). It has been shown, however, that cystic lesions greater

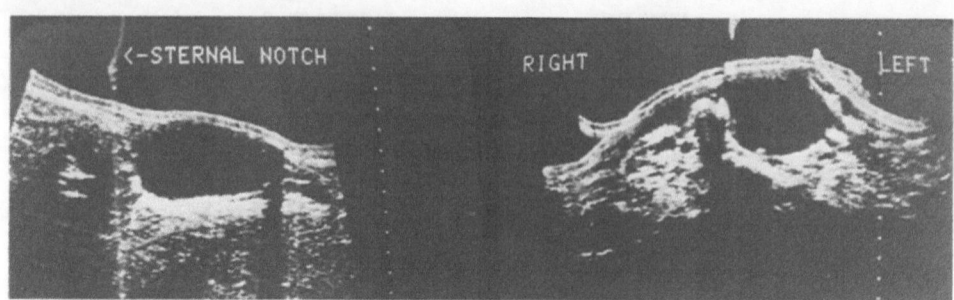

A

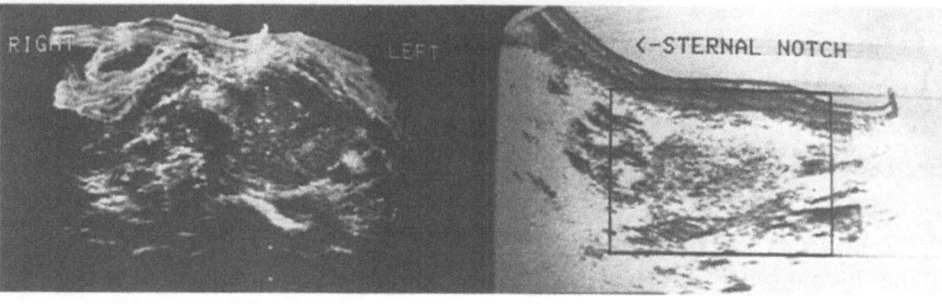

B

Fig. 2-12. **Thyroid ultrasonograms.** **A.** Predominantly cystic nodule. **B.** Solid thyroid nodule. Ultrasound has been essentially superseded by percutaneous needle aspiration, which provides the same information much more expeditiously and at considerably less cost (38).

than 4 cm in diameter are degenerative malignancies in 20%–30% of cases (41,42). For this reason, thyroid cysts greater than 4 cm in diameter should be excised.

Other imaging techniques—fluorescence scanning, lymphography, and arteriography of the thyroid—have no practical role in the evaluation of solitary thyroid nodules. Plain x-ray films of the neck may reveal the characteristic dense, course calcification of a benign degenerative nodule, or irregular flecks of calcium (psammoma bodies) typical of a papillary or medullary cancer; but in the vast majority of patients plain x-ray films yield no useful information. This study is therefore rarely ordered.

Trial of Thyroid Hormone–Suppressive Therapy. As originally proposed by Astwood et al. (43), treatment of hypofunctioning thyroid nodules with thyroid hormone over a 3–6 month period should bring about a reduction in nodule size when there is relatively normal endocrine control compatible with benign hyperplasia. Failure of the nodule to shrink has been conventionally interpreted as suggesting the autonomous, unregulated growth characteristics of a neoplasm. The original favorable reported experience with this form of treatment, however, has not been shared subsequently by others. McConahey and colleagues (44) from the Mayo Clinic found no reduction in the size of thyroid nodules in two-thirds of cases treated by thyroid hormone; in the remaining one-third, the decrease was modest and appeared to result from shrinkage of the extranodular tissue rather than of the nodules themselves. Of more concern was the recognition that on occasion malignant nodules may also shrink during thyroid hormone suppression of TSH.

Thyroid Needle Biopsy. When conventional clinical risk factor analysis has been combined with standard thyroid imaging tests to select nodules for excision, only 10%–30% have subsequently proved at operation to be malignant (21,35,45). This means that for every patient found to have a thyroid cancer, up to nine others have undergone operation only to remove benign lesions. For some time now, thyroid surgeons have recognized an obvious need for a better diagnostic discriminant to sort out more accurately the relatively few cancers from the far more numerous benign nodules. Several techniques utilizing percutaneous thyroid needle biopsy have been developed as a means of obtaining more direct definitive diagnostic information about thyroid nodules without subjecting the patient to surgery.

In *percutaneous core-needle biopsy* a 14-gauge Vim-Silverman or Tru-Cut needle is used to obtain a cylindrical core of parenchyma from the thyroid for histologic examination (Fig. 2-13). This method requires local anesthesia and may cause potentially severe complications such as puncture of the trachea and local hemorrhage and hematoma formation as well as laryngeal nerve injury (46). Moreover, nodules smaller than 1.5–2 cm in diameter may be difficult to impale accurately for biopsy (21,47,48).

Fine-needle aspiration (FNA) biopsy employs a 21–25 gauge needle to aspirate a very small amount of tissue fluid and cells for cytologic examination (Fig. 2-14). A smear is made of the aspirate in much the same manner as a blood smear. The smear is then either immediately wet-fixed in alcohol and stained with Papanicolaou's stain, or it is allowed to dry and then it is stained with May-Grünwald-Giemsa stain. FNA biopsy can be used to sample very small lesions (less than 0.5 cm in diameter) with great accuracy and is virtually risk free. It causes little or no pain and patients readily tolerate multiple biopsies, if necessary, to obtain an adequate sample. Implantation of malignant cells along the needle tract has never been reported after FNA biopsy of the thyroid (20,48).

FNA biopsy cytology is highly accurate in the diagnosis of papillary, medullary, and anaplastic carcinomas (including malignant lymphoma, Fig. 2-15). Similarily, the cytologic diagnosis of colloid nodules—which make up 80% of the lesions subjected to FNA biopsy—and thyroiditis is highly reliable (47–49). However, FNA cannot as yet differentiate between malignant and benign follicular neoplasms (we would include among the latter unusually hypercellular, microfollicular areas of hyperplasia that one occasionally encounters in an adenomatous goiter). This is because the criteria of capsular and vascular invasion are critical to the diagnosis of follicular carcinoma, and this information can only be obtained by histologic examination of the entire excised tumor. FNA biopsy has somewhat limited value in the evaluation of cystic nodules because of the dilution of cells by fluid (20,50,51).

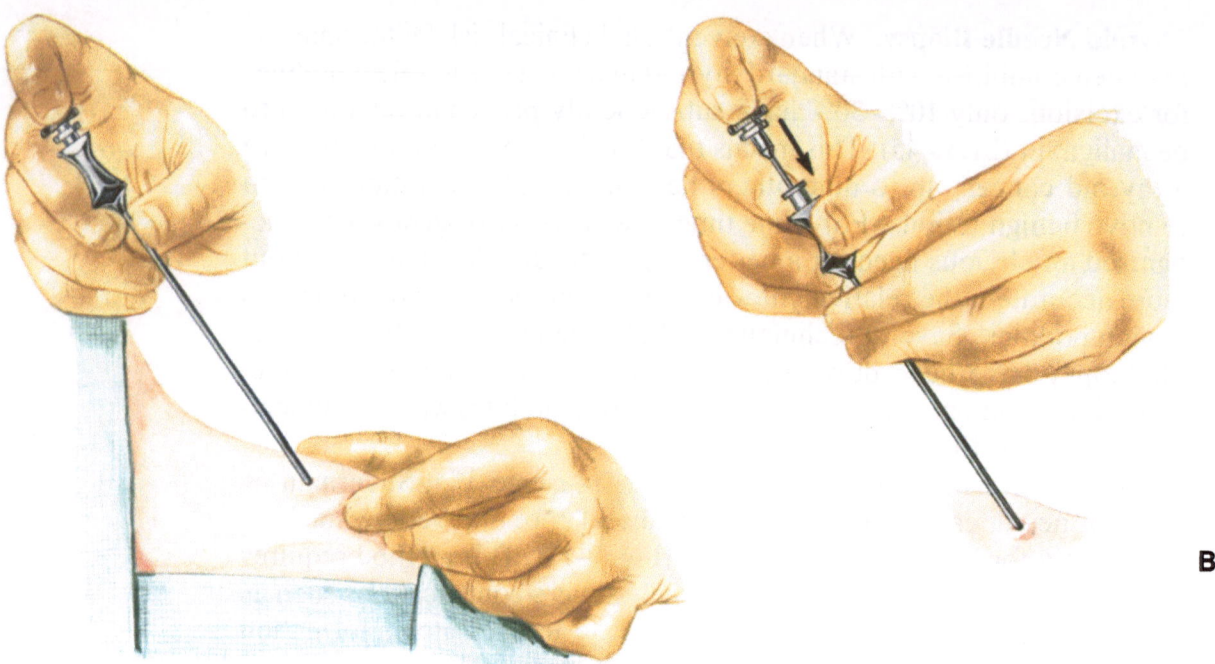

A

B

Fig. 2-13. Core-needle biopsy of the thyroid gland. The use of a Vim-Silverman needle is shown, although today most surgeons would prefer to use a Tru-Cut needle. A pillow is placed under the shoulders to provide adequate extension of the
neck. The skin is prepared with antiseptic and the area is draped with sterile
towels. The skin and subcutaneous tissues overlying the most prominent part of
the goiter are then infiltrated with 1–2 ml 1% lidocaine. **A.** After nicking the
skin, the needle (containing its stylet) is held at an angle of 45° to the skin and
is inserted parallel to the longitudinal axis of the neck into the underlying thyroid gland. The surgeon holds the goiter steady with his left hand (as shown).
Entry of the needle into the thyroid can be confirmed by asking the patient to
swallow; the needle will move up and down with the gland. The stylet is removed. **B.** The cutting blade is now inserted and advanced through the substance of the thyroid gland. **C.** The needle sheath is then pushed and rotated
down over the cutting blade to capture a core of tissue. **D.** The entire needle
assembly containing the specimen is removed. Pressure is applied over the biopsy site for approximately 10 minutes. Significant bleeding is rare, although
one occasionally sees some ecchymotic discoloration of the overlying skin. Tracheal puncture and injury to the recurrent laryngeal nerve have been recorded,
but these complications are very uncommon.

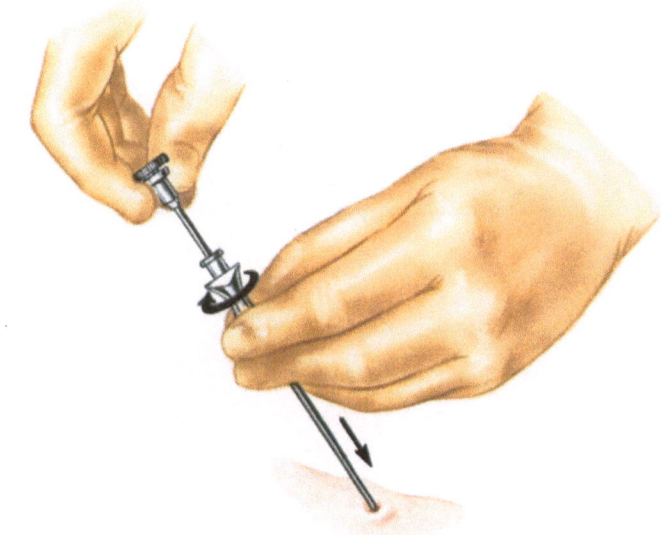

C

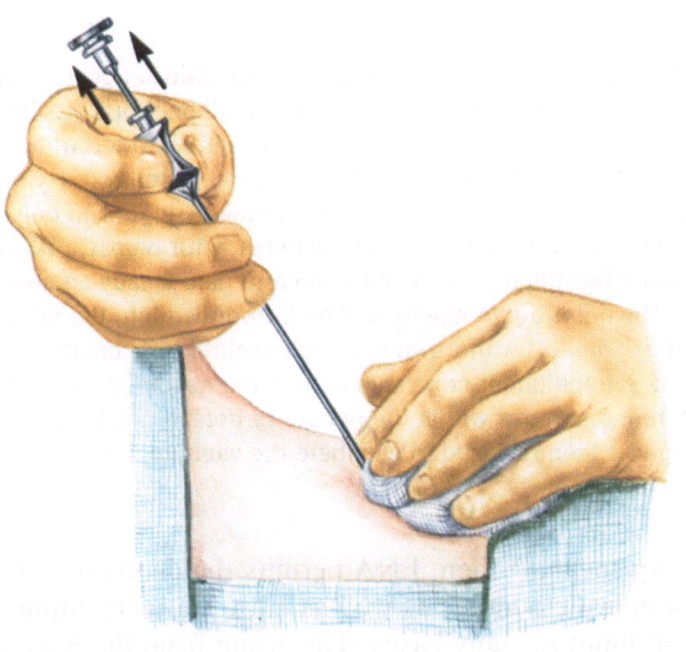

D

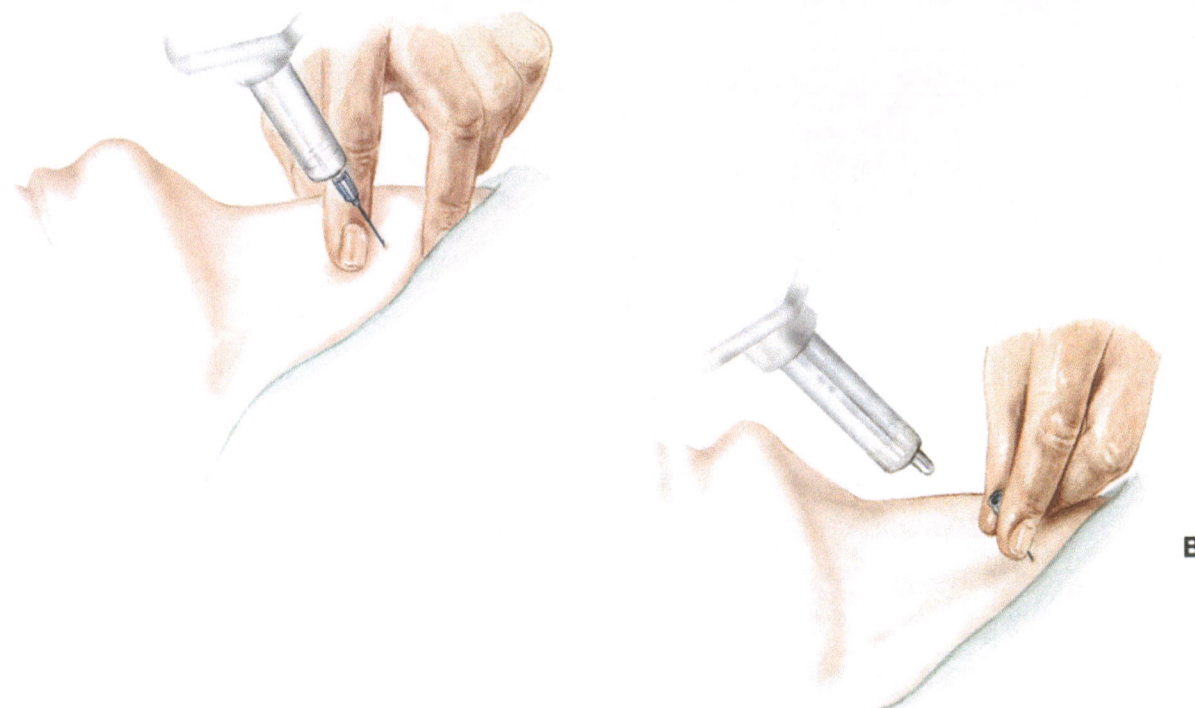

Fig. 2-14. **Fine-needle aspiration biopsy of the thyroid gland.** Local anesthesia is not required; the skin is prepared simply with an alcohol or Betadine wipe. The apparatus consists of a disposable 10-ml plastic syringe fitted with a 21–25 gauge needle. The syringe itself is held in a special pistol-grip device (Cameco) which enables the operator to apply suction to the syringe with only one hand, thereby freeing the other to hold the nodule steady for biopsy. **A.** The nodule is fixed between two fingers of the left hand and held steady against the side of the trachea. The point of the needle is then introduced into the nodule and the plunger of the syringe is withdrawn to its full excursion to create a high vacuum. With the syringe under constant suction, the needle is moved back and forth in different directions within the nodule to detach tiny tissue fragments. **B.** The plunger is then released to eliminate the vacuum, the syringe is disen-

Generally speaking then, FNA permits the distinction of neoplastic from nonneoplastic nodules as well as allowing recognition of the specific type of tumor in many cases. The group from the Karolinska Hospital in Sweden have performed over 20,000 FNA biopsies during the past 25 years and they have convincingly documented the diagnostic value of the method (48). They recommend surgical excision of nodules with a "malignant" cytomorphology and also all those with a hypercellular pattern characteristic of follicular neoplasms. Patients with nodules described as "benign" on FNA smear (typically, colloid goiter or thyroiditis) can be managed expectantly on T4-suppressive treatment with repeat FNA biopsy from time to time (e.g., recheck in 6 months and then annually thereafter). Of course, in view of the fact that false-

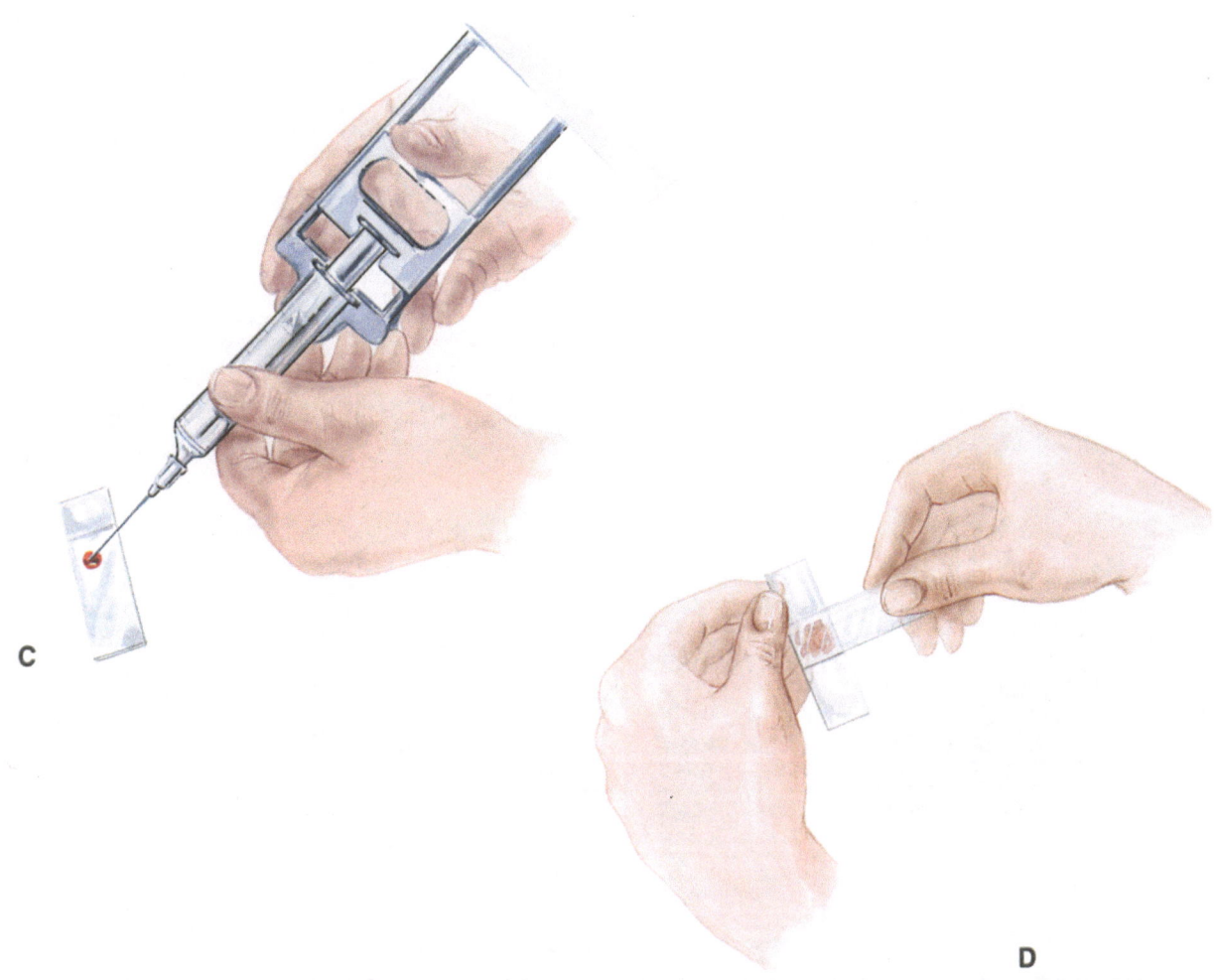

gaged from the needle, and the needle is withdrawn from the neck. **C.** A little air is then drawn up into the syringe and the needle is reattached; the contents of the needle (comprising the total biopsy specimen) is then expressed onto a microscope slide. **D.** A smear is then made of the aspirate in much the same manner as a blood smear.

negative smears can occur—albeit in less than 5% of cases (20,52)—a benign or nonneoplastic smear should not change the therapeutic decision to operate if a neoplasm is otherwise strongly suspected on clinical grounds. In the authors' experience, this situation is encountered very rarely. In this context, FNA biopsy has a supplementary role in further refining the selection of thyroid nodules for excision. Reports from several groups (20,38,47) indicate that its routine use in the evaluation of thyroid nodules maximizes the chance for the diagnosis of thyroid cancer and minimizes the number of patients with benign nodules subjected to a surgical procedure; in general, it can potentially halve the number of unnecessary operations on benign thyroid nodules.

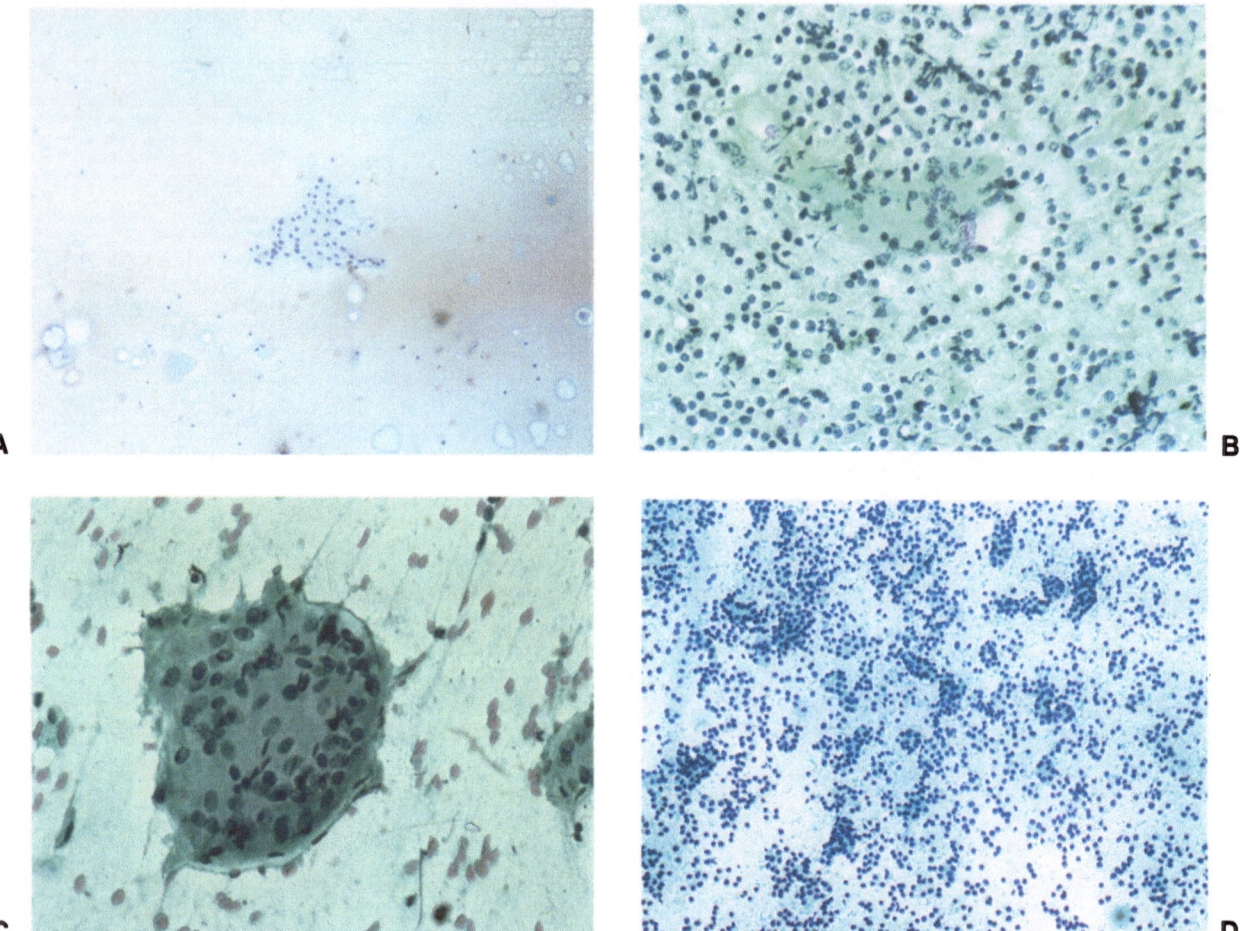

Fig. 2-15. **Representative cytologic smears obtained by FNA biopsy.** **A.** Colloid nodule. The aspirate is relatively acellular with abundant colloid and blood; hemosiderin-laden macrophages are plentiful. **B.** Hashimoto's thyroiditis. There are few follicular epithelial cells, with the Hürthle cell type predominating; abundant lymphocytes form sheetlike infiltrate with occasional elongated, tadpolelike forms. **C.** Granulomatous thyroiditis. The obligatory cytologic feature is the presence of multinucleated histiocytic giant cells of the Langhan's type. There are occasional lymphocytes, macrophages, and elongated fibrocyte-like cells, which are epithelioid cells. **D.** Follicular tumor (from a hyerplastic follicular nodule, follicular adenoma, or well-differentiated follicular carcinoma). The smear is very cellular and the follicular cells appear in small, equi-sized circular clusters or so-called "footprints." Little or no colloid is found. **E.** Papillary carcinoma. As with all malignant tumors, these aspirates are cellular and there is usually very little colloid (if present, it has a viscid, stringy appearance). The follicular cells are usually present in tight sheets and clusters with sharp "community" margins. Often, a characteristic papillary pattern is reproduced, as in this example. **F.** Papillary carcinoma. The cell nuclei in papillary carcinoma are often pleomorphic and have a typical washed-out appearance—the so-called Orphan Annie nuclei. Intranuclear inclusion bodies or "pseudonuclei" are found in 70%–80% of these smears and psammoma bodies may be seen occasionally. High-power, ×400. **G.** Medullary carcinoma. The aspirate is very cellular, and

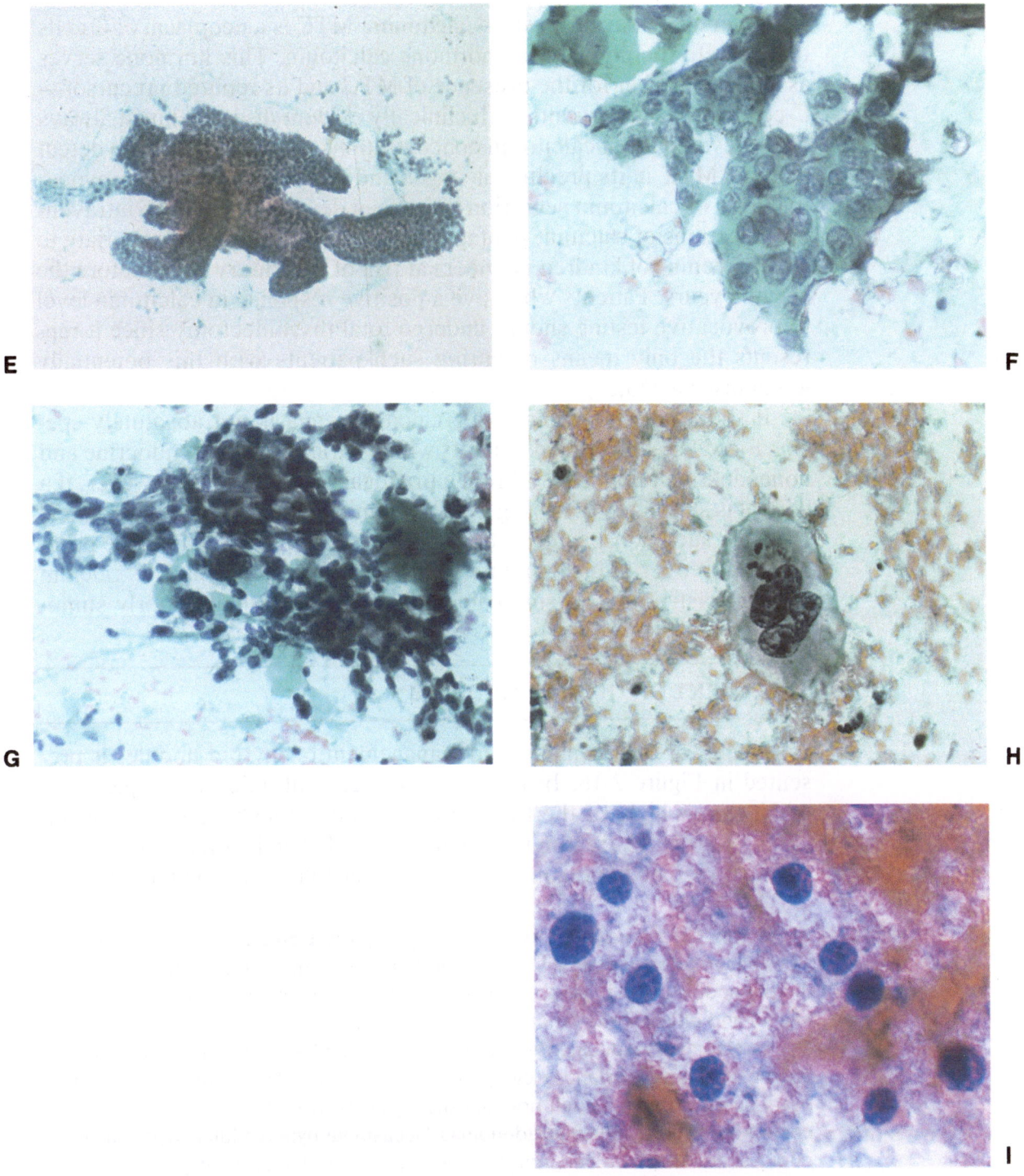

the cells are typically spindle shaped with oval, eccentric nuclei and occasional intranuclear inclusion bodies. Amorphous material is amyloid. **H.** Anaplastic carcinoma. The aspirate is characterized by the presence of large, bizarre pleomorphic tumor cells. **I.** Lymphoma. Dispersed, immature cells, and scattered lymphocytes are seen. In May-Grünwald-Giemsa–stained smears, the background contains numerous small cytoplasmic fragments.

Radioimmunoassay of Plasma Calcitonin. MTC is a neoplasm of C cells that secrete the polypeptide hormone calcitonin. This hormone serves as a tumor marker for the presence of MTC and its reputed precursor—C-cell hyerplasia. Patients with clinically evident disease almost always have elevated basal calcitonin concentrations (53,54). In order to detect minimal MTC in its preclinical stages and C-cell hyperplasia, provocative tests of calcitonin secretion have been developed that use intravenous injections of calcium, pentagastrin, or both (55). It is appropriate to start screening of kindred members at risk of hereditary MTC before the age of 5 years. Patients who have a positive response in calcitonin level to provocative testing should undergo total thyroidectomy since it represents the only means of curing such patients with this potentially lethal disease (53,56).

It should be noted that hypercalcitoninemia is not absolutely specific for MTC. It occurs in patients with a variety of other endocrine and nonendocrine tumors (57). From a practical point of view, however, if a patient is suspected of having MTC by family history or on other clinical grounds, such nonspecificity does not cause significant diagnostic problems. Moreover, if one administers provocative agents such as calcium or pentagastrin, the plasma calcitonin levels are usually poorly stimulated.

TREATMENT OF THYROID NODULES

A schema for the diagnosis and management of thyroid nodules is presented in Figure 2-16. In general, if the clinical index of suspicion of carcinoma is high, or the FNA biopsy result is "malignant" or "suspicious," operative treatment is indicated. Other indications for surgical treatment of nodular goiter include hyperthyroidism, symptoms and

Fig. 2-16. **Algorithm for management of solitary thyroid nodule.** FNA biopsy provides accurate diagnostic discrimination between nonneoplastic and neoplastic thyroid nodules, and it is appropriate to proceed directly to this test after the history and physical examination. "Malignant" smears are obtained from papillary carcinomas, medullary thyroid carcinoma, anaplastic carcinoma, and lymphoma. With an experienced cytopathologist, false-positive results are almost never encountered; all such nodules should be excised. "Suspicious" smears come from cellular follicular adenomas, occasional hypercellular hyperplastic nodules, and follicular carcinomas; it is not yet possible to distinguish between these lesions cytologically. At the present time, it would seem reasonable to recommend that all patients with suspicious smears undergo surgical treatment, although selection of cases could possibly be further refined by ^{99m}Tc scanning. Patients with nodules described as "benign" on FNA cytology (usually colloid nodules) can be managed expectantly usually on T4 suppressive treatment, with repeat FNA biopsy from time to time (e.g., recheck in 6 months and then annually thereafter). Virtually all of the "unsatisfactory" smears will come from cystic lesions (although rebiopsy of the residual nodule following aspiration of the

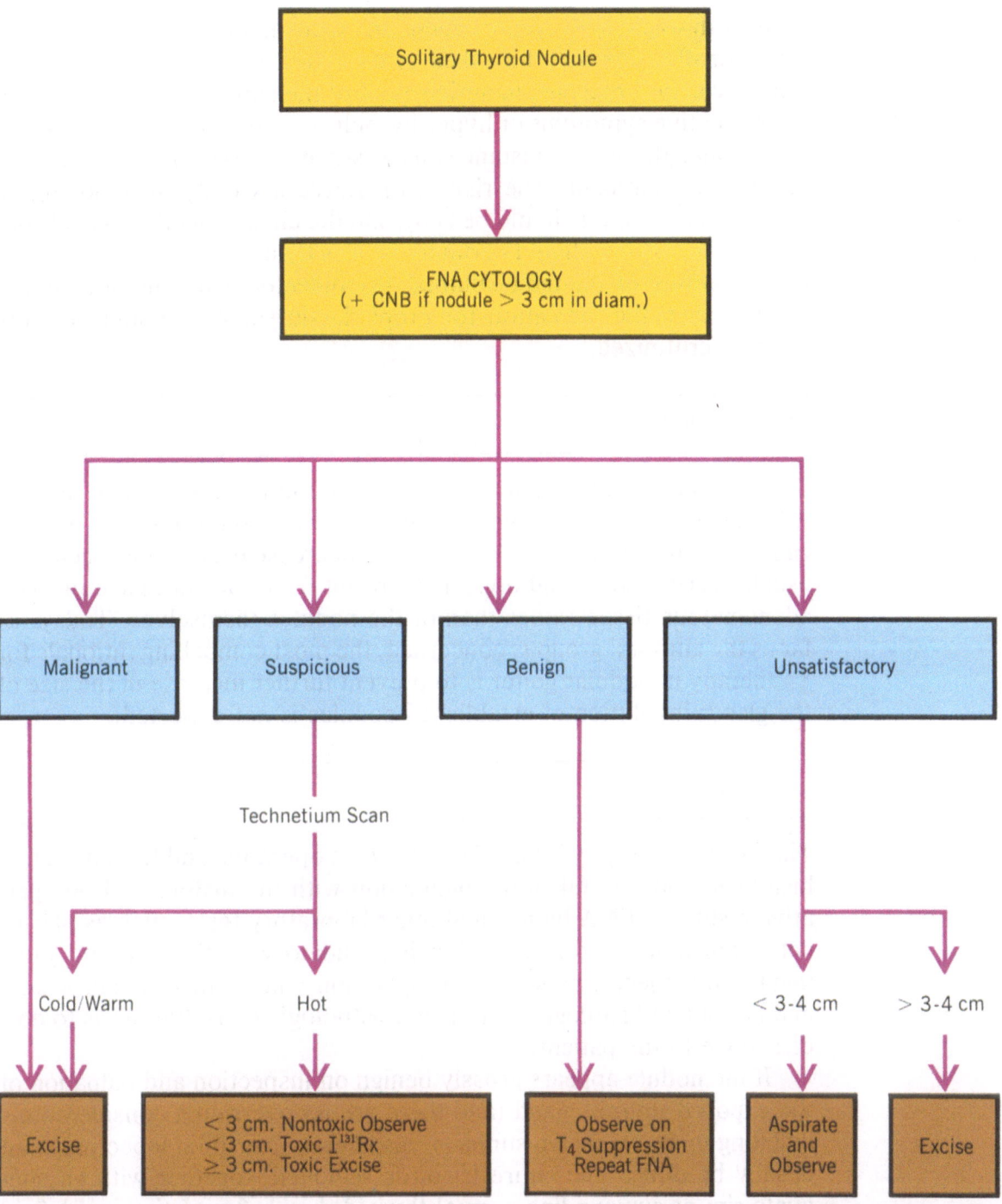

fluid will often provide an adequate sample). Based on the work of Walfish et al. (41,50), we would recommend excision of cystic lesions greater than 3–4 cm in diameter because of the risk of underlying malignancy (20%–30%). Another practical reason for recommending excision of such nodules is that they almost invariably will recur after aspiration. Cystic nodules less than 3 cm in diameter, on the other hand, are rarely malignant (2% or less) and are usually curable by needle aspiration.

signs of thoracic inlet compression, and a cosmetically unsightly lump. Occasionally, one may be asked to remove a large nodular goiter for "prophylactic" reasons, in anticipation of the subsequent development of obstructive symptoms or hyperthyroidism. To recommend thyroidectomy under these circumstances necessitates an extremely safe record of surgical treatment. The risk of operative mortality in removing an asymptomatic goiter should be zero, and the chance of either vocal cord paralysis or tetany should certainly be less than 1%. If the potential for complications of bilateral subtotal thyroidectomy in this situation is greater, then the indication for prophylactic surgery should be more closely scrutinized.

NONSURGICAL

There is general agreement that thyroid hormone–suppressive therapy will usually not bring about a significant regression in the size of clinically discrete solitary nodules. Where a decrease in size does occur it is usually very modest and appears to result from the shrinkage of extra adenomatous tissue rather than of the nodules themselves. Today, as far as the authors' group is concerned, the most compelling rationale for T4 therapy in nodular goiter is to prevent further increase in the size of the gland; involution of established nodules is not expected.

SURGICAL

The extent of surgery is based on the gross operative and frozen-section histologic findings, taken in conjunction with the history and preoperative results of FNA biopsy and other laboratory tests, such as plasma calcitonin assay. Frozen section is mandatory in the authors' judgment—to subject a patient to an operation when cancer is suspected, and not obtain histologic section and pathologic consultation, is to do a disservice to the patient.

If the nodule appears grossly benign on inspection and palpation of the exposed thyroid gland (and there are no overriding considerations dictating more extensive surgery), ipsilateral, near-total lobectomy can usually be done. The entire lesion is removed, together with an adequate rim of surrounding normal thyroid, but 1–2 g of tissue is left in place posteriorly to preserve the parathyroids and avoid damaging the recurrent laryngeal nerve. Bilateral subtotal thyroidectomy is performed if multiple benign nodules are found at operation.

If the nodule is suspected of being a carcinoma, a total lobectomy should be performed. The specific pathologic findings on frozen-section examination of the specimen dictate the extent of further thyroid resection (see the discussion of the treatment of the various forms of thyroid cancer in the next section).

After surgery for benign thyroid nodules, lifelong treatment with thyroid hormone (0.1–0.15 mg T4 per day) is usually advocated to prevent recurrence of nodules and to guard against the possible development of myxedema (58). Although there are no controlled long-term studies that document the effectiveness of such treatment in the prophylaxis of recurrent goiter (59), the authors believe the evidence from their own clinical experience supports continuation of this practice.

TREATMENT OF THYROID CANCER RELATED TO PATHOLOGIC TYPE

There is general agreement that thyroid cancer can be subdivided clinically into a large group of well-differentiated neoplasms of slow growth and high curability, and a small group of highly anaplastic tumors with a uniformly fatal outlook. The simplest and probably the best pathologic classification is that first advanced by Woolner et al. (60) and subsequently adopted by the American Thyroid Association, and with few modifications by the World Health Organization (61). It classifies thyroid cancer into four main types according to their morphology and biologic behavior: papillary, follicular, medullary, and anaplastic. Primary lymphoma of the thyroid can be considered as a separate, fifth entity, of rare occurrence. This classification has an advantage over those based purely on histologic patterns in that it relates morphology to methods of treatment and prognosis. Table 2-1 is a breakdown of the relative frequencies of occurrence of the various types of thyroid cancer encountered in 1146 patients with thyroid malignancies seen at the Mayo Clinic between 1946 and 1971.

Types of Thyroid Cancer in 1146 Patients (Mayo Clinic, 1946–1971)   Table 2-1.

Malignancy	No.	Percent
Papillary	820	70
Follicular	174	15
Pure follicular	130	11
Hurthle cell	44	4
Anaplastic	88	8
Medullary	56	5
Lymphoma	8	<2

Data from McConahey et al. (62).

PAPILLARY CARCINOMA

Papillary carcinoma (Fig. 2-17A and B) is the most common type of thyroid cancer, accounting for 80% of malignant thyroid tumors in children and adults less than 40 years of age, and for about 70% of thyroid

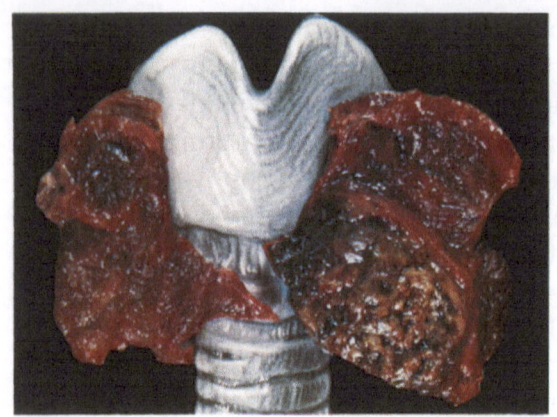

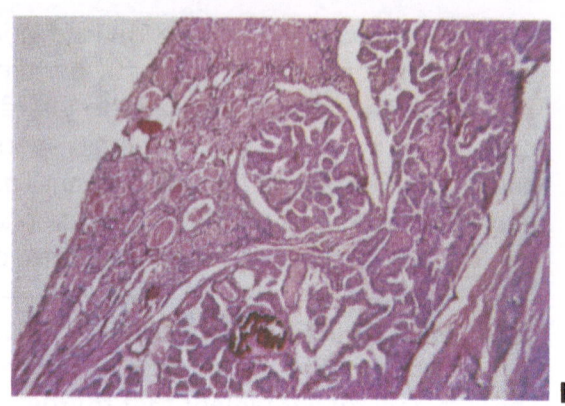

A   B

└───┘ 1 cm

Fig. 2-17. **Papillary carcinoma.** **A.** Papillary carcinoma in the left lobe of the thyroid. The patient had undergone external therapeutic radiation of the neck some 15 years previously. **B.** Histologic appearance of a typical papillary carcinoma. The tumor is composed of papillary projections and of neoplastic but well-differentiated follicles in varying proportions. Calcified areas (psammoma bodies) probably represent necrotic or hyalinized epithelial cells. **C.** Survivorship curves for papillary carcinoma and for normal persons of comparable age and sex. (Used with permission from Woolner LB, Beahrs OH, Black BM, et al: Thyroid carcinoma: general considerations and follow-up data on 1181 cases. *In* Young S, Inman DR (eds): Thyroid Neoplasia. New York, Academic Press, 1968, pp 51–77.)

cancers overall. It is approximately twice as common in females as in males (60,62,63).

These cancers may occur as "minimal" foci of microscopic (often sclerosing) carcinoma that are usually detected incidentally at the time of pathologic examination of thyroid tissue removed at operation for other reasons or at routine autopsy. The incidence of such tiny carcinomas ranges as high as 28% of all thyroid glands examined at routine necropsy and is a function of the number of pathologic sections taken (64) and the geographic area (65); the highest rate has been recorded among the Japanese; one U.S. study reported a prevalence of 13% (66). Interestingly, no relationship seems to exist between the autopsy prevalence of microcarcinomas of the thyroid and the prevalence or death rates from clinically detected thyroid cancer (67). As mentioned earlier, radiation therapy to the head and neck during childhood or young adult life increases the incidence of these microscopic cancers, but there is no evidence to indicate that these radiation-related carcinomas behave any differently from lesions not associated with radiation (68,69).

Papillary cancers are classified with regard to prognosis as follows: *occult* (35%) (69), when the primary lesion is less than 1.5 cm in diameter, with or without associated regional lymph node metastases; *Intrathyroidal* (60%) (69), when the primary lesion is greater than 1.5 cm

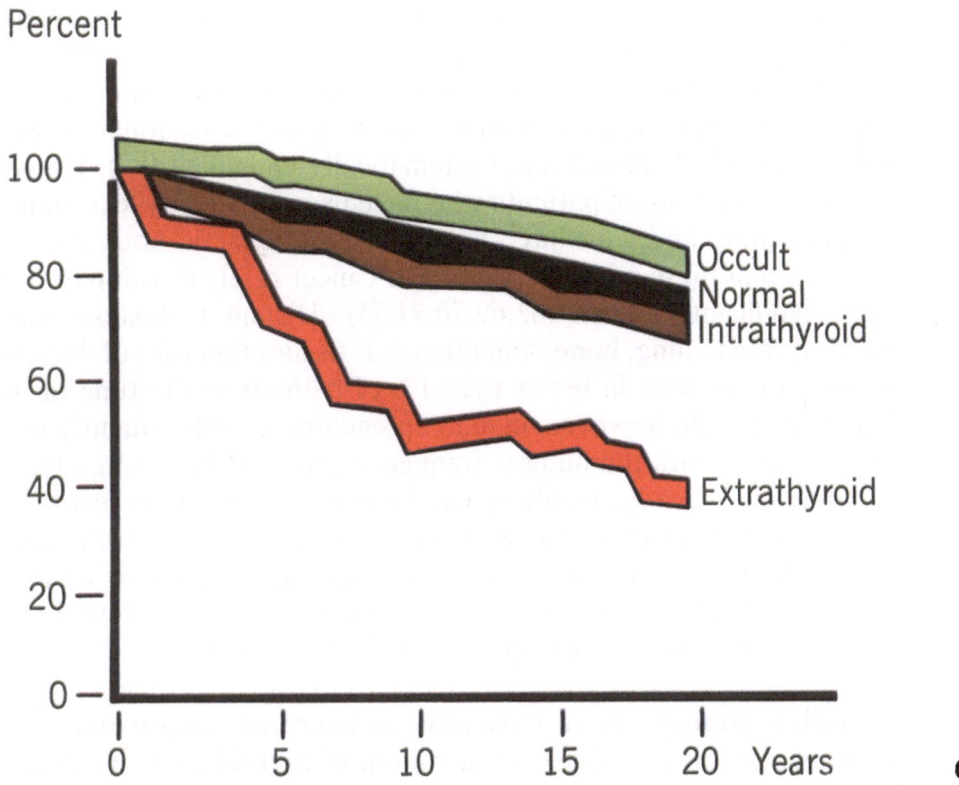

c

in diameter but has not broached the capsule of the thyroid to invade surrounding anatomic structures; and *extrathyroidal* (5%) (69), comprising a small group of advanced cancers that have extended beyond the thyroid to invade adjacent structures. In describing these so-called extrathyroidal cancers, Woolner et al. (70) implied that most such lesions are locally inoperable.

> Paradoxically, the presence of cervical lymph node metastases does not appear to adversely influence the prognosis. Survivorship is determined principally by the size of the primary tumor and the age of the patient. Thus occult lesions, with or without nodal metastases, can be regarded for all practical purposes as almost completely curable by surgical excision. However, when the primary tumor is larger, particularly when it broaches the thyroid capsule to invade surrounding anatomic structures, cancer deaths do occur. Recent studies have also emphasized the important influence of age on prognosis (62,69,70,71). There is a consistent, direct relationship between age at the time of diagnosis and mortality from papillary thyroid carcinoma—with the disease having a materially worse prognosis in patients over age 40 years. Some series report higher mortality rates in men than in women (62,71,72).

In about 20% of cases of papillary cancer there is gross evidence of multicentricity in the gland at operation (63,70), and about one-half of the patients have obvious cervical lymph node metastases palpable at the time of initial surgery (63,70,72). Clark et al. (73) have shown that microscopic foci of multicentric papillary cancer can be found in up to 90% of cases subjected to whole organ section at 50-μm intervals. Similarly, microscopic regional lymph node metastases are found in 90% of nodes routinely removed and systematically examined (74). However, long-term follow-up of patients who have been treated by less than total thyroidectomy and who have not had a prophylactic node dissection indicates that these microscopic foci of cancer rarely develop into clinically significant cancers (62,69,70,71,75). Distant metastasis via the blood stream to lung, bone, and other soft tissues (in order of decreasing frequency) are seen in fewer than 1% of patients at the time of initial diagnosis (69,70); however, distant spread occurs subsequently in 5%–20% of cases, with the highest frequency reported in children (63,70).

Characteristically, papillary carcinomas are low-grade lesions. Occasionally, they can become aggressive and cause death within a matter of months by undergoing transition to anaplastic thyroid carcinoma (76). This transformation appears to be an inherent characteristic of the tumor rather than the consequence of ^{131}I therapy (63).

Operative Strategy. If a *clinically unsuspected microcarcinoma* is found on careful pathologic examination of thyroid tissue resected for benign conditions such as Graves' disease, adenoma, thyroiditis, or adenomatous goiter, reoperation is not required since curative resection has already been accomplished (77).

There is now general agreement that *occult papillary carcinoma* of the thyroid, with or without local metastasis, is curable by means of conservative surgical treatment (62,70,75,77,78)—i.e., less than total thyroidectomy (unless bilateral gross disease is present). Specifically, this will usually involve total lobectomy on the side of the lesion with contralateral subtotal lobectomy and a "modified" neck dissection if there are any palpably enlarged metastatic lymph nodes. A modified neck dissection differs from a classical neck dissection fundamentally in that the cosmetically important sternocleidomastoid muscle is preserved along with the internal jugular vein and spinal accessory nerve. Long-term follow-up studies indicate that more extensive surgery, with its attendant increased potential morbidity (9,69,70,71), is unnecessary for cure.

For *intrathyroidal (greater than 1.5 cm in diameter) and invasive extrathyroidal papillary carcinoma,* the consensus of opinion today would favor total or near-total thyroidectomy with modified neck dissection if metastatic lymph nodes are palpable preoperatively or at the time of operation. In their classic review of 576 patients with papillary thyroid carcinoma, Mazzaferri and Young (69) found twice as many recurrences following subtotal thyroidectomy (20%) versus total thyroidectomy (10%). Of course, total thyroidectomy should not be pursued to the point that one endangers parathyroid function or the recurrent laryngeal nerves. If necessary, a small vestige of thyroid tissue can be left to protect these structures, if the anatomy does not permit a safe total thyroidectomy. In such cases a near-total thyroidectomy with ^{131}I ablation of the remnant is preferable to total thyroidectomy complicated by permanent hypoparathyroidism or recurrent nerve damage. With due attention to important technical details—such as meticulous dissection, careful hemostasis, and preservation of intact parathyroids; autotransplantation of unavoidably devitalized parathyroids; and dissection and preservation of the recurrent laryngeal nerve throughout its course—it should be possible to carry out adequate surgical treatment of papillary cancer without significant morbidity. The risk of permanent hypoparathyroidism under these circumstances should be less than 1%, and the instance of inadvertant recurrent laryngeal nerve injury causing permanent vocal cord paralysis, similarly should be rare (79).

The results of surgical treatment of papillary cancer according to type are shown in Figure 2-17C.

FOLLICULAR CARCINOMA

These carcinomas comprise approximately 15% of all thyroid cancers. The sex and age distribution is similar to that of papillary carcinoma, with a peak occurrence in the third and fourth decades, where it is two to three times more frequent in females (70,80). Follicular thyroid cancers are usually single and encapsulated (Fig. 2-18A and B), and they exhibit a marked tendency to vascular invasion. Their distinctive mode of spread, therefore, is via the blood stream to distant sites, especially the bone and lungs [3%–12% of cases at the time of presentation (80,81)] (Fig. 2-18C). Metastasis to regional lymph nodes is highly unusual and, when present, should lead one to examine the possibility that the primary lesion is a predominantly follicular form of papillary cancer.

Like papillary tumors, their growth is slow, and consequently they are frequently curable; prognosis is related very closely to the extent of capsular or vascular invasion. A 40-year follow-up study carried out some years ago at the Mayo Clinic (70) revealed that when there was minimal angioinvasion or invasion of the tumor capsule, survival did not differ significantly from that of normal individuals of comparable age and sex (Fig. 2-18D). However, when invasion of vessels or the capsule was "moderate or severe," with extensive involvement of the surrounding thyroid parenchyma and vessels outside the capsule, survival decreased to only one-half that of the normal population. More recent reviews indicate a somewhat better overall survival for patients with extensive local invasion, provided distant metastases are not present. This has been attributed to the adjuvant use of ^{131}I and thyroid hormone (80,82).

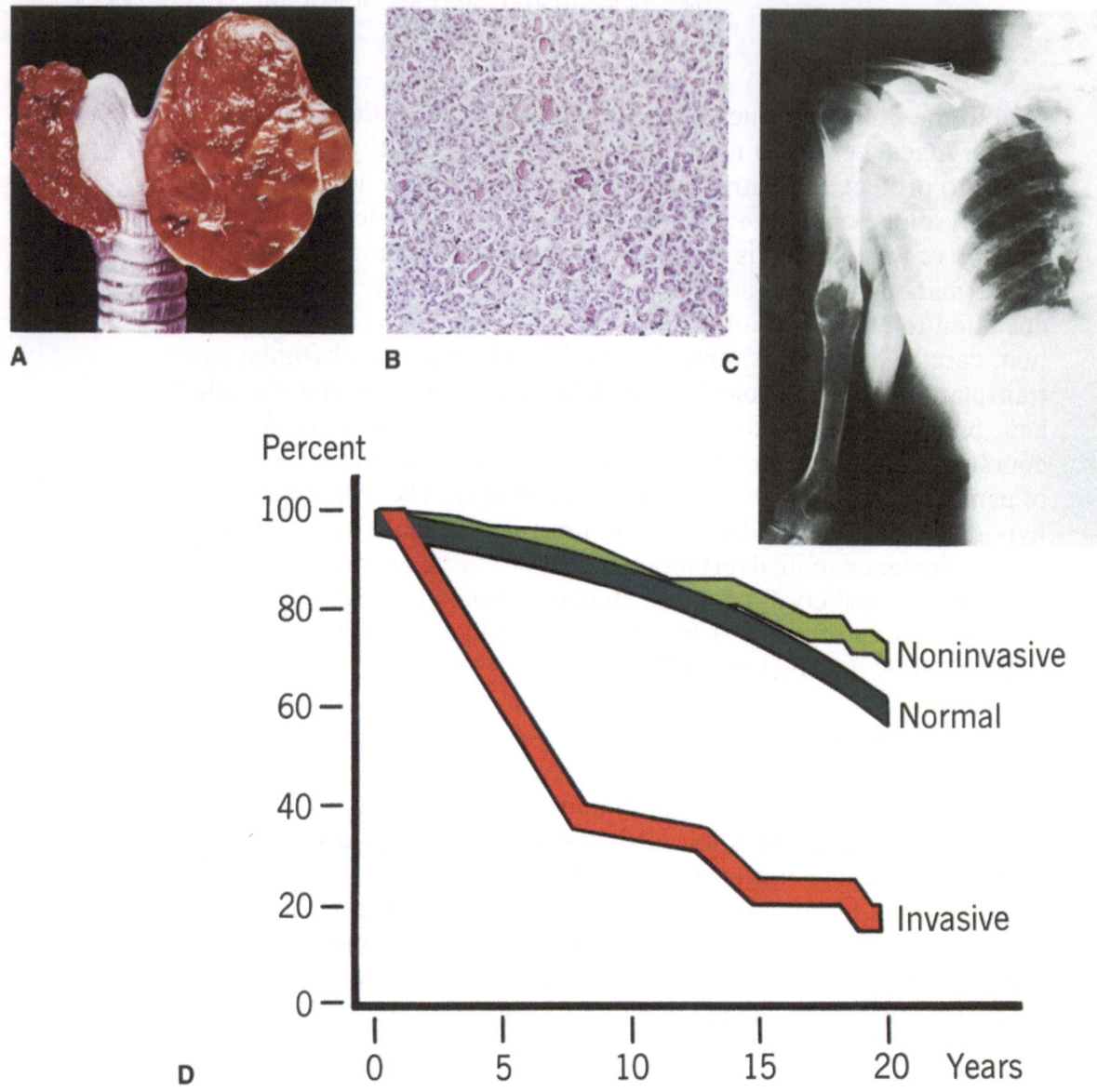

Percent

Noninvasive

Normal

Invasive

Years

D

Fig. 2-18. Follicular carcinoma. A. Encapsulated follicular carcinoma involving the left lobe of the thyroid. The cut surface of the tumor is typically fleshy. **B.** Microscopic appearance of a follicular carcinoma showing the predominantly microfollicular pattern with some colloid production; other examples may show a solid sheet of cells. Note the complete absence of any papillary structures. (Some 20% of follicular carcinomas are comprised largely of Hürthle cells, which have a characteristic voluminous acidophilic cytoplasm. They are considered follicular cancers because of their similar biologic behavior (60).) **C.** A metastasis of follicular carcinoma to the right humerus. Distant metastases, especially to bone, portend a poor outcome. **D.** Survivorship curves for follicular carcinoma and for normal persons of comparable age and sex. Curves highlight the importance of vascular invasion in determining prognosis. Tumors exhibiting moderate or severe invasion (*invasive*) are serious lesions with a 10-year survival of only 30% in this series, whereas tumors showing only slight or equivocal vascular invasion (*noninvasive*) are virtually completely curable. (Used with permission from Woolner LB, Beahrs OH, Black BM, et al: Thyroid carcinoma: general considerations and follow-up data on 1181 cases. *In* Young S, Inman DR (eds): Thyroid Neoplasia. New York, Academic Press, 1968, pp 51–77.)

Operative Strategy. The preferred *operative treatment* of follicular carcinoma today is total or near-total thyroidectomy followed by total ablation of all remaining tissue that concentrates [131]I. Only by removing the thyroid iodine "sink" can one detect ^{131}I uptake in occult metastatic deposits (82). Likewise, a total thyroidectomy sets the stage for effective postoperative radioiodine therapy when distant metastases have been identified (21,63,83,84). Lymph node spread is so rare that neck dissection is almost never indicated in cases of follicular thyroid carcinoma.

MEDULLARY CARCINOMA

MTC represents 5% of all thyroid malignancies (53,62) (Fig. 2-19A and B). It arises from the parafollicular or C cells, which originate embryologically from the neural ectoderm (specifically, from the neural crest; see Fig. 2-1), in common with other cells of the APUD or Neuroendocrine system. Presumably as a result of some genetically determined dysplasia of the APUD system, MTC may be found in association with hyperplasia or neoplasia of the adrenal medulla and parathyroid glands; this particular clinical syndrome is referred to as MEN-II (85,86). The syndrome is further divided into two subtypes—a and b (87). Patients with MEN-IIa have a normal phenotype, whereas patients with MEN-IIb have a distinctive marfanoid habitus and diffuse ganglioneuromatosis of the eyelids, lips, and gastrointestinal tract (86,88,89) (Fig. 2-20). These syndromes, together with familial non-MEN MTC (MTC without other associated endocrinopathies), are inherited as autosomal dominant traits; together they make up about 20% of all patients with MTC. The sporadic, nonfamilial form of MTC makes up the remaining 80% (53,86,90).

It is obviously important to recognize patients with the hereditary form of MTC because if pheochromocytomas are present they should be dealt with prior to thyroidectomy to circumvent the potential physiologic hazards of excessive catecholamine release during the neck operation. Moreover, if there is coexistent hyperparathyroidism, this will require special attention when the thyroid malignancy undergoes surgical treatment. It is also important from the standpoint of detecting disease in other affected members of the same family group by screening for increased concentrations of calcitonin in the plasma. Wells et al. (56) have confirmed that early detection of MTC, either in its precursor form (C-cell hyperplasia) or as subclinical MTC, correlates with higher cure rates.

About 30% of patients with MTC develop watery diarrhea. The diarrheal agent is not known; it may be calcitonin, but other agents, including prostaglandins, serotonin, and vasoactive intestinal polypeptide, have also been implicated. Other paraneoplastic syndromes, such as carcinoid syndrome and ectopic adrenocorticotropic hormone

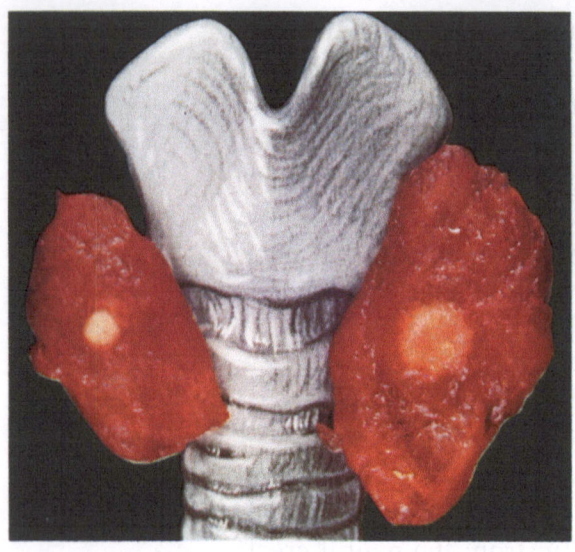
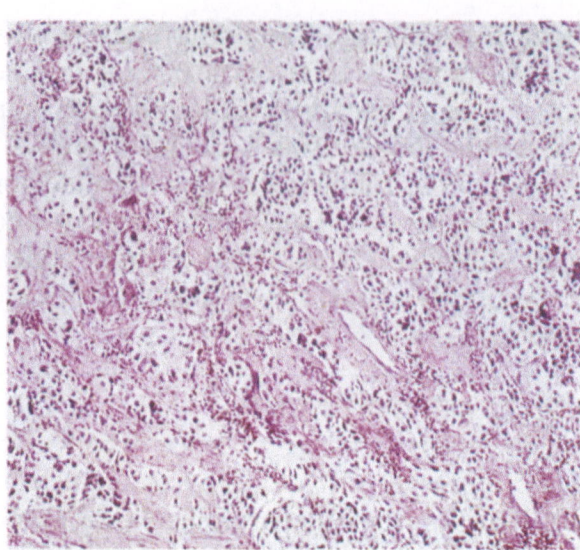

A   B

Fig. 2-19. **Medullary carcinoma.** **A.** MTC from a patient with MEN-IIa. Typically, MTC lesions appear well demarcated from surrounding normal tissues, but they typically infiltrate the adjacent thyroid; the cut surface is usually firm and sclerotic, often with focal calcification. The tumor is usually situated in the upper two-thirds of the thyroid lobe. **B.** Microscopic appearance of MTC showing nests of small epithelial cells in an abundant amyloid stroma. Although amyloid is common, its presence is not necessary for the diagnosis of MTC. Although not shown in this figure, psammoma bodies may be present. **C.** Survivorship curves for MTC. The 10-year survival rate for patients without nodal metastasis closely approximates the rate for normal individuals of comparable age and sex.

(ACTH) syndrome, have been described in association with MTC—usually in patients with advanced disease. Carcinoembryonic antigen and histaminase are other tumor-associated products which, like calcitonin, have been used as tumor markers for detection of MTC and in the postoperative follow-up of treated patients (53,56,86,90).

MTC generally shows a more aggressive biologic behavior than papillary and noninvasive follicular forms of thyroid carcinoma. The pathologic stage of tumor at the time of initial clinical presentation is influenced by patient age and "type." Older patients have a greater likelihood of tumor spread beyond the confines of the thyroid gland, both to regional lymph nodes and to distant sites. In the Mayo Clinic series, extrathyroidal tumor was present in approximately 65% of patients with sporadic disease, 60% of MEN-IIb patients, and only 25% of MEN-IIa patients. Within the MEN-IIa group, the presence of lymph node metastases was closely correlated with the size of the primary tumor (53,86,90).

Prognosis can be linked to a number of factors. Included among those having a negative affect on survival are inadequate primary operation, lymph node metastasis, sporadic type of MTC, the MEN-IIb phenotype, and age over 50 years (86,90). At 10 years, the survival rate for

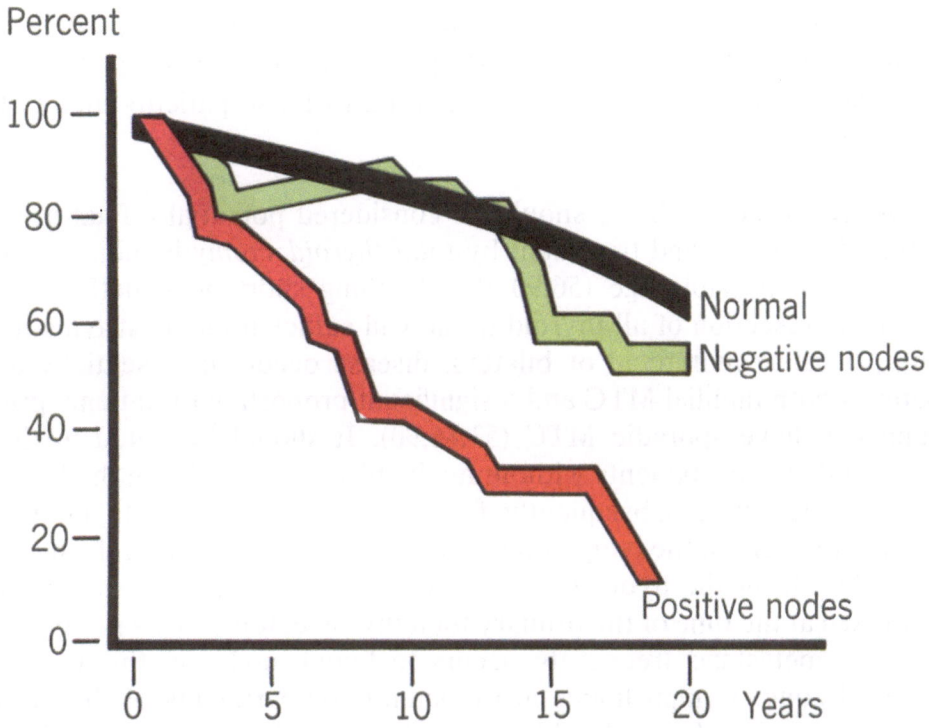

The 10-year survival rate for patients with positive nodes is approximately 45%. (Used with permission from Woolner LB, Beahrs OH, Black BM, et al: Thyroid carcinoma: general considerations and follow-up data on 1181 cases. *In* Young S, Inman DR (eds): Thyroid Neoplasia. New York, Academic Press, 1968, pp 51–77.)

patients without nodal metastasis is close to that expected in normal subjects—86%. In contrast, the survival rate is reduced to 45% for those patients with nodal metastasis (Fig. 2-19C). The frequency of persistence of MTC after primary operation (as evidenced by increased

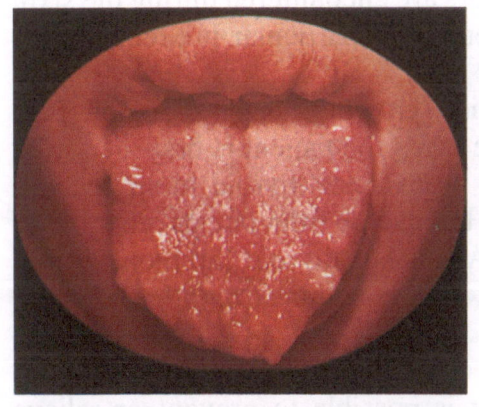

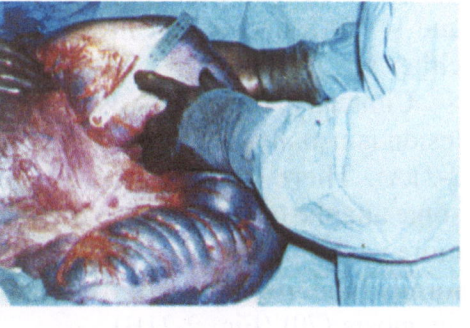

Ganglioneuromas in a patient with MEN-IIb. **A.** Lesions of the lips and tongue. These lesions are also seen on the eyelids. **B.** Megacolon. This is associated with ganglioneuromas in the gastrointestinal tract.

Fig. 2-20.

basal or provoked levels of CT) is greater in MEN-IIb patients than in patients with sporadic disease or MEN-IIa. The 5-year survival is worse in patients over 50 years of age compared to those patients under 50 years.

Operative Strategy. MTC should be considered potentially fatal in all affected subjects, and treatment by *total thyroidectomy* is indicated at the earliest possible age (56,90–93). Nothing short of a methodical, complete resection of all thyroid tissue will suffice if one is striving for cure, because multifocal or bilateral disease occurs in essentially all patients with familial MTC and a significant proportion of patients presumed to have sporadic MTC (53,86,90). It should be noted in this context that 1 in 5 patients without family histories of MTC in the Mayo Clinic series were subsequently found to be index cases to familial disease (53). All of the lymph nodes in the midcompartment of the neck, extending from the hyoid bone to the innominate vessels, should be dissected at the time of the primary total thyroidectomy. This is advised because metastasis frequently occurs to lymph nodes in this central cervical zone. Lymph nodes in the lateral compartments of the neck (internal jugular chain) should be sampled and, if positive, a modified neck dissection should be done (86,91–93). Unlike papillary carcinoma, lymph nodes involved with metastatic MTC are frequently matted and fixed to surrounding structures; thus, they do not lend themselves to a "node-picking" type of dissection, and it may be necessary, on occasion, to remove the internal jugular vein if it is involved.

ANAPLASTIC CARCINOMA

This form of thyroid cancer constitutes less than 10% of all cases in most recent series. It is a rapidly growing lesion that spreads early into the adjacent neck structures by direct invasion and to distant sites via the blood stream. Most of these tumors are encountered during the sixth and seventh decades of life and there is no particular predeliction for either sex (60).

Clinically, the diagnosis of a rapidly growing cancer is obvious; the lesion is usually clearly unresectable when the patient is first seen (Fig. 2-21A). There may be a history of preexistent thyroid lump because some anaplastic cancers are thought to develop from one or other of the more well-differentiated types (76). Anaplastic thyroid carcinoma is uniformly fatal, regardless of treatment, usually within 36 months following diagnosis (70) (Fig. 2-21B).

Operative Strategy. Occasionally, it is possible to prevent or relieve airway obstruction by a palliative debulking of the tumor, but most often the surgeon can do no more than simply biopsy the lesion. External radiation therapy can be of some help in providing palliation for the

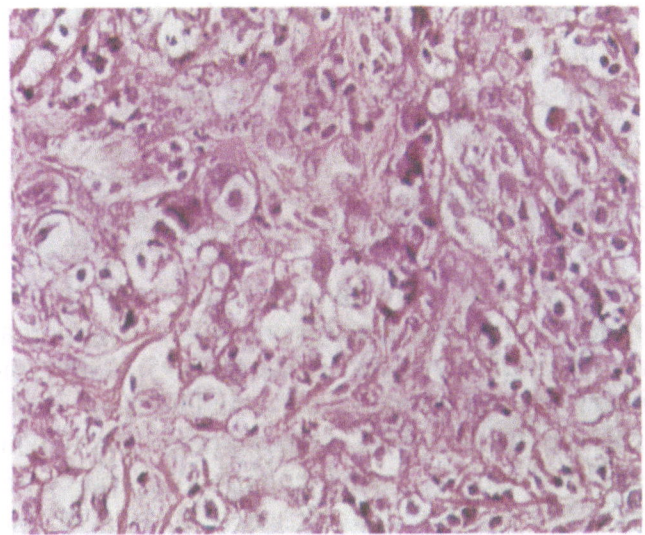

A

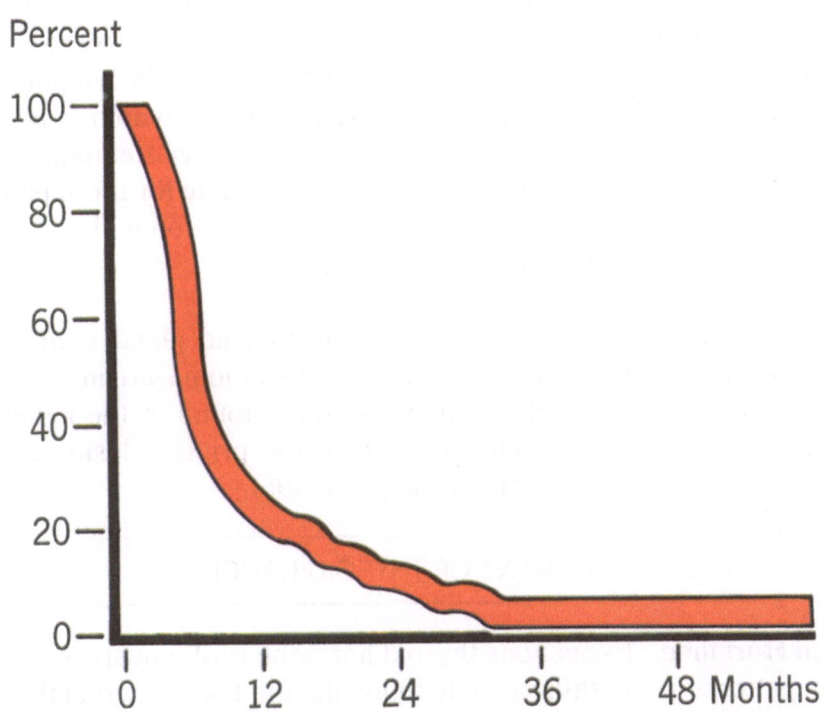

B

Anaplastic carcinoma.   **A.** Histologic specimen. The microscopic pattern   **Fig. 2-21.**
may vary greatly, but all variants are characterized by pronounced anaplasia.
B. Survivorship curve for anaplastic carcinoma plotted in months. (Used with
permission from Woolner LB, Beahrs OH, Black BM, et al: Thyroid carcinoma:
general considerations and follow-up data on 1181 cases. *In* Young S, Inman
DR (eds): Thyroid Neoplasia. New York, Academic Press, 1968, pp 51–77.)

patient and delaying progress of the disease, but it is difficult to find any satisfactory documentation of this in the literature (94). Most, if not all cases of so-called small cell anaplastic carcinoma for which radiotherapy was reportedly effective were probably cases of thyroid lymphoma.

OTHER THYROID MALIGNANCIES

Primary Lymphoma of the Thyroid. Lymphoma of the thyroid may occur as a primary extranodal form of malignant lymphoma. It constitutes less than 1% of all thyroid malignancies (95). The typical clinical profile of primary thyroid lymphoma is a middle-aged to older woman who presents with a fairly rapidly enlarging (and usually painless), firm thyroid mass. The diagnosis can be confirmed by percutaneous core-needle or FNA biopsy of the thyroid; where there is any doubt, open biopsy should be performed.

If there is no evidence of extrathyroid involvement, then resection of the tumor by thyroidectomy should be performed, with subsequent local irradiation. The 5-year survival in such cases can be expected to be around 85% (95). In those patients in whom the thyroid lymphoma is locally invasive into surrounding soft tissues, or in whom it also involves regional lymph nodes, no purpose is served by attempting surgical resection. The 5-year survival figures are the same for these patients whether they are treated by combined surgical resection with radiotherapy or with radiotherapy alone (38%) (95).

Metastatic Carcinoma of the Thyroid. The thyroid gland is an infrequent site of metastatic involvement from carcinoma arising in other organs. Most commonly, the primary lesion is found in the kidney or breast. Thyroidectomy is indicated only if the primary lesion is controlled and there are no secondary deposits (96).

POSTOPERATIVE MANAGEMENT OF THYROID CANCER

Thyroid Hormone. Exogenous thyroid hormone is obviously necessary to keep patients in a euthyroid state following total or near-total thyroidectomy, but there is also considerable evidence to suggest that it helps prevent tumor recurrence and improves survival in patients treated for papillary or follicular carcinoma (63,97). Certainly, the experimental evidence is clear that TSH can stimulate differentiated thyroid cancers to grow (98). There is no good reason to doubt that the same applies in the clinical setting. In the study by Mazzaferri and Young (69), patients with papillary thyroid cancer treated with thyroid hormone had less than a 20% cumulative recurrence rate, whereas patients not receiving thyroid hormone had more than a 40% recurrence rate—a highly significant difference ($p < 0.0001$). Staunton and Greening (99) confirmed a dramatic improvement in survival rates in patients with either papillary or follicular thyroid cancer treated with thyroid hormone. In general, TSH-suppressive therapy has not been helpful in treating patients with undifferentiated or medullary thyroid cancer, although there have been several anecdotal reports of regression of these tumors. Such treatment is probably worthwhile in these cases, since other methods of treatment are quite ineffective. Thyroid hormone should be given in doses sufficient to suppress TSH to low or undetectable levels that will not rise in response to TRH (98).

Radioiodine. In recent studies published by Mazzaferri et al. (69,80), the lowest recurrence rates after surgical treatment of both papillary and follicular carcinomas were observed in those patients treated with near-total thyroidectomy, ^{131}I ablation, and thyroid hormone. The beneficial effect of radioiodine was best observed in those patients with papillary cancers that were larger than 1.5 cm in diameter, bilateral, and metastatic or invasive beyond the thyroid capsule, and those patients with follicular carcinomas exhibiting extensive histologic invasion. There have been isolated reports of objective response of MTC to treatment with ^{131}I but, to date, the authors' group has not had success in employing this treatment.

The protocol calls for a total-body ^{131}I scan following total or near-total thyroidectomy in all patients with papillary and follicular carcinomas, except where the papillary lesion is less than 1.5 cm in diameter. The scan is done with 2–5 mCi, 6 weeks postoperatively, after the patient has been allowed to become hypothyroid. In an alternative program, T3, 25 μg three times daily, is given for 4 weeks, then discontinued for 2 weeks before the scan (100). Under these circumstances, TSH levels are high and there is minimal or no competition by residual thyroid tissue for uptake of ^{131}I by metastatic tumor. If there is significant ^{131}I uptake in the thyroid bed (greater than 2% of the dose at 24 hours), it is ablated with [131]I. Usually a dose of less than 30 mCi can be used for this purpose, but some patients must be given considerably more (up to 150 mCi) if there is a substantial remnant. Patients with significant uptake of ^{131}I in metastatic deposits are routinely treated with 150–200 mCi [131]I. Following this, the patient is given a suppressive dose of 0.2–0.3 mg L-thyroxine. Subsequent scans are done at 6-month intervals with repeated therapeutic doses of ^{131}I, as required, until all residual abnormal uptake is ablated or adverse effects of ^{131}I are detected. Thyroid hormone in full suppressive doses is given between scans. Once the patient has been shown by scan to be free of disease, radioiodine scans can be repeated at 3- and then 5-year intervals (63,101). A reported alternative is to follow the patient using serum thyroglobulin (TG) measurements at half-yearly intervals (102).

Although assay of serum TG is not of any value in establishing the diagnosis of thyroid cancer (elevated concentrations have also been shown in various benign thyroid diseases), it may be helpful in monitoring the course of the disease and its response to treatment. Serum TG levels return to normal in successfully treated patients but remain elevated in those with metastases (102–104). Comparison between whole-body iodine scan and simultaneous sequential serum TG measurements in patients who have undergone total ablation for differentiated thyroid cancer shows an excellent correlation between the two methods for the detection of residual tumor tissue. Serum TG levels remain valid as a marker of tumor occurrence even when patients are receiving T4 therapy (102). On the basis of these results, it might now seem reasonable to measure TG at intervals postoperatively while suppressive thyroid hormone treatment is continued, and to perform scans only when the patient's serum TG concentration increases above a certain level or when there is clinical evidence suggesting occurrence. Monitoring of TG allows more frequent testing and, in most patients, obviates the need for complex and costly investigations.

NONSURGICAL TREATMENT OF THYROID CANCER

External radiation is used as the primary form of therapy or as an adjunct to therapy in the treatment of primary lymphoma of the thyroid (94,95). Its role in the treatment of other types of thyroid malignancy has been essentially limited to the control of locally unresectable undifferentiated thyroid cancer (94). There is a paucity of controlled data concerning its efficacy. Occasionally, patients with MTC have been treated with *chemotherapy* (105,106), but response rates have been disappointing.

Hyperthyroidism

The most common form of hyperthyroidism is Graves' disease. Plummer's disease (hyperfunctioning adenomatous goiter), the only other form of hyperthyroidism likely to be encountered by the surgeon, is much less common; it may present as a single toxic nodule or as a multinodular toxic goiter (107).

Other Types of Hyperthyroidism. (a) Hyperthyroidism (usually transient) may occur in association with thyroiditis, either viral or autoimmune. (b) Hydatidiform mole or choriocarcinoma may produce hyperthyroidism by secreting a thyroid-stimulating factor (probably human chorionic gonadotropin). (c) Widespread functioning metastatic thyroid carcinoma is a rare cause. (d) It may occur in acromegaly and with other TSH-secreting pituitary tumors. (e) It also occurs secondary to ingestion of large amounts of iodine by goitrous individuals (Jod Basedow effect). (f) Another cause is thyrotoxicosis factitia, that is, surreptitious ingestion of thyroid hormone (108).

PATHOLOGY

Graves' disease is a systemic disease process of autoimmune etiology causing hyperthyroidism (Fig. 2-22), either alone or in association with infiltrative ophthalmopathy and dermopathy (pretibial myxedema). This disease is currently thought to result from a specific genetic defect in immunologic surveillance (109). This permits a "forbidden" clone of thyroid-directed lymphocytes (which normally would be suppressed) to survive, interact with an antigen on the thyroid cell membrane, and then produce a number of thyroid autoantibodies, including antibodies directed against the TSH receptor on the thyroid cell membrane. These antibodies are referred to as thyroid-stimulating immunoglobulins because the interaction with the TSH receptors on the thyroid cell membrane appears to stimulate the follicular cells in a manner indistinguishable from TSH. Included among the known thyroid-stimulating immunoglobulins are long-acting thyroid stimulator (LATS), LATS protector, and human thyroid stimulator. It is thought that the infiltrative ophthalmopathy, which occurs in about 10% of cases of Graves' disease, represents a separate autoimmune disorder that is not directly related to the thyroid disease itself (110, 111). It may precede, accompany, or follow the onset of hyperthyroidism.

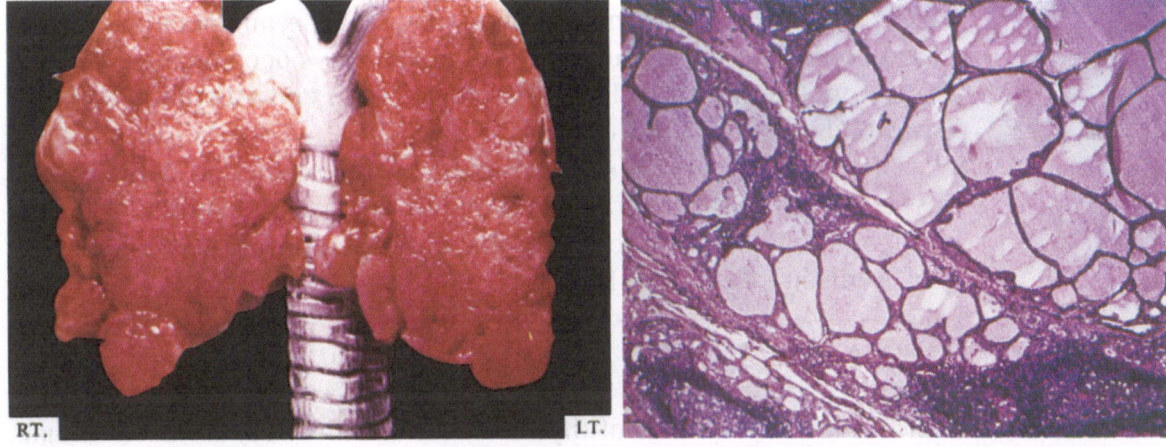

Graves' disease. A. Gross specimen. The thyroid gland is usually moderately and diffusely enlarged, with a meaty texture on cut section. **B.** Microscopic appearance of operative specimen showing the effects of pretreatment with iodine. There is diffuse hypertrophy and hyperplasia of the follicular cells, resulting in papillary infoldings into the follicles. The colloid is thin and scalloped and stains poorly. Lymphocytic infiltration is found to a varying degree throughout the gland. (It should be noted that preoperative treatment with iodine causes a flattening of the epithelial cells and an apparent increase in the size of the follicles, with diminution in the number and size of the papillary infoldings).

Fig. 2-22.

DIAGNOSIS

CLINICAL FEATURES

Graves' disease may occur at any age but is seen most commonly in young women in the third and fourth decades of life (112). There seems to be a strong familial tendency in its development and the condition is thought to be genetically induced (109,110), but the exact nature of the inheritance pattern is not clear.

The symptoms and signs of hyperthyroidism (Fig. 2-23) are associated with a thyroid gland that is usually diffusely enlarged about two to three times normal size. Vascularity of the gland is increased, as evidenced by a bruit (and sometimes a palpable thrill), best demonstrated over the upper poles.

Noninfiltrative ophthalmopathy occurs in approximately 50% percent of patients with Graves' disease. This results from the excess of thyroid hormones, which stimulates sympathetic nervous activity to the levator palpabrae to cause upper lid retraction and a stare. Infiltrative ophthalmopathy, which is specific to Graves' disease, occurs in about 10% of cases, to produce proptosis, soft tissue swelling (lid and conjunctival edema) and ophthalmoplegia (diplopia and blurred vision). These changes result from cellular infiltration and mucopolysaccharide deposition in the posterior orbital tissues and extraocular muscles, secondary to autoimmune processes (113). Pretibial myxedema presents as large, indurated, nonpitting confluent plaques. It is an uncommon manifestation of Graves' disease and is almost always accompanied by infiltrative ophthalmopathy (114). Histologically, it consists of a mucinous, hydrophilic infiltrate in the skin.

Other autoimmune diseases that occur in association with Graves' disease are myasthenia gravis, pernicious anemia, rheumatoid arthritis, vitiligo, idiopathic thrombocytopenic purpura, chronic active hepatitis, and Addison's disease (110).

LABORATORY STUDIES

Various laboratory tests of thyroid function (115–117) are used to diagnose Graves' disease. Measurement of serum T4 and free T4 concentration (or T3 uptake) should be the first step in the laboratory confirmation of the diagnosis of hyperthyroidism. If these concentrations are high, the diagnosis is confirmed. If the results are normal or equivocal, serum T3 should be determined since the patient may have just T3 thyrotoxicosis (118). In the typical case of Graves' disease, the thyroidal uptake of radioiodine is increased and cannot be suppressed by exogenous administration of T3. The T3 suppression test is of special value in the diagnosis of mild thyrotoxicosis in patients with marginal clinical findings and laboratory test results. Another useful study in such patients is the TRH

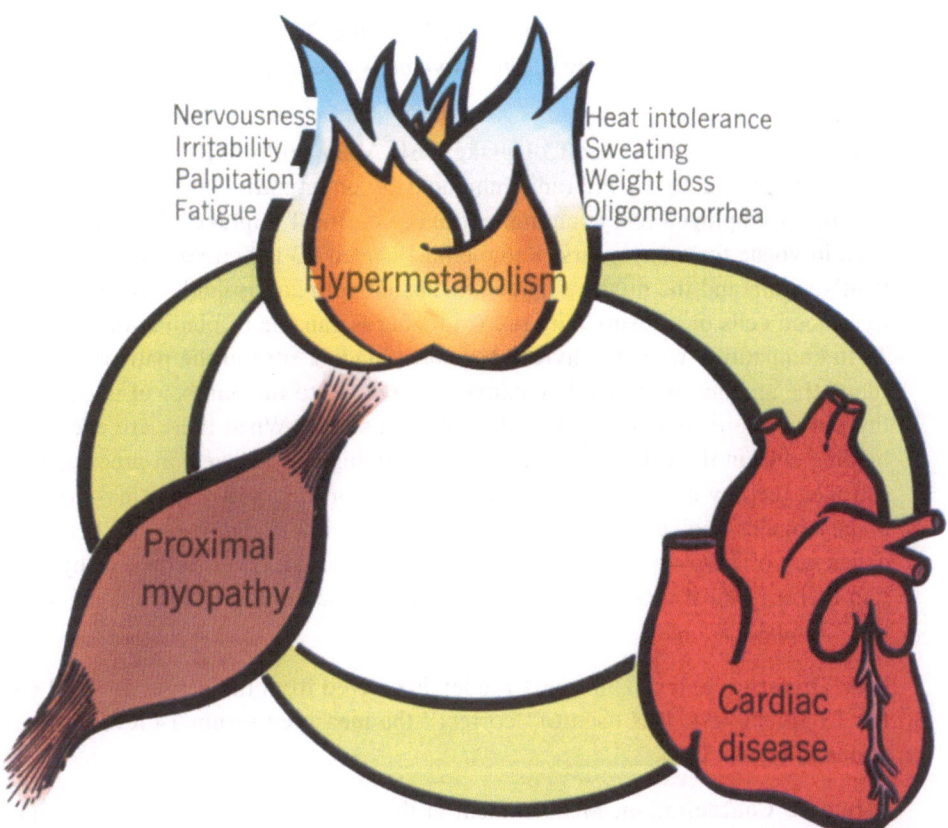

Nervousness
Irritability
Palpitation
Fatigue

Heat intolerance
Sweating
Weight loss
Oligomenorrhea

Hypermetabolism

Proximal myopathy

Cardiac disease

Clinical features of hyperthyroidism. The symptoms of hypermetabolism are heat intolerance, increased perspiration, palpitations, weight loss despite increased appetite, emotional lability and irritability, tremor, and fatigue. The skin, especially the hands, is hyperemic, warm, and moist. Tachycardia is almost invariably present, and about 20% of patients manifest atrial fibrillation; older patients may experience angina, and congestive cardiac failure may supervene. A proximal muscle weakness is quite common and is well demonstrated by the patient's inability to get up from the squatting position. Some patients may exhibit a wasting syndrome characterized by marked weakness and atrophy of proximal muscles, which may mimic the cachexia of malignancy (so-called apathetic hyperthyroidism).

Fig. 2-23.

test. In the near future, assays for thyroid-stimulating immunoglobulins may become widely available and should be of use both in the diagnosis and in the detection of immunologic remissions in patients with Graves' disease undergoing antithyroid drug treatment.

Serum Thyroxine. Both T4 and T3 are transported in the circulation bound to binding proteins, of which the most important is thyroxine-binding globulin (TBG); only 0.01% of T4 and T3 circulates as free, unbound hormone. The serum free T4 concentration can be measured by a dialysis technique or by radioimmunoassay. The serum total T4 concentration can also be measured by radioimmunoassay or by competitive protein binding. Because the total T4 concentration is dependent on the amount of circulating TBG, an assessment of

TBG is usually combined with the serum T4 value. This enables one to determine whether a high or a low serum T4 value is due to a variation of TBG or to thyroid dysfunction.

Thyroxine-Binding Proteins: T3 Uptake Test. Although the TBG level itself can be measured directly by the radioimmunoassay or saturation analysis, the most commonly employed test is an indirect one, i.e., the T3 uptake test, which has been in vogue for many years. Radioiodine-labeled T3 is first added to the patient's serum and the mixture is then incubated with an insoluble second binder (red blood cells or a resin). The second binder is capable of binding the labeled T3 in competition with the thyroid hormone–binding sites in the patient's serum—the amount of uptake being inversely related to the number of unoccupied thyroid hormone–binding sites in the patient's serum. When there are excess binding sites in the patient's serum—e.g., with high TBG levels in pregnancy, estrogen therapy or contraceptive pill regimens, or in hypothyroidism—the secondary binder uptake of labeled T3 (T3 uptake) is low. Conversely, if there is a deficiency of TBG—as in liver disease, or with steroid, testosterone, or hydantoin therapy—or if there is hyperthyroidism with saturation of the binding sites, the T3 uptake is high.

Free Thyroxine Index. The free T4 index is derived from the serum T4 level and the T3 uptake test. It is used to "correct" the measured serum T4 level for variations in serum TBG.

Serum T3 Concentration. Measurement of the level of bound T3 by radioimmunoassay is very useful in the diagnosis of hyperthyroidism since it is elevated in the early stages of the disease, when T4 is still within the normal range. In some patients hypermetabolism can only be ascribed to elevated serum T3, the serum T4 level being normal (so-called T3-toxicosis). Like serum T4, serum T3 concentration is also greatly influenced by the serum concentration of TBG. Free T3 can also be measured by an expensive dialysis procedure.

Radioiodine Uptake. This test involves oral administration of ^{131}I, or more recently, ^{123}I, and then determination of the fraction of radioactivity accumulated by the thyroid in a specified period, usually 24 hours. The normal range of 24-hour thyroid uptake in most areas of the United States is now about 5%–35%. This test is of relatively little usefulness in the diagnosis of hyperthyroidism but is of considerable value in determining the underlying cause, when there is any doubt. Thyroid RAIU is typically high or high normal in hyperthyroidism due to Graves' disease or nodular goiter. (Except where the patients have ingested or have received parenteral iodine, iodide, or iodine-containing drugs). Thyroid uptake is suppressed in hyperthyroid patients whose hyperthyroidism is a result of subacute thyroiditis or thyrotoxicosis factitia caused by a surreptitious ingestion of thyroid hormone.

Thyroid Uptake Suppression Test. In normal individuals, administration of exogenous thyroid hormone suppresses TSH secretion and thyroid uptake of radioiodine. In a patient with autonomous thyroid hyperfunction, as in Graves' disease or hyperfunctioning adenomatous goiter, thyroid hormone administration causes little or no suppression of RAIU. This test is of special value in the diagnosis of mild thyrotoxicosis in patients with marginal clinical findings and laboratory results.

Serum TSH Concentration. An elevated TSH level is quite specific for the diagnosis of primary hypothyroidism, even in its subclinical, borderline stage. In hypothyroidism due to pituitary dysfunction (secondary hypothyroidism) the serum TSH level may be normal or low. In hyperthyroidism, TSH is suppressed and it is usually undetectable in the serum by routine assays.

TRH Stimulation Test. In normal individuals, the serum TSH level doubles within 20–30 minutes after injection of a standard intravenous dose of synthetic TRH. This increase of TSH can be inhibited by even a minute increase in the level of circulating thyroid hormone. This is the basis for the use of the TRH stimulation test in the diagnosis of cases of clinically occult hyperthyroidism that are not detectable by other means. The TRH test is also useful to check for complete suppression of TSH in patients who have been treated for thyroid cancer and are taking thyroid hormone to achieve therapeutic suppression.

Other Tests. A thyroid scan (using ^{131}I, ^{125}I, ^{123}I, or ^{99m}Tc-pertechnetate) can assist in the differential diagnosis of thyrotoxicosis. If the thyroid gland is diffusely enlarged and the scan shows uniformly increased uptake throughout (which is not suppressible by T4 administration), then the diagnosis is Graves' disease; in subacute thyroiditis and thyrotoxicosis factitia the thyroid isotope uptake is blocked. In patients with nodular goiter and thyrotoxicosis the scan assists in the differential diagnosis of solitary toxic adenoma (a single "hot" nodule with perinodular tissue showing suppressed uptake), multinodular goiter (increased uptake corresponding to the nodules), and Graves' disease with coincidental nonfunctioning nodules (increased uptake in the perinodular tissue). Scintigraphy is also undoubtedly helpful in localizing hyper-functioning thyroid tissue in extrathyroidal sites (e.g., substernal goiter, metastatic thyroid carcinoma, or struma ovarii).

Thyroid-stimulating immunoglobulins (including LATS, LATS protector, and human thyroid stimulator) can be detected in the serum of patients with Graves' disease. Approximately 20% also have antithyroglobulin antibodies, and about 70% have antimicrosomal antibodies.

Serum calcium, phosphorus, and alkaline phosphatase may be elevated due to increased bone turnover in Graves' disease (114).

TREATMENT

Three methods are available today for the treatment of hyperthyroidism due to Graves' disease: antithyroid drugs (119), radioiodine (120), and surgery (121–123) (Fig. 2-24). The role of each form of therapy continues to be debated, as no one form of treatment is ideal; each has its advantages and disadvantages (124,125). In the United States, nonsurgical methods of treatment have all but replaced subtotal thyroidectomy, except in certain circumstances discussed below.

NONSURGICAL

Antithyroid Drugs. The two main groups of specific antithyroid drugs currently used in the therapy of hyperthyrodism are the thiourea

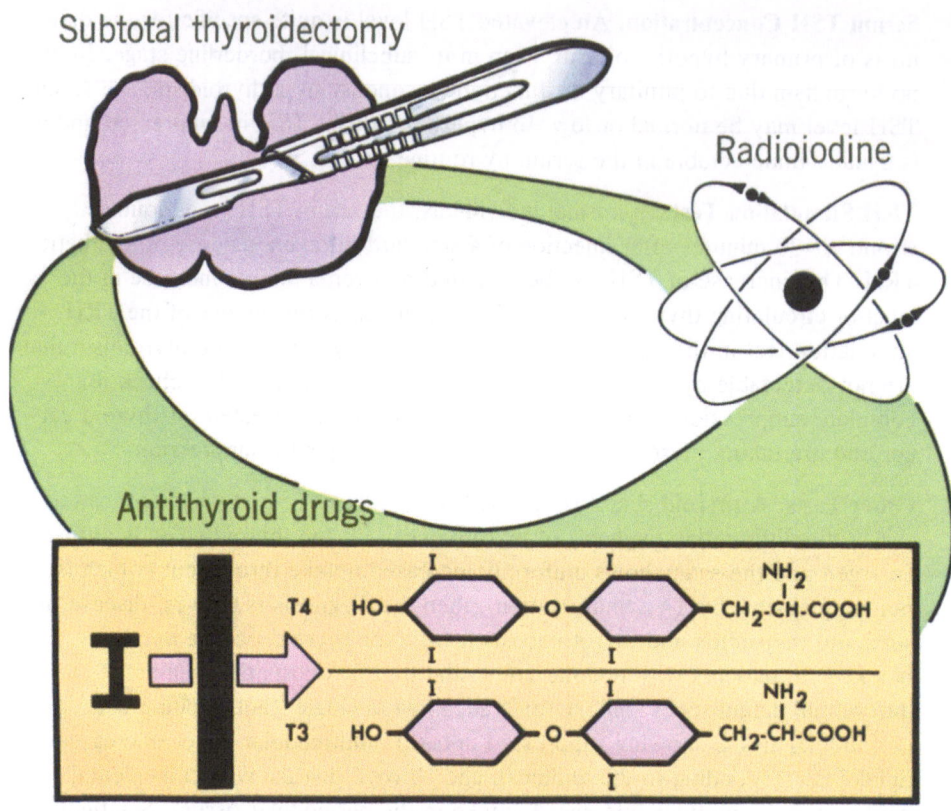

Fig. 2-24.   **Treatment modalities in Graves' disease.**

group—including propylthiouracil (PTU) and carbimazole (Neomerca-zole)—and the imidazole group, including methimazole (Tapazole). The former drugs act principally by inhibiting the incorporation of iodine, already trapped by the thyroid, into thyroid hormone; PTU has the valuable additional property of inhibiting peripheral conversion of T4 to T3. The imidazole drugs appear to act by preventing oxidation of trapped iodide by inhibiting the peroxidase enzyme system. There is, however, little to distinguish the two groups in terms of clinical response. The duration of action of these drugs is approximately 8 hours; however, once patients are under control, a once-daily regimen may be used.

The optimum duration of antithyroid drug therapy is controversial. The objective of therapy is to attain control of the hyperthyroidism and maintain a euthyroid state until the disease undergoes remission. In a recent report, 90% of patients who took carbimazole for less than 2 years relapsed (112); relapse rates in patients treated for longer than 2 years are as high as 50%–80% (126). In general, those patients who fail to undergo remission after a course of antithyroid drug therapy, or who suffer recurrence after cessation of the medication, will require ablative therapy either with surgery or with radioiodine. Remission is more likely to occur with (a) disease of short duration, (b) a small goiter, (c) a reduction in the size of the goiter during the course of treatment, and (d) disappearance of thyroid-stimulating immunoglobulins.

The chief disadvantages of antithyroid drug therapy therefore are the high rate of recurrence of hyperthyroidism after therapy is discontinued, the extended period of treatment required, the necessity for assiduous dose compliance and regular monitoring of treatment, and the adverse reactions that occur in about 2% of patients, consisting mainly of rash, arthralgia, and neutropenia (in decreasing order).

Other Drugs. A potent beta-adrenergic blocking agent, *propranolol*, has a prominent role in the treatment of hyperthyroidism. While it has no effect on thyroid hormone secretion, it will decrease the tachycardia and other signs and symptoms of beta-adrenergic stimulation. Recent evidence indicates that propranolol blocks the peripheral conversion of T4 to T3 and thus might also have some effect on the metabolic rate. Thus, rapid heartbeat is controlled, nervousness declines, and sweating and tremor are reduced. Propranolol has proved particularly useful in providing rapid control of symptoms during initial treatment with antithyroid drugs or radioactive iodine, and in preparing patients for thyroidectomy.

A massive supraphysiologic dose of *iodine* has the immediate effect of blocking the secretion of preformed thyroid hormone; eventually, the thyroid will "escape" from the iodine effect, but this probably takes several weeks. Thus, iodine is very useful in the initial treatment of severe thyrotoxicosis and in the preparation of patients for subtotal thyroidectomy.

Lithium carbonate has effects similar to those of iodide. As yet, its place in the treatment of hyperthyroidism remains to be properly defined.

Radioactive Iodine. This is by far the simplest and least expensive therapy for Graves' disease, and in many centers it has become the treatment of choice for adult hyperthyroidism. It has many advantages: treatment is usually definitive, there is no surgical scar, there is no period of hospitalization or time lost from work, and there is no significant risk (only rarely is ^{131}I administration followed by radiation thyroiditis, with an increase in hyperthyroid symptoms, and this problem can be prevented by pretreatment with antithyroid drugs).

Earlier fears about the possible carcinogenic effects of ^{131}I treatment have been largely dispelled. There has been no increased incidence of thyroid carcinoma or hematologic malignancy since ^{131}I therapy for hyperthyroidism was introduced over 35 years ago (127,128).

One explanation for the absence of radiation-induced thyroid carcinoma is that the dose of radiation to the thyroid cells (7000–10,000 rads) is much higher than the dose required to induce cancer (50–1500 rads); the higher radiation dose apparently impairs the ability of the cells to replicate (124).

There has been no increased incidence of mutation secondary to gonadal radiation by radioactive iodine. In fact, the radiation dose to the gonads is no more than that received during an intravenous pyelogram or colon x-ray. However, lingering concern about possible delayed mutagenic effects and induction of malignancy still influences many physicians today to recommend alternative treatment for children and women of child-bearing age.

The major complication of radioactive iodine treatment is hypothyroidism. Within 1 year of treatment approximately 5%–20% of patients become hypothyroid, and there is an annual increase in incidence thereafter—so that about 50% are hypothyroid within a decade (129–131). Lower hypothyroidism rates, achieved by using smaller doses of radioactive iodine, can only be achieved at the expense of treatment failures. Follow-up after radioiodine therapy must be lifelong—first to detect the onset of hypothyroidism, which may be subtle; then to ensure that the patients continue taking their replacement T4 therapy. Semicomputerized review systems have been successfully employed to ensure close, long-term follow-up of large groups of treated patients (132).

One minor practical disadvantage of ^{131}I therapy is the time necessary to control hyperthyroidism: it usually takes about 6 weeks, although in some cases it may take up to 6 months. Antithyroid drug therapy is usually employed to achieve control of hyperthyroidism during the "lag" period.

SURGICAL

Operative Strategy. Depending on the treatment philosophy, subtotal thyroidectomy may leave as little as 2–4 g or as much as 8–10 g of thyroid tissue. It provides rapid control of hyperthyroidism, and in expert hands, the risk of serious postoperative complications, such as vocal cord paralysis or permanent hypoparathyroidism, is less than 1%, and mortality is virtually zero (122,133–135). The object of the operation is to cure the patient's hyperthyroid state. Patients who develop recurrent thyrotoxicosis will almost invariably require treatment with radioactive iodine because reoperation is fraught with hazard to the recurrent laryngeal nerves and parathyroids.

A number of factors have been implicated in determining thyroid status after surgical treatment of Graves' disease, but the most important one is unquestionably the size of the thyroid remnant (136,137). The incidence of postoperative hypothyroidism is inversely related to remnant size; recurrent thyrotoxicosis is a direct function of remnant size. It is apparent from a review of the published data that if the rate of recurrent thyrotoxicosis is to be kept below 5%, then the remnant size should be no greater than 5–8 g; under these circumstances, the cumulative incidence of postoperative hypothyroidism will probably approach that seen after radioactive iodine therapy. However, in contradistinction to the gradual, progressive, and cumulative increase in the incidence of posttreatment hypothyroidism following radioactive iodine, the vast majority of cases of hypothyroidism developing after subtotal thyroidectomy occur within the first 6–12 months of operation (122,136,138,139). This early onset of posttreatment hypothyroidism has been cited as one of the advantages of surgical therapy over radioactive iodine therapy. Recent work also suggests that up to 70% of cases of postoperative hypothyroidism after surgical treatment of Graves' disease are temporary, with thyroid function returning to normal or near normal 6–12 months after surgery (140,141). This temporary postoperative hypothyroidism can be prevented by short-term thyroid replacement therapy without increasing the eventual frequency of permanent hypothyroidism (141).

Indications. The authors favor surgical treatment of Graves' disease in children and women of child-bearing age in whom therapy is either impracticable (poor drug compliance, adverse reactions, large goiters) or has failed to produce a lasting clinical remission. Hyperthyroidism rarely occurs in pregnant women (0.2% of pregnancies) (142), but when this complication occurs, subtotal thyroidectomy is probably the treatment of choice after initial control with Lugol's iodine, antithyroid drugs and/or short-term β-blocking agents.

> The principal problem with antithyroid drug therapy in pregnancy is that these agents cross the placenta and, if given in excess, may cause fetal goiter and, occasionally, fetal hypothyroidism with subsequent mental retardation (143). These complications cannot be prevented by administration of thyroid hormone to the mother since neither T4 nor T3 cross the placenta in appreciable concentration. If antithyroid drugs are used to treat Graves' disease in pregnancy, PTU is preferred over methimazole because the latter has been associated with producing scalp defects in the offspring of treated mothers (143). Radioiodine therapy should never be administered during pregnancy because of the dangers of irradiation to the conceptus (before the 12th week) or to the fetal thyroid when it begins to trap iodine after the 12th week (143, 144).

Preoperative Preparation. The use of iodine, which acts by inhibiting the synthesis and release of thyroid hormones, was first introduced by Plummer in 1923, to prepare patients with Graves' disease for surgery (145). Prior to the introduction of preoperative iodine preparation, the mortality for thyroidectomy for Graves' disease was at least 5% percent and as high as 20%–30% in some reports. Preoperative preparation with Lugol's iodine, 10 drops three times daily for 7–10 days, essentially eliminated the problem of postoperative thyroid crisis and reduced the mortality for thyroidectomy in these cases to less than 1%. Later, the introduction of antithyroid drugs and propranolol made it possible to have even more effective preoperative preparation.

It is still standard practice at many institutions to prepare patients preoperatively with Lugol's iodine (122). If the patient is already receiving an antithyroid drug, iodide may be added to the regimen. If the patient is severely toxic, iodide pretreatment is supplemented with propranolol at a dose of 40–80 mg every 8 hours for 7–10 days before operation to obtain a resting heart rate of 90 beats/minute (135). The propranolol is continued throughout the day of operation and for 3–5 days postoperatively to ensure that beta-adrenergic blockade is maintained until circulating levels of thyroid hormone are no longer elevated—the half-life of T4 in the periphery is normally about 6–7 days (146).

Treatment of Graves' Ophthalmopathy. Mild exophthalmos can be managed conservatively with methylcellulose eyedrops, dark glasses, and elevation of the head at night. Severe progressive exophthalmos can lead to serious ocular discomfort, profound cosmetic disfigurement, diplopia secondary to ocular muscle palsy, and loss of vision. Thyroidectomy has no predictable effect on the eye condition (147)—the exophthalmos may deteriorate or improve but most often it remains unchanged after operation—and the surgeon should specifically point this out to the patient prior to operation.

In serious cases of exophthalmos the first line of treatment is administration of large doses of glucocorticoids. If steroid therapy fails to produce a remission within several weeks, then one can consider either high-voltage orbital irradiation, as described by Donaldson et al. (148), or surgical decompression of the orbit via the transantral approach (149).

Plummer's Disease

HYPERFUNCTIONING ADENOMATOUS GOITER: TOXIC NODULAR GOITER

PATHOLOGY

Plummer's disease differs fundamentally from Graves' disease in that the basic pathologic process is confined to the thyroid gland (150). The term usually refers to the development of hyperthyroidism in a multinodular adenomatous goiter (Fig. 2-25). A single toxic "hot" nodule may result from localized hyperplasia to form a single encapsulated nodule and is thus a special example of Plummer's disease (others are true follicular adenomas in an otherwise normal thyroid gland).

DIAGNOSIS

CLINICAL FEATURES

Plummer's disease comprises about 10% of all cases of hyperthyroidism referred to the surgeon. As a general rule, patients who develop hyperthyroidism due to adenomatous goiter are in the older age groups, usu-

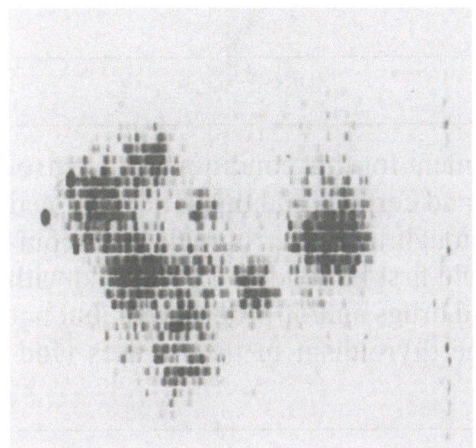

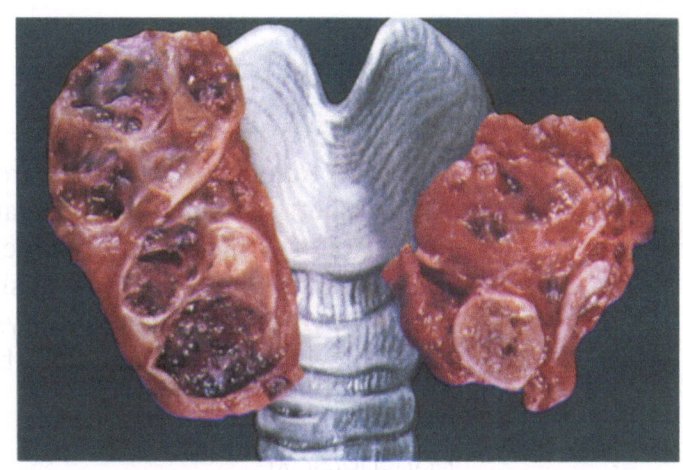

A   B

Plummer's disease. **A.** Thyroid scintiscan showing multiple areas of increased uptake in a toxic multinodular goiter. **B.** Gross operative specimen.   **Fig. 2-25.**

ally in their 50s or 60s, and have had their goiters for many years. Plummer believed that practically all adenomatous goiters would eventually become toxic given enough time, and that the average interval from the time the goiter was first noted to the subsequent development of symptoms of hyperthyroidism was approximately 15 years (150). The percentage of patients with adenomatous goiter who eventually develop hyperthyroidism is probably less than 10% overall. Like Graves' disease, this condition is many times more common in women than in men.

The hyperthyroidism that accompanies nodular toxic goiter is usually characterized by cardiovascular disturbances (Fig. 2-23). There may be incipient or overt congestive cardiac failure with dyspnea and edema; cardiac arrythmias (usually atrial fibrillation) are often present. Nervous manifestations that characterize the young patient with Graves' disease are usually less prominent in Plummer's disease, although emotional lability may later be quite pronounced. Patients with Plummer's disease may also exhibit a wasting syndrome characterized by marked weight loss and weakness, with atropy of proximal muscles which may mimic the cachexia of malignancy (so-called apathetic hyperthyroidism). Noninfiltrative eye signs (lid lag and stare) may occur but are rare.

LABORATORY STUDIES

The serum T4, free T4, and T3, and the various suppression and stimulation tests described in the preceding section on thyroid function tests can be used to confirm the clinical suspicion of thyroid hyperfunction. A thyroid scintiscan (Fig. 2-25A) reveals multiple areas of increased uptake or a single area of increased uptake with suppression of the remaining gland in cases of solitary toxic nodule. A specific histologic diagnosis can be obtained by FNA cytology.

TREATMENT

SURGICAL

Thyroidectomy is the preferred treatment for this condition (3). Control of the hyperthyroidism is immediate and certain, and the patient is freed of the goiter, which is often large enough to cause thoracic inlet compressive symptoms. The patient should first be rendered euthyroid with drug therapy—in this case antithyroid drugs and/or propranolol, but not iodides, which may exacerbate hyperthyroidism in these cases (Jod-Basedow).

NONSURGICAL

Treatment with *radioiodine* is generally considered inferior to thyroidectomy because the goiter usually persists after treatment, several months must elapse before treatment is effective, and the radiation dosage is highly variable (variations in the size of the gland and the percentage of uptake of ^{131}I may require that multiple courses of treatment be given over several months). In the case of solitary toxic adenomas, there is some concern that if radioiodine is used, the surrounding normal tissue will be exposed to a sufficient radiation dosage to induce subsequent thyroid cancer (151). The use of radioiodine in the treatment of hyperfunctioning adenomatous goiter is usually reserved for elderly patients who are considered too ill to tolerate thyroidectomy.

Treatment with *antithyroid drugs* has never been widely attempted because lifetime therapy would be required (3); unlike Graves' disease, which tends to remit spontaneously, the hyperthyroidism of nodular goiter probably continues indefinitely.

Thyroiditis Causing Hyperthyroidism

"Hashitoxicosis." Some patients with the typical clinical features of Graves' disease (with or without associated ophthalmopathy) are found on biopsy or at surgery to have thyroid glands that show the histologic picture of Hashimoto's thyroiditis alone or a mixture of both parenchymatous hypertrophy of Graves' disease and extensive lymphocytic infiltration. It is now generally accepted that Hashimoto's thyroiditis and Graves' disease are interrelated disorders of similar etiology that may occasionally coexist in the same patient (152).

Subacute Thyroiditis with Transient Hyperthyroidism. It has long been recognized that some patients with painful, viral subacute thyroiditis will manifest transient clinical thyrotoxicosis in association with an elevated circulating thyroid hormone level and very low thyroid RAIU (153). Recently, however, a number of reports have appeared also describing transient clinical hyperthyroidism (usually lasting about 4–6 weeks) with blocked RAIU and nontender diffuse thyroid enlargement due to lymphocytic thyroiditis (154,155). A temporary phase of hypothyroidism often follows the hyperthyroidism; subsequent recurrent episodes of transient hyperthyroidism may occur in 10% or more of the patients (155).

This disorder can be mistakenly diagnosed as Graves' disease unless the very low thyroid RAIU is noted. Since all of these patients can be expected to have a spontaneous remission of their thyrotoxicosis within a few weeks, it is important that the differential diagnosis from Graves' disease be made, so that long-term antithyroid drug therapy or thyroidectomy can be avoided. All patients with a diffuse goiter and a clinical diagnosis of thyrotoxicosis should have RAIU measured; those with low values can be observed with only supportive therapy; propranolol is the preferred treatment as it allows the process of spontaneous resolution to be easily monitored (156).

PREVENTION AND MANAGEMENT

RARE COMPLICATIONS

Complications of Thyroid Surgery

Mortality. Mortality from thyroid surgery is virtually negligible today. Even before the turn of the century, without the benefit of blood transfusion, antibiotics, or endotracheal anesthesia, Theodor Kocher was able to perform thousands of thyroidectomies (often for huge goiters) with a mortality of only 0.5% (157).

Thyroid Crisis. Prior to the introduction of preoperative iodine preparation for Graves' disease by Plummer in 1923, the principal cause of death in patients undergoing thyroidectomy was postoperative thyroid crisis. As Pemberton and Haines, Mayo Clinic physicians of that era described it,

> Often, within a few hours after the goiter had been resected successfully, an acute explosive reaction would follow, characterized by extreme tachycardia, high temperature, nausea and vomiting, marked restlessness and prostration, mental stimulation or delerium and frequently coma; often death supervened within from 12 to 48 hours (158).

With Lugol's iodine, antithyroid drugs, and propranolol available for preoperative preparation of patients with Graves' disease, thyroid crisis as a complication of thyroidectomy today is entirely preventable. This exceedingly rare complication is treated with high doses of antithyroid drugs (PTU 600–1000 mg loading dose, then 200 mg every 8 hours) followed by iodide (10 drops of Lugol's iodine every 8 hours by mouth or 1 g sodium iodide by intravenous infusion every 8 hours) and/or propranolol (1–2 mg) intravenously with electrocardiographic control, followed by 10–40 mg by mouth every 8 hours) along with other general supportive measures (fluids, ice packs, hypothermic blanket). Corticosteroids have also been used empirically to treat this condition.

Postoperative Hemorrhage with Airway Obstruction. This should be an exceedingly rare postoperative complication. Bleeding will usually be heralded by an unusual degree of postoperative pain, apprehension, swelling of the neck, and excessive blood drainage through the skin incision or via any drains that may have been used. Once recognized, an expanding hematoma should be evacuated by reopening the wound, preferably under sterile conditions in the operating room. If the hematoma has gone unrecognized too long and has progressed to the point of causing laryngeal compression and airway obstruction with stridor and hypoxia, then the skin and deep fascial sutures should be removed post haste at the bedside to release the hematoma. If this maneuver does not restore an adequate airway immediately, endotracheal intubation will be necessary. Bedside tracheotomy should be required rarely, if ever (159).

Bilateral Recurrent Laryngeal Nerve Injury. This may be a rare consequence of definitive surgery for extensive malignant disease of the thyroid. It results in the vocal cords assuming a flaccid, paralyzed intermediate position; the airway may or may not be adequate. Bilateral cord paralysis should always be suspected in patients in whom stridor and cyanosis develop shortly after extubation. Immediate reintubation must be carried out, but one does not always need to do an emergency tracheotomy. The problem may be simply one of recurrent nerve neuropraxia or even simple laryngeal edema—both of which are reversible with time. The patient may be subsequently safely extubated after 1 or 2 days of parenteral steroid therapy (2–4 mg dexamethasone every 6 hours intramuscularly). Of course, if the cords are paralyzed and the airway is compromised, tracheotomy will ultimately be necessary.

If there is no return of cord function during the subsequent 6–12 months, transoral arytenoidectomy can be performed to enlarge the airway by laterofixation of one cord. Attempts at delayed nerve repair (160) or nerve–muscle pedicle implants (161) have generally not been successful in restoring cord function. In those patients in whom the airway is initially adequate despite bilateral cord paralysis, the voice is hoarse and breathy at first; later its quality improves. This may mean that nerve function has recovered, but it may also have a more ominous significance, signaling impending airway compromise. This is because when the cords remain paralyzed, the glottic aperture becomes progressively more narrow as atrophy, fibrosis, and contraction in the intrinsic laryngeal muscles draw the cords into a tense midline position.

Injury to the External Branch of the Superior Laryngeal Nerve. This complication is frequently discussed, and much is made of the vulnerability of this branch when the superior vascular pedicle of the thyroid is clamped. There is no simple way to document such injury, however, and therefore its true frequency is unknown. Gross changes that occur are usually of a subtle nature and will probably go unnoticed by the patient unless he or she is a professional singer or public speaker. The patient may be aware of an inability to reach high-pitched sounds (this is because the superior laryngeal nerve innervates the cricothyroid muscle, which is a tensor of the vocal cord) or easy fatigability of the voice when speaking to crowds. Injury to this nerve can best be avoided by leaving division of the superior pole vessels until after the isthmus has been divided and the lobe has been substantially mobilized. The adventitial tissue attaching the upper pole of the thyroid to the larynx is then separated by blunt dissection. This leaves the pole suspended by the superior vascular pedicle. Now the thyroid lobe can be swung away from the larynx in order to clamp, suture-ligate, and divide the superior thyroid vessels, leaving the superior laryngeal nerve medially and safe from injury.

Other Rare Neurologic Complications. Complications of thyroid surgery also include the following: injury to the cervical sympathetic trunk (it is vulnerable when the inferior thyroid artery is ligated), causing Horner's syndrome; damage to the phrenic nerve (which is liable to be injured in the course of a modified neck dissection for metastatic thyroid cancer), causing paralysis of the hemidiaphragm; and transection of the spinal accessory nerve during nodal dissection of the posterior triangle, causing a shoulder droop and winging of the scapula due to paralysis of the trapezius muscle.

Injury to the Right Lymphatic Duct or Thoracic Duct. Such an injury can occur in the course of a modified neck dissection. Leakage of chyle will usually be obvious during operation, at which time it is an easy matter to ligate the duct. Attempted repair of this friable, thin-walled vessel is inadvisable, because a persistent leak will almost certainly result, with the subsequent development of a chylous fistula. Reoperation will then be required to ligate the duct in the neck or, if this fails, in the chest.

MORE FREQUENT COMPLICATIONS

Unilateral Paralysis of the Recurrent Laryngeal Nerve. Indirect laryngoscopy should be performed routinely, both preoperatively and postoperatively. In these times of heightened medicolegal sensibility, it is important to document normal vocal cord function before operation, even if there is no previous history of neck surgery. In such cases, cord paralysis may be related to the thyroid disease itself [either benign (162) or malignant] or to unsuspected intrathoracic pathology, such as a tracheal neoplasm or aortic aneurysm. Occasionally, one will also encounter so-called idiopathic vocal cord paralysis, for which there is no apparent cause (163). In patients who have had previous thyroid or parathyroid surgery, it is doubly important to know of the presence of cord paralysis before operation, not only because of the potential medicolegal implications, but also because of concern about possible injury to the remaining functioning nerve causing bilateral cord paralysis and airway compromise.

The best way to avoid injuring the recurrent nerves at operation is to conscientiously expose and identify them and to refrain from handling them directly with instruments. Transient cord paresis may occur in up to 5% of cases, even in the best of hands, presumably due to stretching or edema of the nerve occasioned by dissection of adjacent tissues; this seldom lasts more than 4–6 weeks. The surgeon should also be aware that trauma from the endotracheal tube cuff can cause temporary cord paralysis (164). Even bilateral vocal cord paralysis can occur as a direct result of endotracheal intubation (165).

If the nerve is severed in the course of dissection and the injury is recognized at the time, one should attempt to reapproximate the cut ends immediately with the use of meticulous microsurgical technique. Unfortunately, there is not much hope that full recovery will occur (166). Delayed nerve repair is essentially worthless (160).

Unless routine indirect laryngoscopy is performed, many cases of cord paralysis will never be discovered. This is because compensatory overadduction of the uninvolved cord narrows the glottic chink to produce a normal voice (generally within 4–6 weeks). When symptoms occur, they are usually those of hoarseness and an ineffective nonexplosive type of cough, but even in these patients, a normal speaking voice will almost always return in time as fibrotic changes in the paralyzed muscles move the cord from a paramedian position to the midline. If after 6–12 months there has not been spontaneous recovery of nerve function, the quality of the voice can often be improved by injection of Teflon paste into the paralyzed cord (167). The incidence of inadvertant unilateral recurrent nerve injury causing permanent cord paralysis should be less than 1% (0.5% of nerves exposed to risk after subtotal or total thyroidectomy).

Postoperative Hypocalcemia. The serum calcium level should be checked routinely following bilateral subtotal or total thyroidectomy. Despite attempts to implicate other factors (168), hypocalcemia following thyroidectomy almost always results from injury to the parathyroid glands or interference with their blood supply. If the damage is severe enough, overt hypoparathyroidism will result, usually within 1–7 days. (For treatment of hypoparathyroidism see the section in Chapter 1, Postoperative Hypocalcemia.)

The incidence of permanent hypoparathyroidism following subtotal thyroidectomy should approach zero. After total thyroidectomy it should be possible to keep the risk of permanent hypoparathyroidism to less than 1% by meticulously dissecting the parathyroid glands away from the thyroid and preserving their blood supply intact. Autotransplantation of a parathyroid will be necessary if its blood supply is destroyed (79). (For technique of parathyroid autotransplantation see the section in Chapter 1, Total Parathyroidectomy with Autotransplant.)

TOTAL THYROID LOBECTOMY

Operative Technique

When thyroid carcinoma is suspected (either grossly at the time of operation, or preoperatively on the basis of the needle biopsy findings), total lobectomy should be performed on the side of the lesion. Then, depending upon the frozen-section pathologic findings and the anatomy of the recurrent laryngeal nerve and parathyroid glands, a subtotal, near-total, or total lobectomy is carried out on the opposite side (see section, Thyroid Cancer).

The sequential steps for gaining exposure of the thyroid are similar to those for parathyroid exploration illustrated in Chapter 1 (see Figs. 1-19 to 1-26). With the recurrent laryngeal nerve and one or both parathyroid glands now identified, the thyroid lobe is freed and removed as depicted in Figures 2-26 to 2-31. Note the use of small hemoclips to divide the individual branches of the inferior thyroid artery and to sever the ligament of Berry—the dense condensation of vascular pretracheal fascia that attaches the thyroid posteriorly to the first and second tracheal rings. Division of this ligament releases the lobe. The recurrent laryngeal nerve must be exposed right up to its site of entry into the larynx, deep to the cricopharyngeus muscle and posterior to the cricothyroid articulation and the inferior horn of the thyroid cartilage. At this stage of the operation, the superior parathyroid gland is routinely identified and preserved along with its blood supply.

Before closure, the tissues of the neck are irrigated with saline and residual bleeding points are ligated. Closure is effected as illustrated in Chapter 1 (see Figs. 1-39 to 1-41).

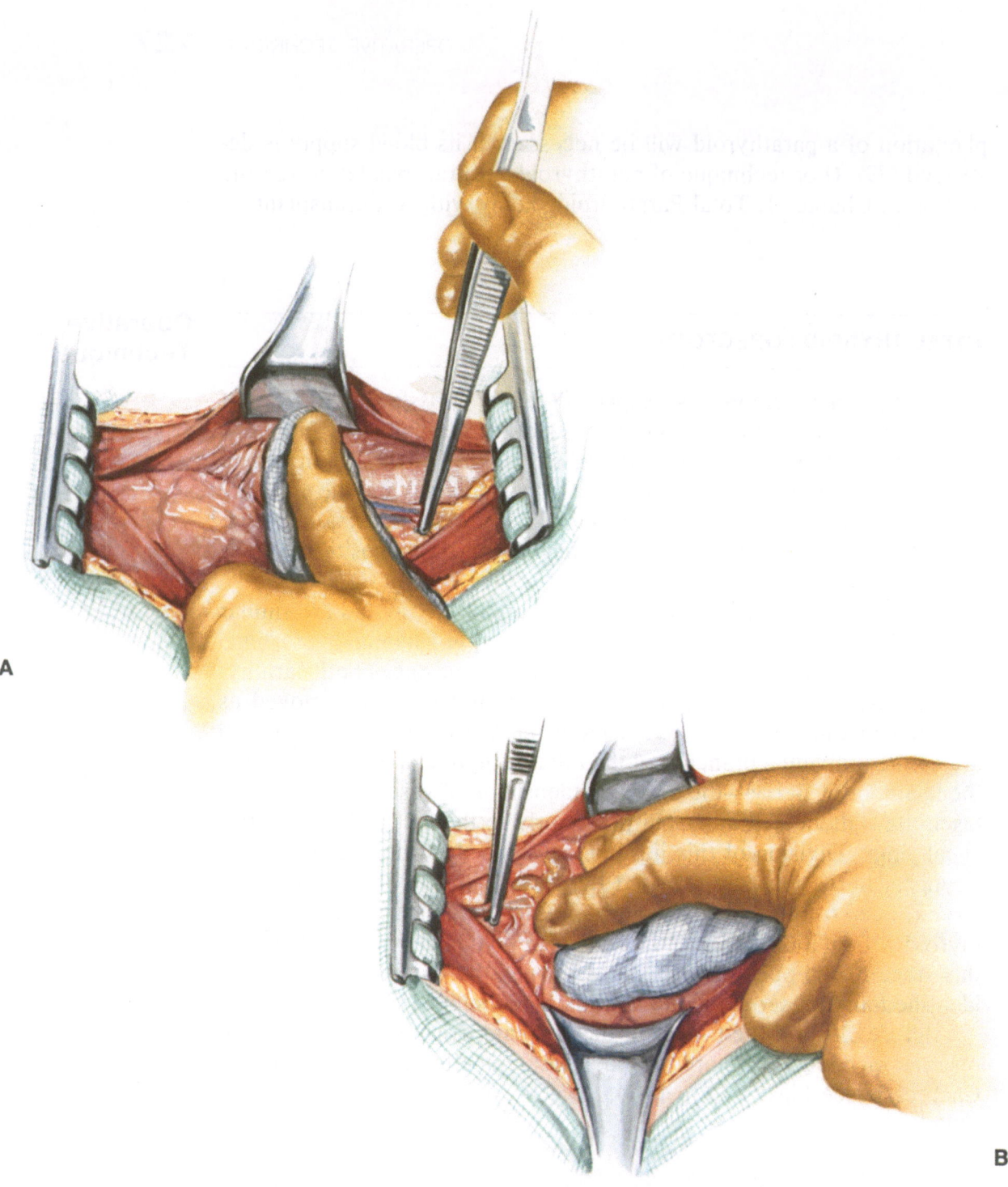

Fig. 2-26. **Freeing of thyroid isthmus.** **A.** The usual collar incision has been made, the midline cervical fascia divided, and the strap muscles retracted laterally. The entire anterior aspect of the thyroid gland now lies exposed. Using a gauze sponge for traction, the surgeon pushes the isthmus of the gland upward, bringing the inferior thyroid veins into taut relief. The subisthmic lymph nodes and fat are stripped upward toward the thyroid, skeletonizing the veins, which are then clamped, divided, and tied. One must exercise care during this step to avoid possible injury to an anomalous anteriorly placed recurrent laryngeal nerve (see Fig. 2-6). **B.** The Delphian lymph nodes, situated in the midline immediately above the isthmus, and the pyramidal lobe (if present) are dissected down off the anterior aspect of the larynx to free the isthmus from above. Small bleeders encountered at this stage are either cauterized or clamped and tied.

128

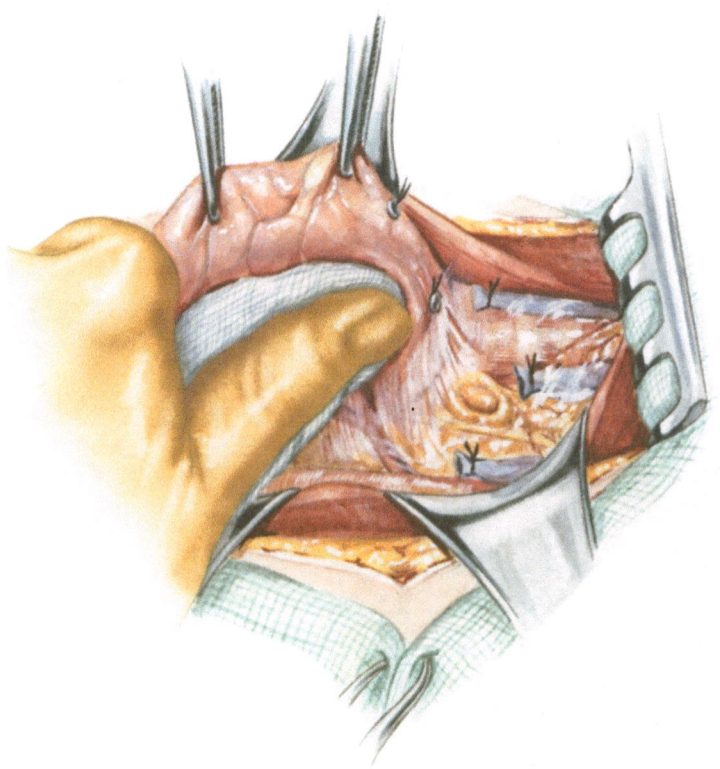

Freeing of thyroid lobe laterally: exposure of the recurrent laryngeal Fig. 2-27.
nerve and inferior thyroid artery (right side). The right lobe of the thyroid
is grasped with Kocher clamps (or Lahey thyroid tenacula) and rotated medially
out of its bed. The areolar planes adjacent to the thyroid are now suffused with
air drawn into the tissues by suction created by traction on the thyroid and
countertraction of the strap muscles. This process is best described as "air dissection" of the tissues and it facilitates the rapid exposure of the inferior thyroid
veins, inferior thyroid artery, recurrent laryngeal nerve, and parathyroid glands;
the areolar tissues are simply stripped away with thumb forceps from these
structures without causing any blood loss. The middle thyroid veins are ligated
(or clipped with hemoclips) and divided. The inferior thyroid artery is identified
and traced medially to its intersection with the recurrent laryngeal nerve, which
usually is deep to the artery. The recurrent nerve often can be palpated before it
is visualized by being gently "popped" with the finger against the lateral aspect
of the trachea (see Fig. 2-31). The inferior parathyroid gland is seen in this figure as a small, tan nodule surrounded by thymic fat beneath the lower pole of
the thyroid.

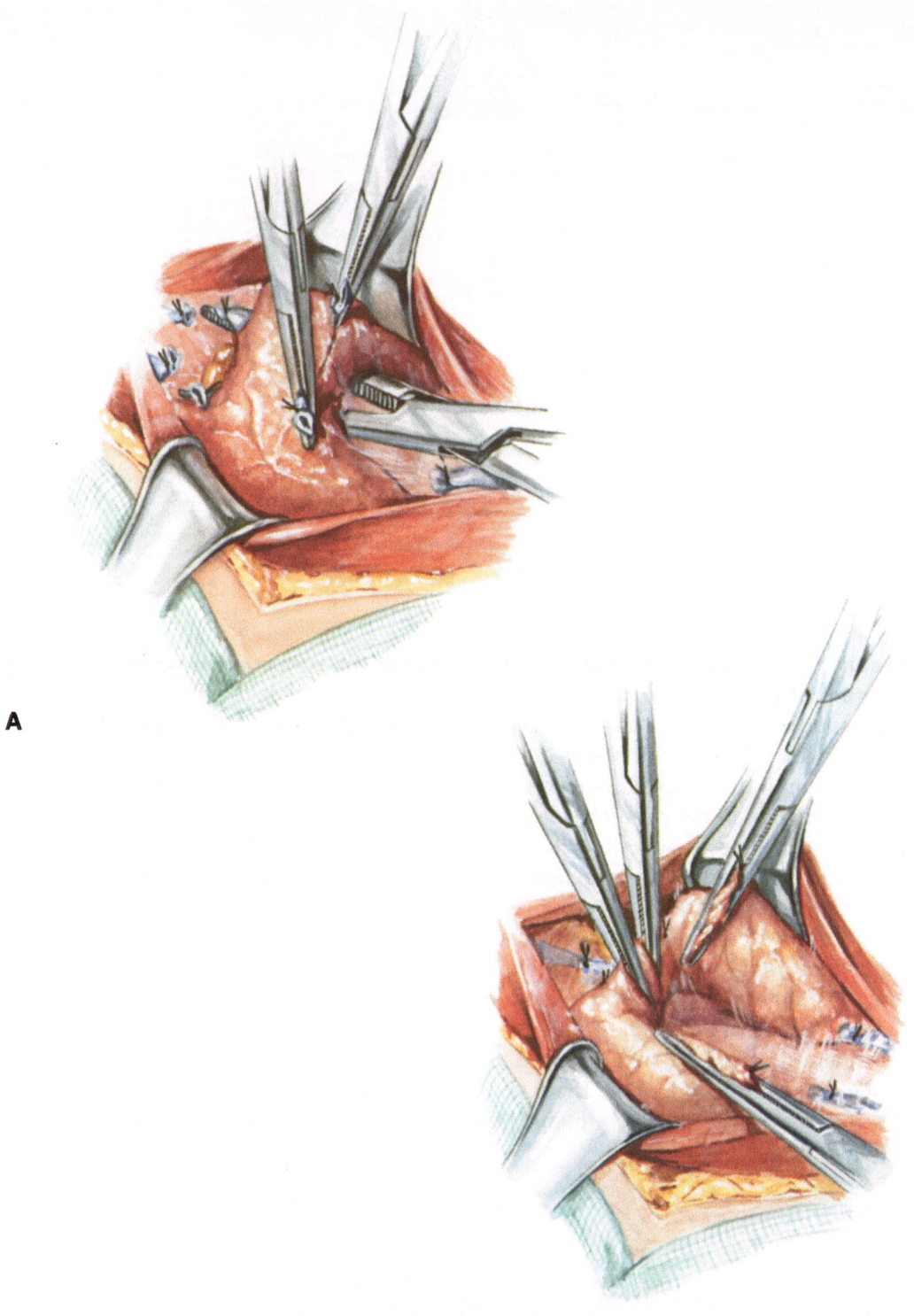

A

B

Fig. 2-28.   Freeing of thyroid lobe medially: division of the isthmus.   A. The thyroid isthmus is separated from the underlying trachea by blunt dissection with a Kocher clamp.   **B.** It is then clamped on either side and divided.

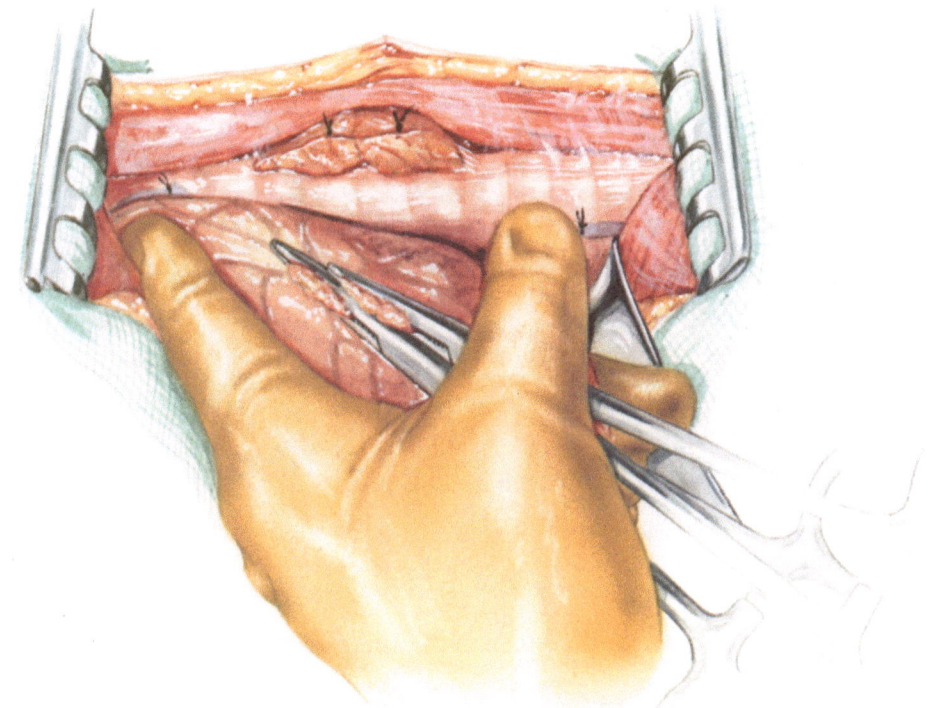

A

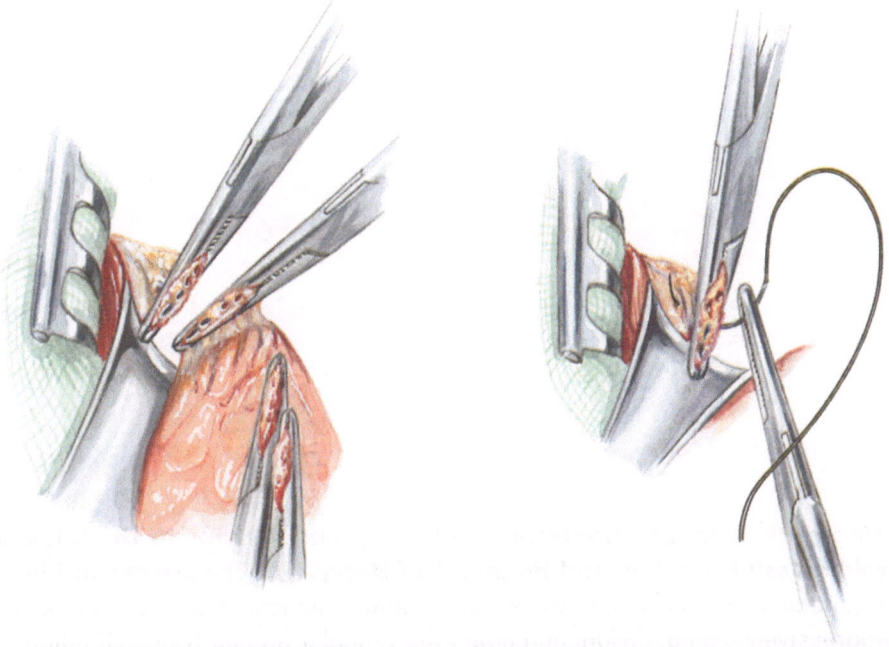

B

C

**Freeing of thyroid lobe superiorly: ligation and division of the superior
thyroid pedicle.** **A.** The lobe, being partially mobilized by division of the isthmus, is pulled laterally and downward away from the side of the larynx. **B.** This
maneuver permits clamping and division of the superior thyroid vascular pedicle
without fear of injuring the external laryngeal nerve. **C.** The stump is secured
with transfixion ligatures.

Fig. 2-29.

131

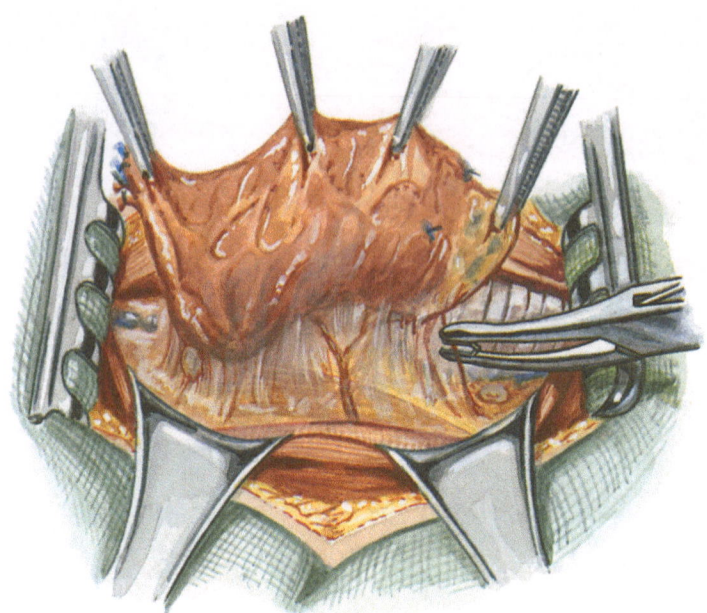

A

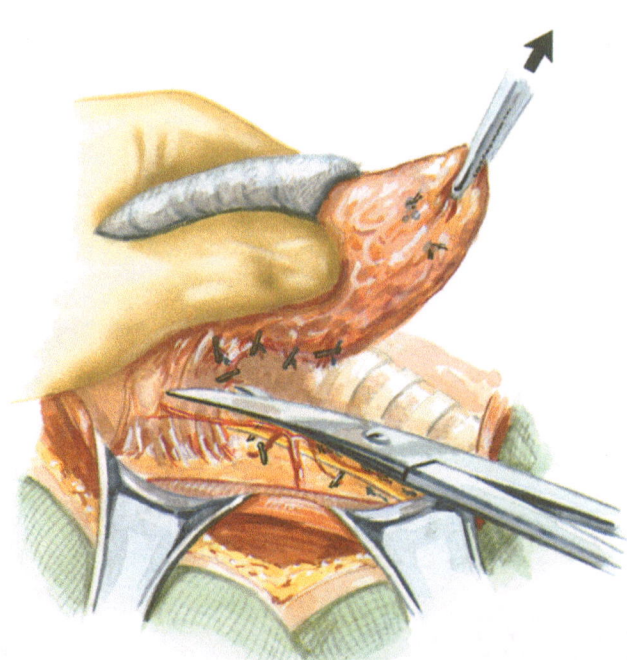

B

Fig. 2-30. **Freeing of thyroid lobe posteriorly: clipping and division of the inferior thyroid artery branches and ligament of Berry.** **A.** The use of small hemoclips facilitates this step, however, fine-pointed hemostats also can be used to progressively clamp, divide, and ligate the vascular areolar tissues binding the thyroid posteriorly to the trachea. **B.** The ligament of Berry, which consists of dense vascular connective tissue, is divided with the scissors; care is taken to stay clear of the recurrent laryngeal nerve and preserve the superior parathyroid gland with its blood supply intact. Individual branches of the inferior thyroid artery are clipped separately.

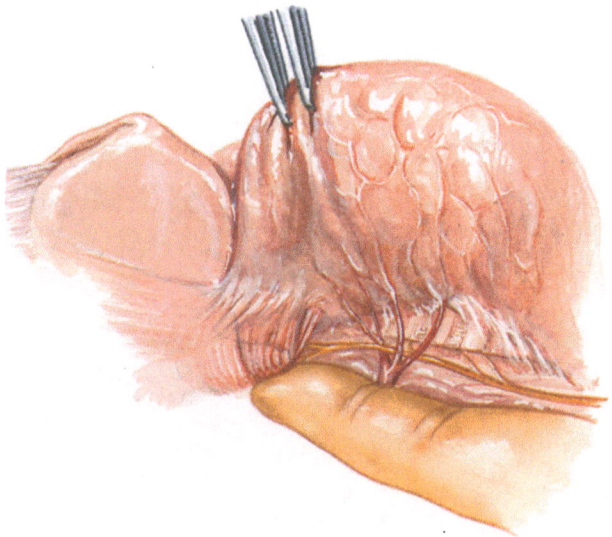

Guide to the identification of the recurrent laryngeal nerve at its entrance to the larynx. The recurrent laryngeal nerve is vulnerable at this level, where it traverses the ligament of Berry; occasionally, it may even lie within the posterior portion of the thyroid gland itself. The course of the nerve must be clearly identified before these fascial bands are severed. The inferior horn of the thyroid cartilage is easily felt and serves as a convenient guide to the position of the nerve at this point, as it enters the larynx deep to the cricopharyngeus muscle and posterior to the cricothyroid articulation and the inferior horn.

Fig. 2-31.

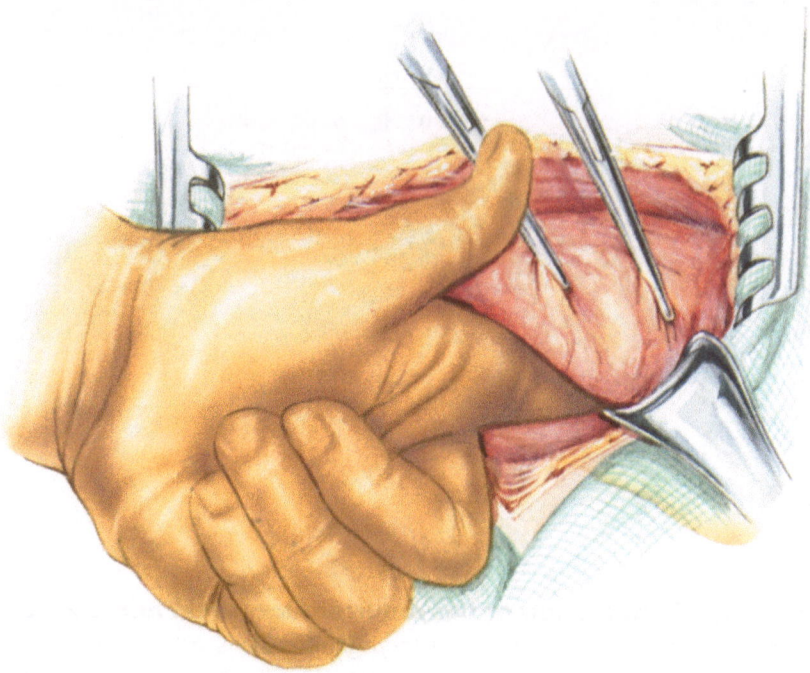

A

Fig. 2-32. **Removal of substernal goiter.** **A.** The cervical portion of the thyroid is mobilized as far as possible. The middle thyroid vein and inferior thyroid artery are secured. A finger is then insinuated downward behind the substernal goiter to free it from the surrounding structures. **B.** Traction from above, aided by pressure with the finger from below, is used to ease the gland upward and deliver it into the neck.

REMOVAL OF A SUBSTERNAL GOITER

Almost all substernal goiters can be removed via a cervical incision. The cervical approach permits control of the blood supply, identification of the recurrent laryngeal nerves, and preservation of the parathyroid glands. The collar incision may be extended by splitting the sternum to give wider exposure, but this step is seldom necessary.

In rare instances, a goiter lies wholly within the thorax. These tumors may arise primarily from ectopic intrathoracic thyroid tissues; more often, they are the residual portion of a goiter that was incompletely removed by previous cervical thyroidectomy. Such cases may be best approached through a primary thoracic incision, either sternum-splitting or posterolateral thoractomy, depending on their location.

Those patients whose airway is compromised by a huge substernal goiter should not receive sedatives until they are under the direct super-

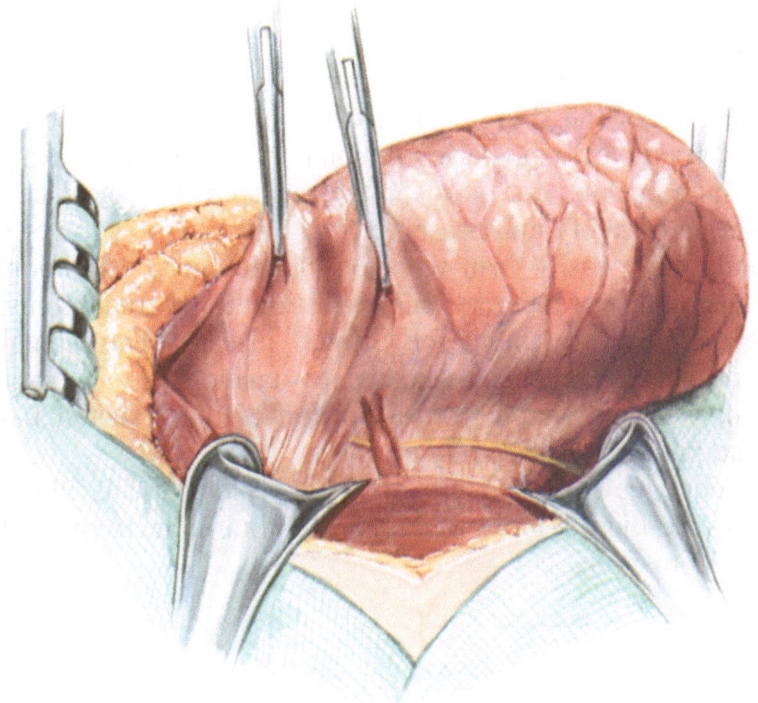

B

vision of the anesthesiologist. It may be preferable to intubate these patients while awake, with topical anesthesia, in order to avoid airway difficulties during induction.

The thyroid is mobilized as shown in Figure 2-32. Occasionally, a very large substernal goiter cannot be delivered in the manner described. In such instances the capsule may be incised and the central portion of the mass removed piecemeal (i.e., by morcellation) with sponge-holding forceps or Russian forceps. This permits removal of the goiter without injury to surrounding structures and, if accomplished expeditiously, with minimal blood loss. Subtotal resection is then carried out (described in Figs. 2-33 to 2-38; see below).

The substernal space is filled with saline and the lungs are hyperinflated to check for any air bubbles, which would indicate a pleural leak. A suction catheter may be left in place for 24–36 hours; it is connected to underwater-seal drainage if a pneumothorax is present.

SUBTOTAL THYROID LOBECTOMY

Benign lesions of the thyroid are treated by subtotal lobectomy. The technique preserves a posterior remnant of several grams of thyroid tissue, which enables one to clear the recurrent laryngeal nerve by a wider margin of safety and preserve both the upper and lower parathyroid glands more easily than with total lobectomy. Multinodular adenomatous goiter is treated by bilateral subtotal thyroidectomy; this is also the definitive treatment for Graves' disease. The weight of the thyroid remnants are best estimated by fashioning a ''template'' of equivalent size and shape from a portion of the resected tissue and having the pathologist carefully weigh it.

The sequence for exposure of the thyroid gland is illustrated in Chapter 1 (see Figs. 1-19 to 1-26). The subtotal lobectomy is shown in Figures 2-33 to 2-38.

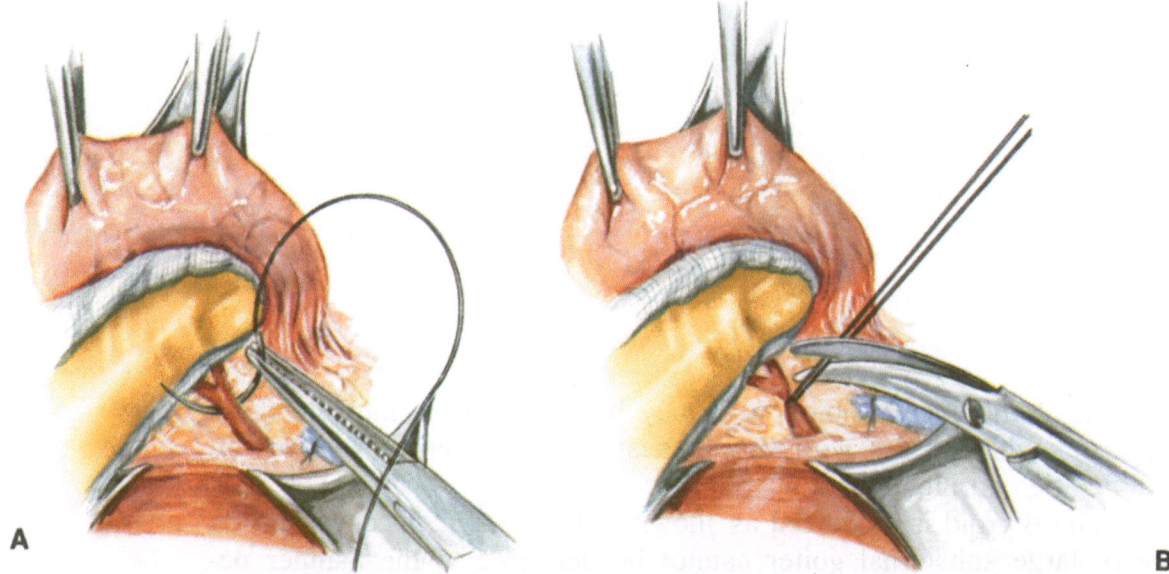

A   B

Fig. 2-33. **Preliminary ligation of the inferior thyroid artery (optional).** The inferior thyroid artery may be ligated in continuity with catgut, silk, or a metal clip. In cases of multinodular goiter, this step is advised as a means of reducing bleeding during the course of the subtotal lobectomy. When operating for Graves' disease, the authors prefer not to ligate the inferior thyroid artery in younger individuals, so as to be certain of preserving optimal blood supply to the parathyroids. Wade et al. (169) have pointed out that the ''functional reserve'' of the parathyroids may be compromised after thyroidectomy with the possibility of frank hypoparathyroidism developing when there is increased demand for calcium—such as with the adolescent growth spurt and in pregnancy.

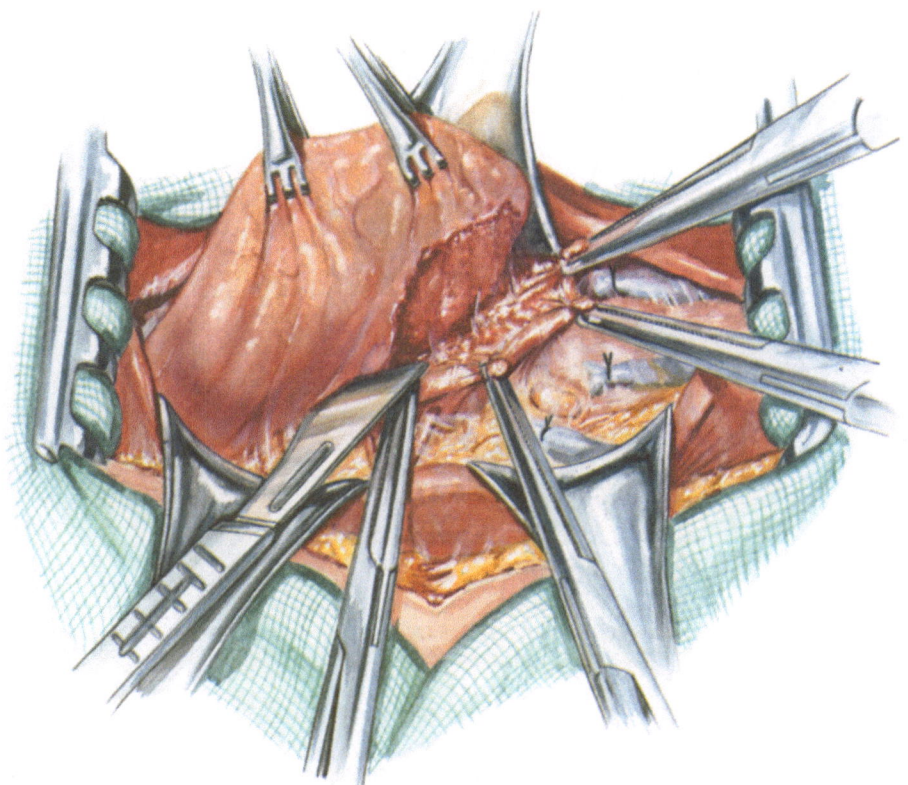

Subtotal resection of the lobe. This is initiated by retracting the thyroid
lobe anteriorly with Lahey tenacula. Beginning medially, the surgeon applies
Kocher clamps successively to the thyroid capsule, working around the circum-
ference of the lobe in a horizontal plane approximately flush with the anterior
surface of the trachea, and constantly checking the position of the recurrent
laryngeal nerve and the parathyroids to avoid injuring them. As each clamp is
applied to the thyroid, the tissues held in the jaws of the clamp are severed
flush with the upper surface of the instrument; in this way, the superficial portion of the lobe is progressively freed. If a parathyroid gland is unavoidably
devascularized in the course of the resection (the inferior parathyroid glands are
most vulnerable because they are frequently situated high on the lateral surface
of the thyroid), then the gland should be diced and autotransplanted into the
sternocleidomastoid muscle (for technique see section in Chapter 1, Total
Parathyroidectomy with Heterotropic Autotransplantation).

Fig. 2-34.

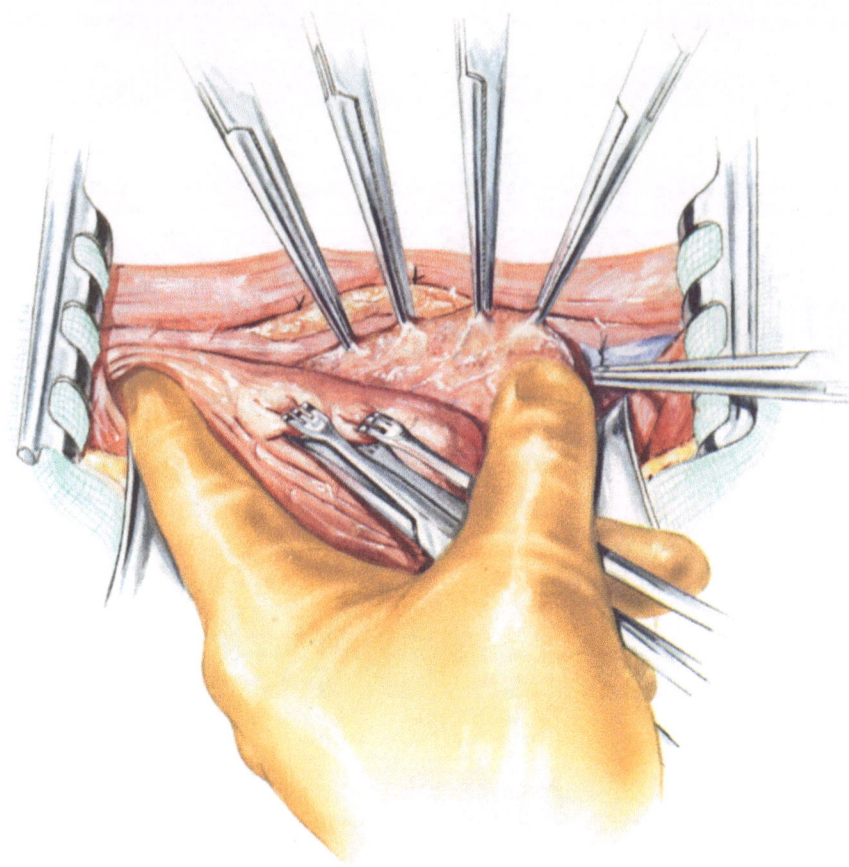

A

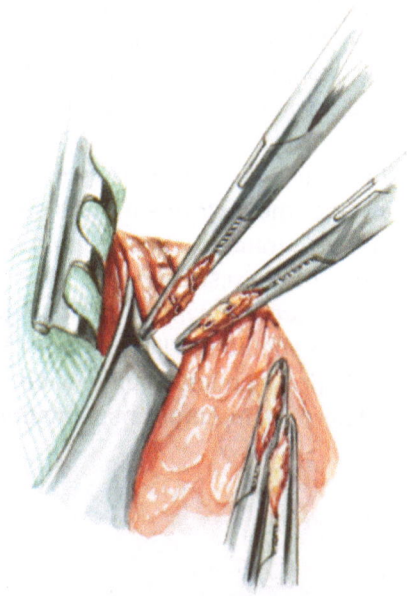

B

Fig. 2-35. **Ligation of the superior thyroid pedicle.** **A.** Once most of the lobe has been partially detached, it is sufficiently mobile to be retracted laterally and downward, thereby bringing the superior thyroid vessels prominently into view. In this way, the vascular pedicle is pulled away from the side of the larynx and the external laryngeal nerve, which at this level turns medially to reach the cricothyroid muscle. **B.** The superior thyroid pedicle is now clamped and divided **138** without fear of catching and injuring the external laryngeal nerve.

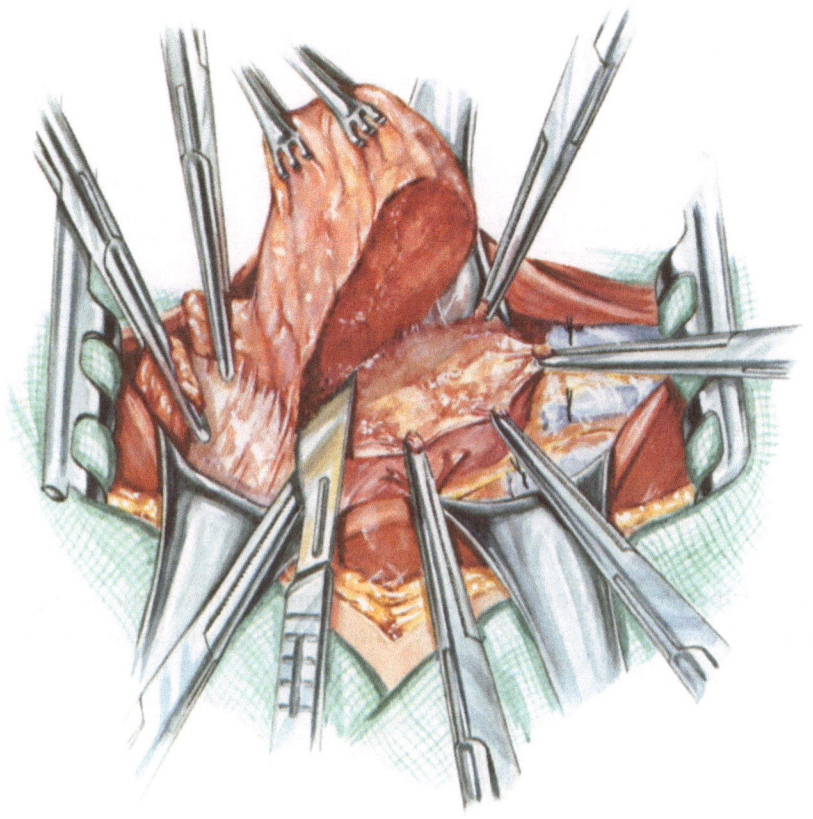

Completion of subtotal resection. Subtotal resection of the lobe is com-   **Fig. 2-36.**
pleted by clamping and dividing the remaining bridges of thyroid tissue. Bleeding points on the cut surface of the gland are best controlled by cautery or
transfixion catgut sutures (care must be taken to avoid deep bites with the needle, which might penetrate the posterior capsule and injure the recurrent laryngeal nerve). All clamps affixed to the thyroid remnant are tied off with 2/0 or 3/0
catgut or silk.

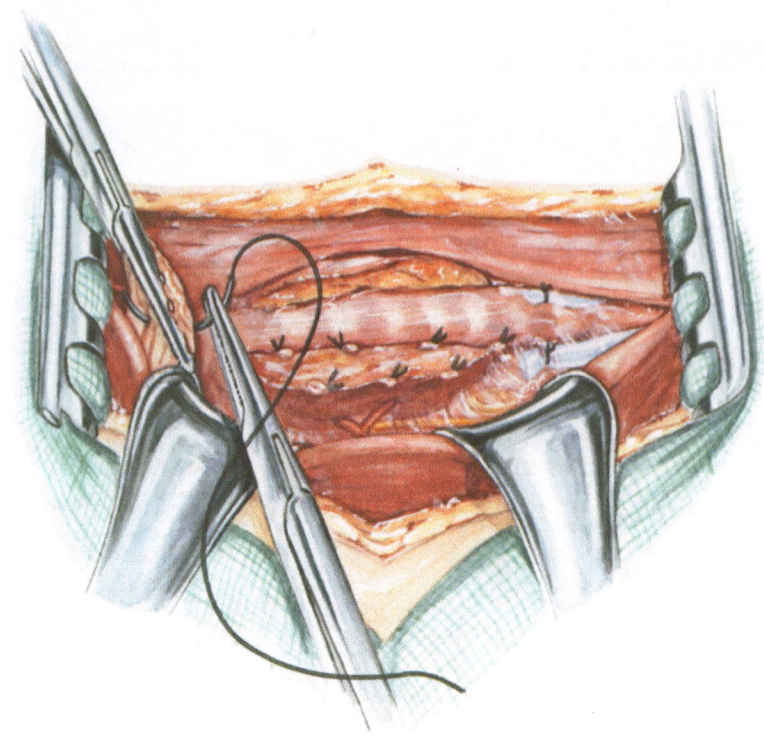

Fig. 2-37. The superior thyroid vascular pedicle is now secured with two suture ligatures of 3/0 chromic catgut, the second suture being left long with the needle attached.

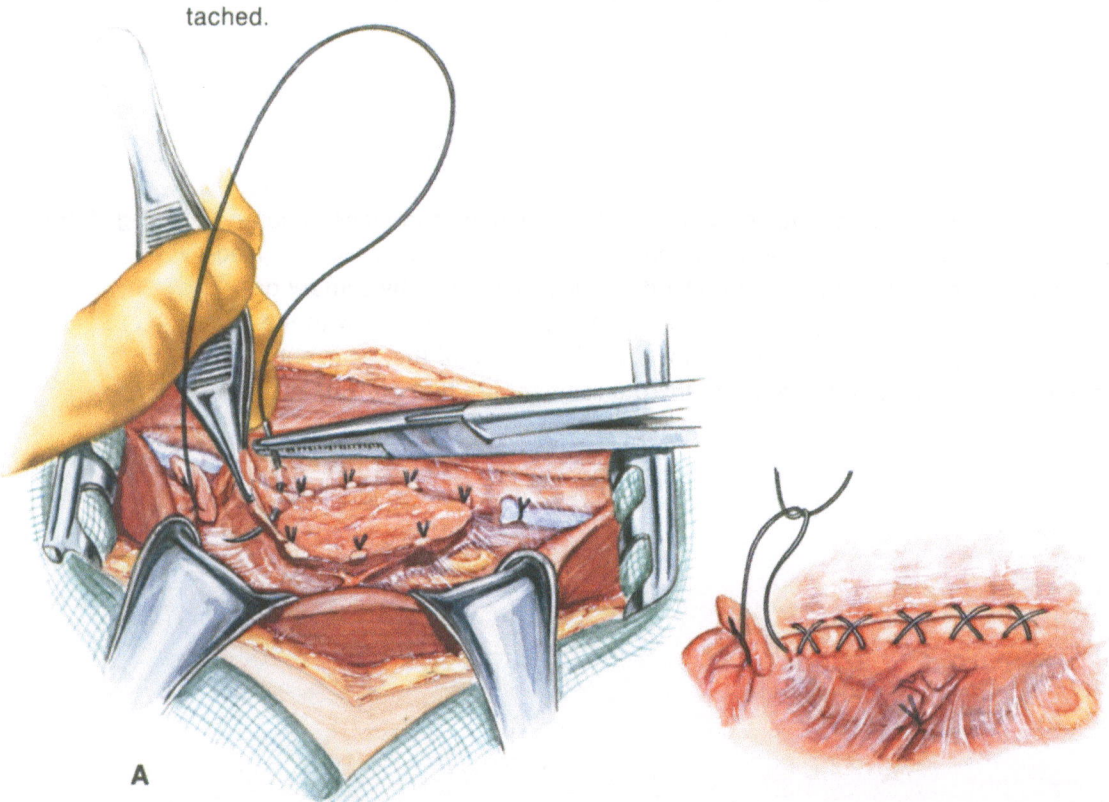

A   B

Fig. 2-38. **A.** The suture is used to oversew the exposed raw surfaces of the thyroid remnant, anchoring the lateral rim of the thyroid capsule to the pretracheal fascia as shown, as a hemostatic stitch. **B.** The stitch returns to its starting point and is tied. The recurrent nerve is carefully inspected once again. If a suture has caught the nerve inadvertently, that stitch must be removed. Recovery of nerve function should return within 6–12 weeks.

140

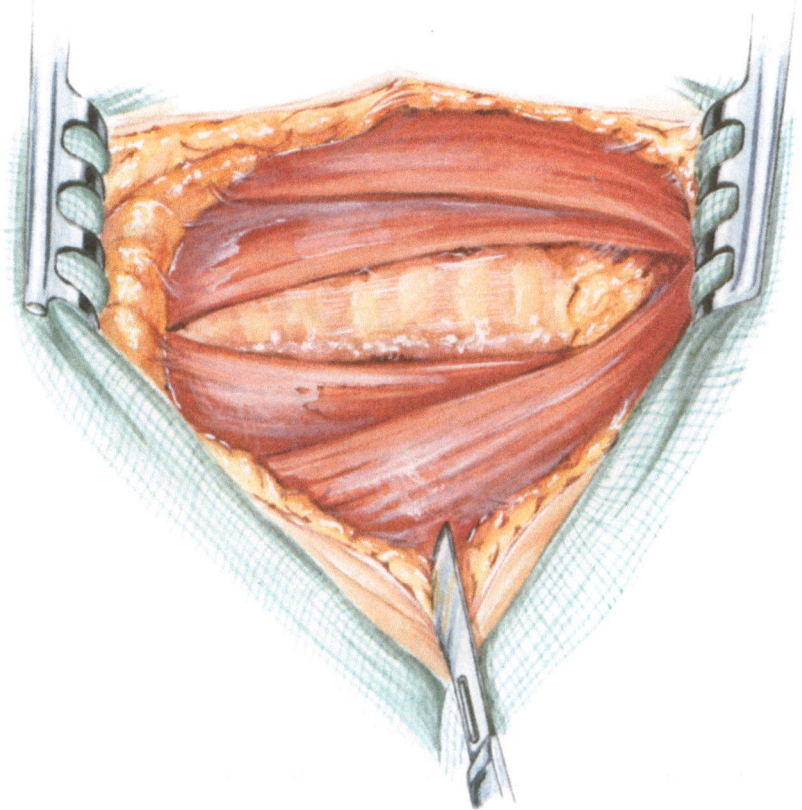

Extended incision for node dissection. The standard collar incision for thyroid-ectomy (see Fig. 1-19) is extended laterally and upward for about 1–2 inches along the posterior border of the sternocleidomastoid muscle.

Fig. 2-39.

MODIFIED NECK DISSECTION FOR PAPILLARY THYROID CARCINOMA

The classical radical neck dissection includes sacrifice of the cosmetically important sternocleidomastoid muscle, the internal jugular vein, and often the spinal accessory nerve supplying the trapezius. The result is a large, disfiguring scar, an asymmetric concave depression of the neck, and drooping of the shoulder on that side. In an operation for papillary thyroid carcinoma that has involved regional cervical lymph nodes by metastasis (as evidenced by palpable enlargement of the nodes), the classical radical neck dissection is modified in such a way as to preserve the important structures alluded to above (Figs. 2-39 to 2-42). The internal jugular chain of lymph nodes, together with the fascia, fat, and lymph nodes of the posterior triangle and the midcompartment of the neck, are removed—preferably in continuity, however, it would appear that thorough piecemeal removal of the nodes achieves the same results (see section, Papillary Carcinoma—Operative Strategy).

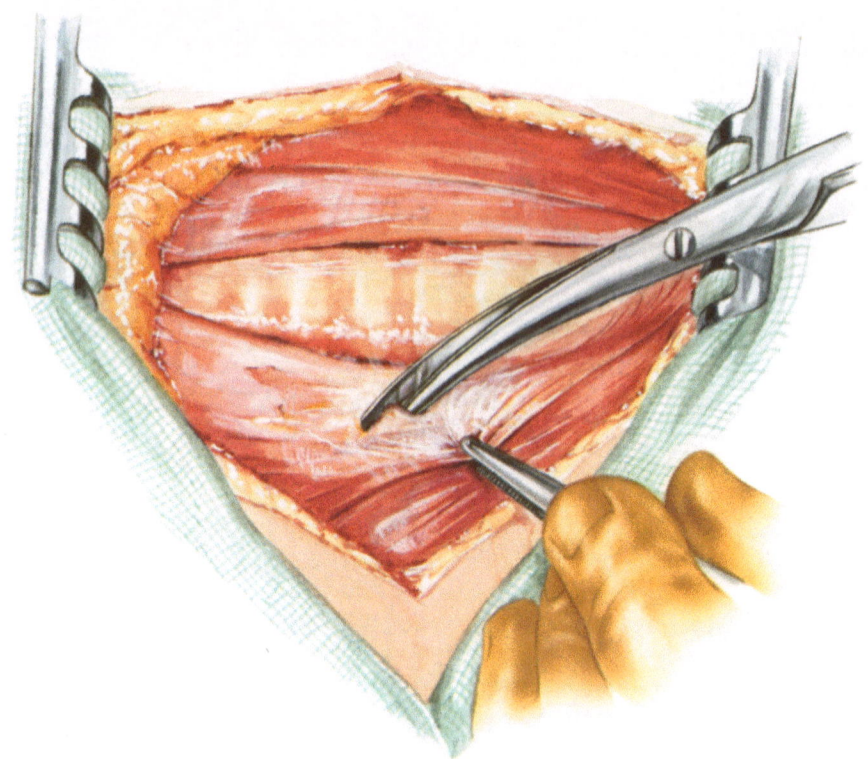

Fig. 2-40.   The areolar space between the sternocleidomastoid and midline strap muscles is opened.

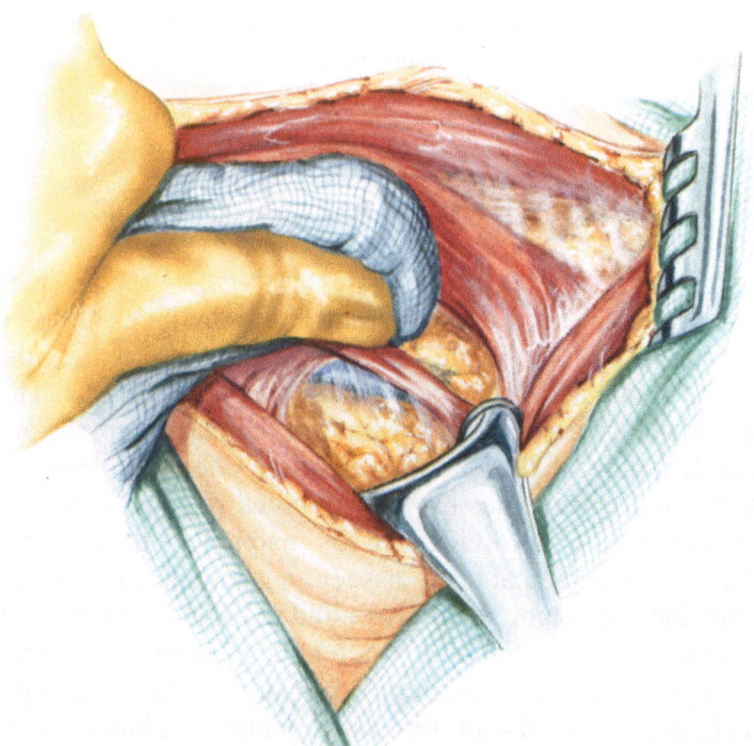

Fig. 2-41.   The muscles are then retracted apart to expose the underlying carotid sheath and internal jugular vein, the omohyoid muscle, and associated lymph nodes.

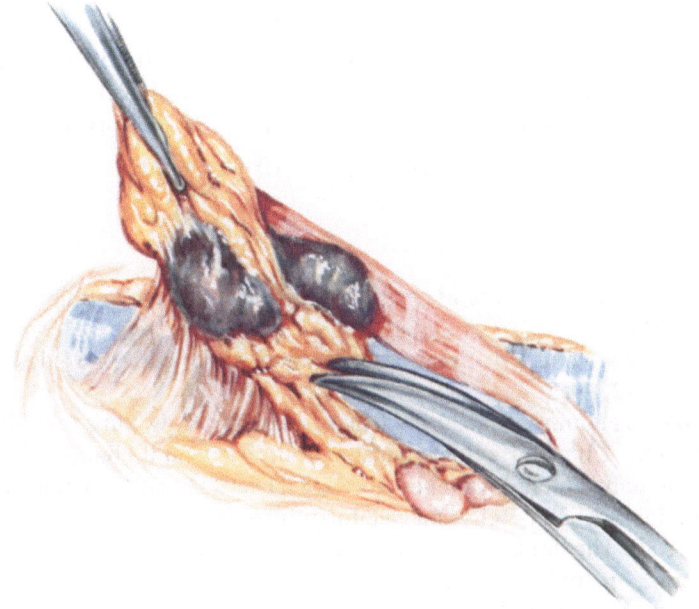

A

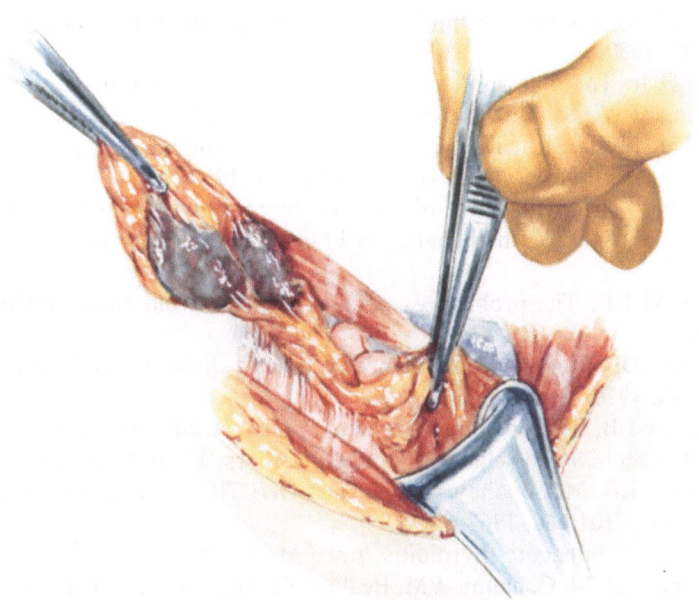

B

Node dissection.   A. The internal jugular nodes are dissected off the vein   **Fig. 2-42.**
and removed en bloc with the surrounding fascia and fat. In this case several of
the lymph nodes are obviously involved with metastatic tumor, being enlarged
and characteristically discolored.   **B.** Node-bearing tissue from the posterior triangle is dissected in continuity with the internal jugular specimen, using thumb
forceps. The omohyoid muscle and transverse cervical vessels may be divided
to facilitate this part of the dissection, carefully preserving the underlying
nerves.

Care should be taken to prevent injury to the vagus, phrenic, and spinal accessory nerves, to the internal jugular vein, and to any of the major lymphatic channels at the root of the neck. If either the thoracic or right lymphatic duct is inadvertently torn, it is better to ligate the main channel rather than attempt suture of the rent.

References

1. Astwood EB: Treatment of hyperthyroidism with thiourea and thiouracil. JAMA 122:78, 1943.
2. Greer MA, Astwood EB: Treatment of simple goiter with thyroid. J Clin Endocrinol 13:1312, 1953.
3. Black BM: The present position of thyroidectomy. Adv Surg 4:73, 1970.
4. Pearse AGE: Common cytochemical and ultrastructural characteristics of cells producing polypeptide hormones (the APUD series) and their relevance to thyroid ultimobranchial C cells and calcitonin. Proc R Soc Lond [Biol] 170:71, 1968.
5. Pearse AGE: The diffuse neuroendocrine system and the APUD concept: related "endocrine" peptides in brain, intestine, pituitary, placenta, and anuran cutaneous glands. Med Biol 55:115, 1977.
6. Pearse AGE, Takor TT: Neuroendocrine embryology and the APUD concept. Clin Endocrinol (Oxf) [Suppl] 5:229s, 1976.
7. Sterling K: Thyroid hormone action at the cell level. N Engl J Med 300:117, 1979.
8. Curtis GM: The blood supply of the human parathyroids. Surg Gynecol Obstet 50:805, 1930.
9. Crile G Jr: The fallacy of the conventional radical neck dissection for papillary carcinoma of the thyroid. Ann Surg 145:317, 1957.
10. Smith I, Murley RS: Damage to the cervical sympathetic system during operations on the thyroid gland. Br J Surg 52:673, 1965.
11. Vander J: The significance of nontoxic thyroid nodules: a 15-year study on the incidence of thyroid malignancy in Framingham Mass. Ann Intern Med 69:537, 1968.
12. Astwood EB: The problem of nodules in the thyroid gland. Pediatrics 18:501, 1956.
13. Baldwin DB, Rowett D: Incidence of thyroid disorders in Connecticut. JAMA 239:742, 1978.
14. Woolner LB, McConahey WM, Beahrs OH: Struma lymphomatosa (Hashimoto's thyroiditis) and related thyroidal disorders. J Clin Endocrinol 19:53, 1959.
15. Woolner LB, McConahey WM, Beahrs OH: The surgical aspects of thyroiditis. Am J Surg 104:666, 1962.
16. Greene JN: Subacute thyroiditis. Am J Med 51:97, 1971.
17. Woolner LB, McConahey WM, Beahrs OH: Granulomatous thyroiditis (de Quervain's thyroiditis). J Clin Endocrinol 17:1202, 1957.
18. Woolner LB, McConahey WM, Beahrs OH: Invasive fibrous thyroiditis (Riedel's struma). J Clin Endocrinol 17:201, 1957.
19. Hay ID, McConahey WM, Woolner LB: Riedel's thyroiditis associated with extra cervical fibrosclerosis. Clin Res 27:627a, 1979.
20. Lowhagen T, Grandberg P-O, Lundell G, et al: Aspiration biopsy cytology (ABC) in nodules of the thyroid gland suspected to be malignant. Surg Clin North Am 59:3, 1979.
21. Thompson NW, Nishiyama RH, Harness JK: Thyroid carcinoma: current controversies. Curr Probl Surg 15:1, 1978.
22. Hayles AB, Johnson LM, Beahrs OH, et al: Carcinoma of the thyroid in children. Am J Surg 106:735, 1963.

23. Favus MJ, Schneider AB, Stachura ME, et al: Thyroid cancer occurring as a late consequence of head-and-neck irradiation: evaluation of 1056 patients. N Engl J Med 294:1019, 1976.

24. Rao SD, Frame B, Miller MJ, et al: Hyperparathyroidism following head and neck irradiation. Arch Intern Med 140:205, 1980.

25. Swelstad JA, Scanlon EF, Oviedo MA, et al: Irradiation-induced polyglandular neoplasia of the head and neck. Am J Surg 135:820, 1978.

26. Van Den Berg CJ, Edis AJ: Multicentric thyroid carcinoma, parathyroid adenomas, and vagal neurilemmoma in a young man with antecedent tonsillar radiation. Mayo Clin Proc 55:648, 1980.

27. Modan B, Baidatz D, Mart H, et al: Radiation induced head and neck tumours. Lancet 1:277, 1974.

28. Crile G Jr, Esselstyn CB Jr, Hawk WA: Needle biopsy in the diagnosis of thyroid nodules appearing after radiation. N Engl J Med 301:997, 1979.

29. Refetoff S, Harrison J, Karanfilski BT, et al: Continuing occurrence of thyroid carcinoma after irradiation to the neck in infancy and childhood. N Engl J Med 292:171, 1975.

30. Schneider AB, Favus MJ, Stachura ME, et al: Incidence, prevalence and characteristics of radiation-induced thyroid tumors. Am J Med 64:243, 1978.

31. Mortenson JD, Bennett WA, Woolner LB: Incidence of carcinoma in thyroid glands removed at 1000 consecutive routine necropsies. Surg Forum 5:659, 1954.

32. Schneider AB, Favus MJ, Stachura ME, et al: Plasma thyroglobulin in detecting thyroid carcinoma after childhood head and neck irradiation. Ann Intern Med 86:29, 1977.

33. Alderson PO, Sumner HW, Siegel BA: The single palpable thyroid nodule. Cancer 37:258, 1976.

34. Shunoako K, Sokal JE: Differentiation of benign and malignant thyroid nodules by scintiscan. Arch Intern Med 144:36, 1964.

35. Beahrs OH, Pasternak BM: Cancer of the thyroid gland. Curr Probl Surg, December: 1–38, 1969.

36. Sisson JC, Bartold SP, Bartold SL: The dilemma of the solitary thyroid nodule: resolution through decision analysis. Semin Nucl Med 8:59, 1978.

37. Nelson RL, Wahner HW, Gorman CA: Rectilinear thyroid scanning as a predictor of malignancy. Ann Intern Med 88:41, 1978.

38. Hamberger B, Gharib H, Melton LJ III, et al: Fine-needle aspiration of thyroid nodules. Impact on thyroid practice and cost of care. Am J Med 73:381, 1982.

39. Crile G Jr: Treatment of thyroid cysts by aspiration. Surgery 59:210, 1966.

40. Miller JM, Zafar SU, Karo JJ: Cystic thyroid nodules—recommendation and management. Radiology 110:257, 1974.

41. Rosen IB, Wallace C, Strawbridge HG, et al: Reevaluation of needle aspiration cytology in detection of thyroid cancer. Surgery 90:747, 1981.

42. Varhaug JE, Segadal E, Heimann P: The utility of fine needle aspiration cytology in the management of thyroid tumors. World J Surg 5:573, 1981.

43. Astwood EB, Cassidy CE, Aurbach GD: Treatment of goiter and thyroid nodules with thyroid. JAMA 174:459, 1960.

44. McConahey WM, Woolner LB, Black BM, et al: Effect of dessicated thyroid in lymphocytic (Hashimoto's) thyroiditis. J Clin Endocrinol 19:45, 1959.

45. Miller JM, Hamburger JI, Kini S: Diagnosis of thyroid nodules: use of fine-needle aspiration and needle biopsy. JAMA 241:481, 1979.

46. Wang CA, Vickery AL Jr, Maloof F: Needle biopsy of the thyroid. Surg Gynecol Obstet 143:365, 1976.

47. Hamburger JI, Miller JM, Kini S: Clinical-Pathological Evaluation of Thyroid Nodules: Handbook and Atlas (limited ed). Private publication, 1979, pp 10–19, 74–84.

48. Lowhagen T, Willems J-S, Lundell G, et al: Aspiration biopsy cytology in diagnosis of thyroid cancer. World J Surg 5:61, 1981.
49. Burrow GN: Aspiration needle biopsy of the thyroid (editorial). Ann Intern Med 94:536, 1981.
50. Walfish PG, Hazani E, Strawbridge H, et al: A prospective study of combined ultrasonography and needle aspiration biopsy in the assessment of the hypofunctioning thyroid nodule. Surgery 82:474, 1977.
51. Gharib H: Fine-needle aspiration biopsy of thyroid nodules. Mayo Clin Proc 56:62, 1981.
52. Gershengorn MC, McClung MR, Chu EW, et al: Fine-needle aspiration biopsy cytology in the preoperative diagnosis of thyroid nodules. Ann Intern Med 87:265, 1977.
53. Sizemore GW, Carney JA, Heath H III: Epidemiology of medullary carcinoma of the thyroid gland: a 5-year experience (1971–1976). Surg Clin North Am 57:633, 1977.
54. Wells SA, Baylin SB, Gann DS, et al: Medullary thyroid carcinoma: relationship of method of diagnosis to pathologic staging. Ann Surg 188:377, 1978.
55. Wells SA, Baylin SB, Linehan WM, et al: Provocative agents and the diagnosis of medullary carcinoma of the thyroid gland. Ann Surg 188:139, 1978.
56. Wells SA, Baylin SB, Leight GS, et al: The importance of early diagnosis in patients with hereditary medullary thyroid carcinoma. Ann Surg 195:595, 1982.
57. Austin LA, Heath H III: Calcitonin. Physiology and pathophysiology. N Engl J Med 304:269, 1981.
58. Goretzki P, Roeher HD, Horeyseck G: Prophylaxis of recurrent goiter by high-dose l-thyroxine. World J Surg 5:855, 1981.
59. Persson CPA, Johansson H, Westermark K, et al: Nodular goiter—is thyroxine medication of any value? World J Surg 6:391, 1982.
60. Woolner LB, Beahrs OH, Black BM, et al: Classification and prognosis of thyroid carcinoma. A study of 885 cases observed in a thirty year period. Am J Surg 102:354, 1961.
61. Histologic typing of thyroid tumors. *In:* International Histological Classification of Tumours, No 11. Geneva, World Health Organization, 1974, p 22.
62. McConahey WM, Taylor WM, Gorman CA, et al: Retrospective study of 820 patients treated for papillary carcinoma of the thyroid at the Mayo Clinic between 1946 and 1971. Presented at the International Colloquium on Thyroid/Neoplasia. Rome, Sept 1981.
63. Mazzaferri EL: Papillary and follicular thyroid cancer: a selective approach to diagnosis and treatment. Ann Rev Med 32:73, 1981.
64. Sampson RG: Prevalence and significance of occult thyroid cancer. *In* DeGroot LJ, Frohnan LA, Kaplan EL, et al (eds): Radiation-Associated Thyroid Carcinoma. New York, Grune & Stratton, 1977, pp 137–153.
65. Fukunaga FH, Yatani R: Geographic pathology of occult thyroid carcinomas. Cancer 36:1095, 1975.
66. Nishiyama RH, Ludwig GK, Thompson NW: The prevalence of small papillary thyroid carcinomas in 100 consecutive necropsies in an American population. *In* DeGroot LJ, Frohnan LA, Kaplan EL, et al (eds): Radiation-Associated Thyroid Carcinoma. New York, Grune & Stratton, 1977, p 123.
67. Sampson RJ, Key CR, Buncher CR, et al: Thyroid carcinoma in Hiroshima and Nagasaki. I. Prevalence of thyroid carcinoma at autopsy. JAMA 209:65, 1969.
68. Edis AJ: Natural history of occult thyroid cancer. *In* DeGroot LJ, Frohnan LA, Kaplan EL, et al (eds): Radiation-Associated Thyroid Carcinoma. New York, Grune & Stratton, 1977, p 155.
69. Mazzaferri EL, Young RL: Papillary thyroid carcinoma: a 10 year follow-up

report of the impact of therapy in 576 patients. Am J Med 70:511, 1981.

70. Woolner LB, Beahrs OH, Black BM, et al: Thyroid carcinoma: general considerations and follow-up data on 1181 cases. *In* Young S, Inman DR (eds): Thyroid Neoplasia. New York, Academic Press, 1968, pp 51–77.

71. Cady B, Sedgwick CE, Meissner WA, et al: Risk factor analysis in differentiated thyroid cancer. Cancer 43:810, 1979.

72. Cady B, Sedgwick CE, Meissner W, et al: Changing clinical, pathologic, therapeutic and survival patterns in differentiated thyroid carcinoma. Ann Surg 183:541, 1976.

73. Clark RL, White SC, Russell WO: Total thyroidectomy for cancer of the thyroid: significance of intraglandular dissemination. Ann Surg 149:858, 1959.

74. Noguchi S, Noguchi A, Murakami N: Papillary carcinoma of the thyroid. II. Value of prophylactic lymph node excision. Cancer 26:1061, 1970.

75. Tollefsen HR, Shah JP, Huvos AG: Papillary carcinoma of the thyroid. Recurrence in the thyroid gland after initial surgical treatment. Am J Surg 124:468, 1972.

76. Nishiyama RH, Dunn EL, Thompson NW: Anaplastic spindle-cell and giant-cell tumors of the thyroid gland. Cancer 30:112, 1972.

77. Cady B: Surgery of thyroid cancer. World J Surg 5:3, 1981.

78. Deleted in proof.

79. Paloyan E, Lawrence AM, Paloyan D: Successful autotransplantation of the parathyroid glands during total thyroidectomy for carcinoma. Surg Gynecol Obstet 145:364, 1977.

80. Young RL, Mazzaferri EL, Rahe AJ: Pure follicular thyroid carcinomas: impact of therapy in 214 patients. J Nucl Med 21:733, 1980.

81. Tollefson HR, Shah JP, Huvos AG: Follicular carcinoma of the thyroid. Am J Surg 126:523, 1973.

82. Varma VM, Beierwaltes WH, Nofal MM, et al: Treatment of thyroid cancer. JAMA 214:1437, 1970.

83. Beierwaltes WH, Nishiyama RH, Thompson NW, et al: Survival time and "cure" in papillary and follicular thyroid carcinoma with distant metastases: statistics following University of Michigan therapy. J Nucl Med 23:561, 1982.

84. Edis AJ: Surgical treatment for thyroid cancer. Surg Clin North Am 57:533, 1977.

85. Steiner AL, Goodman AD, Powers SR: Study of a kindred with pheochromocytoma, medullary thyroid carcinoma, hyperparathyroidism, and Cushing's disease: multiple endocrine neoplasia, type 2. Medicine (Baltimore) 47:371, 1968.

86. Sizemore GW, van Heerden JA, Carney JA: Medullary carcinoma of the thyroid gland and the multiple endocrine neoplasia type 2 syndrome. *In* Kaplan EL (ed): Surgery of the Thyroid and Parathyroid Glands. New York, Churchill Livingstone, 1983, p 76–102.

87. Chong GC, Beahrs OH, Sizemore GW, et al: Medullary carcinoma of the thyroid gland. Cancer 35:695, 1975.

88. Carney JA, Sizemore GW, Hayles B: Multiple endocrine neoplasia, type 2b. Pathobiol Annu 8:105, 1978.

89. Sizemore GW, Heath H III, Carney JA: Multiple endocrine neoplasia type 2. Clin Endocrinol Metab 9:299, 1980.

90. Sizemore GW: Medullary carcinoma of the thyroid gland. Thyroid Today, 5:3, 1982.

91. Russell CF, van Heerden JA, Sizemore GW, et al: The surgical management of medullary thyroid carcinoma. Ann Surg 197:42–48, 1983.

92. Simpson WA, Palmer JA, Rosen IB: Management of medullary carcinoma of the thyroid. Am J Surg 144:420, 1982.

93. Freier DT, Thompson NW, Sisson JC, et al: Dilemmas in the early diagnosis and

treatment of multiple endocrine adenomatosis type II. Surgery 82:407, 1977.

94. Tubiana M: External radiotherapy and radioiodine in the treatment of thyroid cancer. World J Surg 5:75, 1981.

95. Devine RM, Edis AJ, Banks PM: Primary lymphoma of the thyroid: a review of the Mayo Clinic experience through 1978. World J Surg 5:33, 1981.

96. Wychulis AR, Beahrs OH, Woolner LB: Metastasis of carcinoma to the thyroid gland. Ann Surg 160:169, 1964.

97. Crile G Jr: The endocrine dependency of certain thyroid cancers and the danger that hypothyroidism may stimulate their growth. Cancer 10:1119, 1957.

98. Clark OH: TSH suppression in the management of thyroid nodules and thyroid cancer. World J Surg 5:39, 1981.

99. Staunton MD, Greening WP: Treatment of thyroid cancer in 293 patients. Br J Surg 63:253, 1976.

100. Martin ND: Endogenous serum TSH levels and metastatic survey scans in thyroid cancer patients using triiodothyronine withdrawal. Clin Nucl Med 10:401, 1978.

101. Beierwaltes WH: The treatment of thyroid carcinoma with radioactive iodine. Semin Nucl Med 8:79, 1978.

102. Black EG, Cassoni A, Gimlette TMD, et al: Serum thyroglobulin in thyroid cancer. Lancet 2:443, 1981.

103. Van Herle J, Uller RP: Elevated serum thyroglobulin. A marker of metastases in differentiated thyroid carcinomas. J Clin Invest 56:272, 1975.

104. Lo Gerfo P, Stillman T, Colacchio D, et al: Serum thyroglobulin and recurrent thyroid cancer. Lancet 1:881, 1977.

105. Gottlieb JA, Hill CS Jr: Adriamycin therapy in thyroid carcinoma. Cancer Chemother Rep 6:283, 1975.

106. Shimaoka K: Adjunctive management of thyroid cancer: chemotherapy. J Surg Oncol 15:283, 1980.

107. Edis AJ, Beahrs OH: Surgery of the thyroid gland. In Goldsmith HS (ed): Practice of Surgery. Hagerstown, Md, Harper & Row, 1980.

108. Cooper DS, Ridgeway EC, Maloof F: Unusual types of hyperthyroidism. Clin Endocrinol Metab 7:199, 1978.

109. Volpe R: The pathogenesis of Graves' disease: An overview. Clin Endocrinol Metab 7:3, 1978.

110. Volpe R: Autoimmunity in the endocrine system. Monographs in Endocrinology, No 20. Heidelberg, Springer-Verlag, 1981.

111. Solomon DH, Chopra IJ, Chopra U, et al: Identification of subgroups of euthyroid Graves' ophthalmopathy. N Engl J Med 296:181, 1977.

112. Sugrue D, McEvoy M, Feely J, et al: Hyperthyroidism in the Land of Graves: Results of treatment by surgery, radio-iodine and carbimazole in 837 cases. Q J Med 49:51, 1980.

113. Riley FC: Orbital pathology in Graves' disease. Mayo Clin Proc 47:975, 1972.

114. Gorman CA: Unusual manifestations of Graves' disease. Mayo Clin Proc 47:926, 1972.

115. Chopra IJ: Laboratory aids in the diagnosis of hyperthyroidism. Thyroid Today 1:17, Apr/May 1978.

116. Yao Y: A current view of thyroid function tests. Hosp Pract Sept 1981, p 149.

117. Bantle JP, Oppenheimer JH: Laboratory assessment of thyroid function. In Najarian JS, Delaney JP (eds): Endocrine Surgery. Miami, Symposia Specialists, 1981, p 295.

118. Ivy HK, Wahner HW, Gorman CA: Triiodothyronine (T3) toxicosis: its role in Graves' disease. Arch Intern Med 128:529, 1971.

119. Greer MA: Antithyroid drugs in the treatment of thyrotoxicosis. Thyroid Today 3:1, Feb/Mar 1980.

120. Becker DV: Current status of radioactive iodine treatment of hyperthyroidism. Thyroid Today 2:7, Nov 1979.

121. Beahrs OH, Sakulsky SB: Surgical thyroidectomy in the management of exophthalmic goiter. Arch Surg 96:512, 1960.

122. Farnell MB, van Heerden JA, McConahey WM, et al: Hypothyroidism after thyroidectomy for Graves' disease. Am J Surg 142:535, 1981.

123. Irvine WJ, Toft AD: The diagnosis and treatment of thyrotoxicosis, Clin Endocrinol 5:687, 1976.

124. Volpe R: Treatment of Graves' disease: an overview. Thyroid Today 1:1, Aug 1977.

125. Utiger RD: Treatment of Graves' disease (editorial). N Engl J Med 298:681, 1978.

126. Wartofsky L: Low remission after therapy for Graves' disease: possible relation of dietary iodine with antithyroid therapy results. JAMA 237:2089, 1977.

127. Dobyns BM, Sheline GE, Workman JB, et al: Malignant and benign neoplasms of the thyroid in patients treated for hyperthyroidism: a report of the cooperative thyrotoxicosis therapy follow-up study. J Clin Endocrinol Metab 38:976, 1974.

128. Safa AM, Schumacher OP, Rodriguez-Antunez A: Long-term follow-up results in children and adolescents treated with radioactive iodine (^{131}I) for hyperthyroidism. N Engl J Med 292:167, 1975.

129. Goldsmith RE: Radioisotope therapy for Graves' disease. Mayo Clin Proc 47:953, 1972.

130. Nofal MM, Beierwaltes WH, Patno ME: Treatment of hyperthyroidism with sodium iodide I-131. A 16-year experience. JAMA 197:605, 1966.

131. Cevallos JL, Hagen GA, Maloof F, et al: Low-dosage ^{131}I therapy of thyrotoxicosis (diffuse goiter). N Engl J Med 290:141, 1974.

132. Barber SG, Carter DJ, Bishop J: System for long-term review of patients at risk of becoming hypothyroid—further experience. Lancet 2:967, 1977.

133. Beahrs OH, Sakulsky SB: Surgical thyroidectomy in the management of exophthalmic goiter. Arch Surg 96:512, 1968.

134. Michie W: Whither thyrotoxicosis? Br J Surg 62:673, 1975.

135. Feek CM, Sawers JS, Irvine WJ, et al: Combination of potassium iodide and propranolol in preparation of patients with Graves' disease for thyroid surgery. N Engl J Med 302:883, 1980.

136. Toft AD, Irvine WJ, Sinclair I, et al: Thyroid function after surgical treatment of thyrotoxicosis. N Engl J Med 298:643, 1978.

137. Michie W, Beck JS, Pollet JE: Prevention and management of hypothyroidism after thyroidectomy for thyrotoxicosis. World J Surg 2:307, 1978.

138. Michie W, Pegg CA, Bewsher PD: Prediction of hypothyroidism after partial thyroidectomy for thyrotoxicosis. Br Med J 1:13, 1972.

139. Olsen WR, Nishiyama RH, Graber LW: Thyroidectomy for hyperthyroidism. Arch Surg 101:175, 1970.

140. Toft AD, Irvine WJ, McIntosh D, et al: Temporary hypothyroidism after surgical treatment of thyrotoxicosis. Lancet 2:1135, 1976.

141. Wilkin TJ, Gunn A, Isles TE, et al: Short-term triiodothyronine in prevention of temporary hypothyroidism after subtotal thyroidectomy for Graves' disease. Lancet 2:63, 1979.

142. Dailey ME, Benson RC: Hyperthyroidism in pregnancy. Surg Gynecol Obstet 94:102, 1952.

143. Stice RC, Grant CS, Gharib H: The management of Graves' disease during pregnancy. Surg Gynecol Obstet 158:157–160, 1984.

144. Herbst AL, Selenkow HA: Hyperthyroidism during pregnancy. N Engl J Med 273:627, 1965.

145. Plummer HS: Results of administering iodine to patients having exophthalmic goiter. JAMA 80:1955, 1923.

146. Ingbar SH, Woeber KA: The thyroid gland. *In* Williams RH (ed): Textbook of Endocrinology (6th ed). Philadelphia, Saunders, 1981.

147. McGill DA, Asper SP Jr: Endocrine exophthalmos. N Engl J Med 267:188, 1962.

148. Donaldson SS, Bagshaw MA, Kriss JP: Supervoltage orbital radiotherapy for Graves' ophthalmopathy. J Clin Endocrinol Metab 37:276, 1973.

149. Gorman CA, DeSanto LW, MacCarty CS, et al: Optic neuropathy of Graves' disease. Treatment by transantral or transfrontal orbital decompression. N Engl J Med 290:70, 1974.

150. Plummer HS: The clinical and pathological relationship of simple and exophthalmic goiter. Trans Assoc Am Physicians 28:587, 1913.

151. Gorman CA, Robertson JS: Radiation dose in the selection of ^{131}I or surgical treatment for toxic thyroid adenoma. Ann Intern Med 88:85, 1978.

152. Fatourechi V, McConahey WM, Woolner LB: Hyperthyroidism associated with histologic Hashimoto's thyroiditis. Mayo Clin Proc 46:682, 1971.

153. Hamburger JL: Subacute thyroiditis: diagnostic difficulties and simple treatment. J Nucl Med 15:81, 1974.

154. Gorman CA, Duick DS, Woolner LB, et al: Transient hyperthyroidism in patients with lymphocytic thyroiditis. Mayo Clin Proc 53:359, 1978.

155. Nikolai TF, Brosseau J, Kettrick MA, et al: Lymphocytic thyroiditis with spontaneously resolving hyperthyroidism (silent thyroiditis). Arch Intern Med 140:478, 1980.

156. Mazzaferri EL, Reynolds JC, Young RL: Propranolol as primary therapy for thyrotoxicosis. Arch Intern Med 136:50, 1976.

157. Becker WF: Pioneers in thyroid surgery. Ann Surg 185:493, 1977.

158. Pemberton JDeJ, Haines SF: Hyperfunction of the thyroid gland: recent developments in clinical recognition and surgical treatment. Am J Surg 23:399, 1934.

159. Edis AJ: Prevention and management of complications associated with thyroid and parathyroid surgery. Surg Clin North Am 59:83, 1979.

160. Peters LL, Gardner RJ: Repair of recurrent laryngeal nerve injuries. Surgery 71:865, 1972.

161. Tucker HM: Human laryngeal reinnervation: long-term experience with the nerve–muscle pedicle technique. Laryngoscope 88:598, 1978.

162. Deves JR, Tonkin JP: Vocal cord paralysis in benign thyroid disease before operation (letter). Med J Aust 11:632, 1980.

163. Neel HB III, Townsend GL, Devine KD: Bilateral vocal cord paralysis of undetermined etiology: clinical course and outcome. Ann Otol Rhinol Laryngol 81:514, 1972.

164. Minuck M: Unilateral vocal-cord paralysis following endotracheal intubation. Anesthesiology 45:448, 1976.

165. Holley HS, Gildea JE: Vocal cord paralysis after tracheal intubation. JAMA 215:281, 1971.

166. Sato F, Ogura JH: Neurorrhaphy of the recurrent laryngeal nerve. Laryngoscope 88:1034, 1978.

167. Arnold GE: Further experiences with intracordal Teflon injection. Laryngoscope 74:802, 1964.

168. Wilkin TJ, Paterson CR, Isles TE, et al: Post-thyroidectomy hypocalcemia: a feature of the operation or a thyroid disorder? Lancet 1:621, 1977.

169. Wade JSH, Fourman P, Deane L: Recovery of parathyroid function in patients with "transient" hypoparathyroidism after thyroidectomy. Br J Surg 52:493, 1965.

Surgery of the Adrenals

3

The adrenal gland comprises two physiologically and embryologically distinct parts: the cortex and medulla. It produces a wide variety of hormones whose synthesis, secretion, regulation, and end effects are highly complex. Rather dramatic physical changes and symptoms may result from hormonal imbalance.

General Introduction

Hyperplasia or neoplasia of the adrenal cortex produces characteristic syndromes dependent on the "zone" of origin:

Zona glomerulosa: primary aldosteronism
Zona fasciculata: Cushing's syndrome
Zona reticularis: virilism.

A mixture of excess hormonal production is often indicative of an adrenal carcinoma, whereas pure syndromes are typically associated with benign pathologic lesions. These conditions are relatively rare in a clinically overt form, although it is possible (as with primary HPT) that unrecognized subclinical disease may be present in a significant proportion of the general population.

The adrenal medulla functions as a giant presynaptic sympathetic nerve ending that has the capacity to synthesize not only norepinephrine but also epinephrine. Tumors that arise from the adrenal medullary cells are known as *pheochromocytomas*. They secrete huge excesses of catecholamines to produce a characteristic spectrum of cardiovascular and metabolic effects. Hypertension is almost always a prominent feature.

New innovations in diagnostic and localizing technology have refined our ability to specifically select the appropriate, and usually highly successful treatment for patients with adrenal pathology. A number of operative approaches to the adrenals have been described (i.e., translumbar, transabdominal, transthoracic, lateral, and loin), but most surgeons today use either an anterior or a posterior approach. The extraperitoneal posterior approach is preferred in many situations because the adrenals can be exposed with relatively little dissection. Extensive mobilization and retraction of viscera are not necessary, so that inadvertant visceral injury is uncommon and gastrointestinal function usually returns promptly postoperatively. Patients do not appear to have the severe incisional discomfort, occasioned by coughing and deep

151

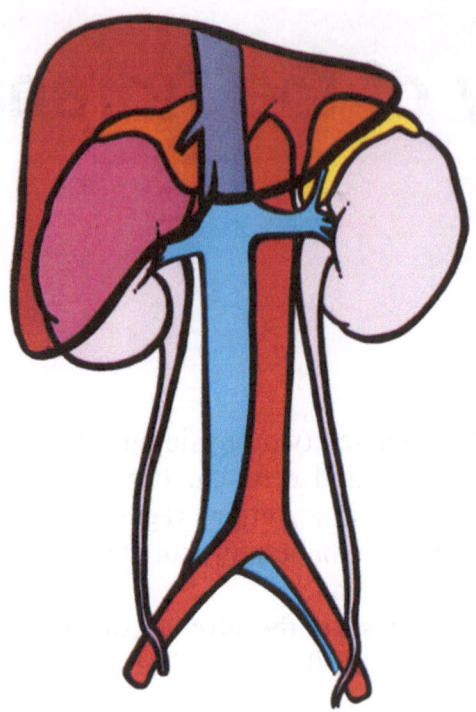

Fig. 3-1. **Normal anatomic relationships of the adrenal glands.** The glands differ in shape: the right is pyramidal and the left crescentic. The medial aspect of the right adrenal gland is often overlapped by the inferior vena cava.

breathing, which is so typical of abdominal wounds; pulmonary atelectasis and pneumonitis are therefore uncommon. Early ambulation and a shortened hospital stay are additional benefits.

Operative mortality and morbidity are generally less when the posterior approach is elected over the anterior transabdominal route. There are three situations, however, in which the anterior approach to adrenalectomy is favored: (a) when operating for pheochromocytoma it is important to thoroughly explore the entire abdominal cavity in order to rule out supernumerary extraadrenal tumors; (b) with a large adrenal carcinoma, the anterior approach with extension of the incision into the chest, if necessary, facilitates the wide exposure required to remove the tumor en bloc; and (c) when one must deal with other intraabdominal pathology the anterior route affords appropriate access.

SURGICAL ANATOMY

ORIENTATION

Each adrenal gland caps the superomedial pole of its corresponding kidney (Fig. 3-1). The right gland is triangular in shape; the left is more flattened and elongated and assumes a somewhat crescentic shape. Av-

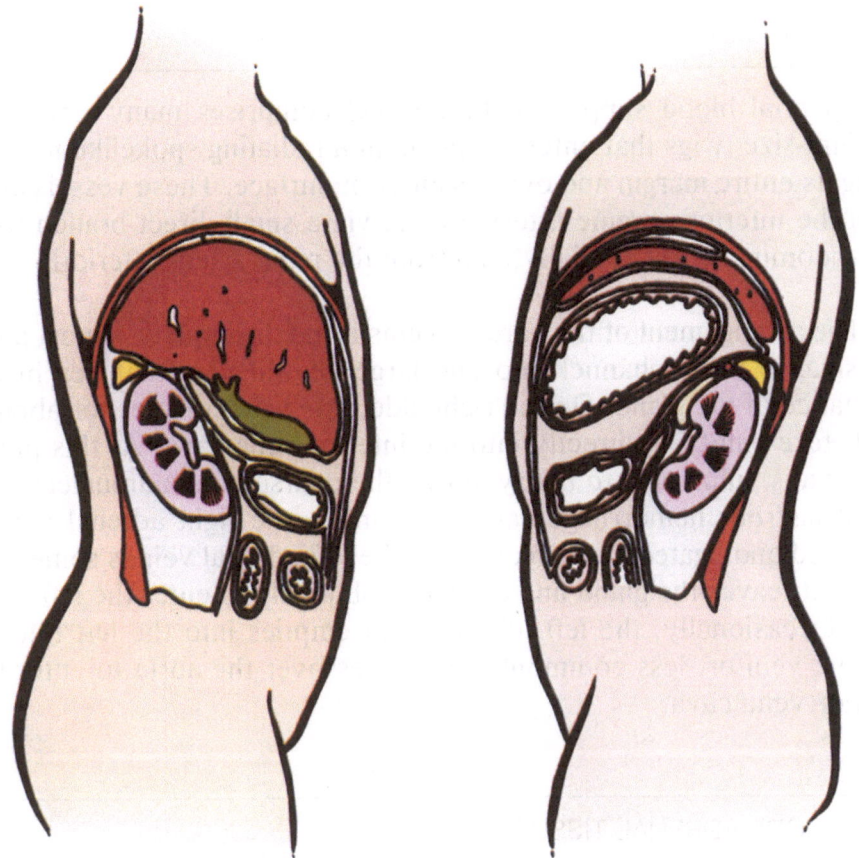

A **B**

Sagittal sections through the right (A) and left (B) adrenal glands. The bare area of the liver is immediately anterior to the right adrenal. On the left, the adrenal is behind the lesser sac and is partially overlapped by the tail of the pancreas and splenic vessels.   **Fig. 3-2.**

erage dimensions in the adult are about 5 × 2.5 × 0.5 cm and each adrenal gland weighs about 3–6 g, the left being slightly larger than the right.

Each gland, together with the kidney, is enclosed by Gerota's (perirenal) fascia and surrounded by fat. The adrenal is easily distinguished from fat by its characteristic chrome-yellow color, firmer consistency, and slightly granular texture.

Posteriorly, each gland lies in close proximity to the diaphragmatic crus; the kidney is inferior. Medially, the right gland is in contact with the inferior vena cava and often tucks behind it; the left abuts on the aorta. Anteriorly, the right adrenal is covered almost completely by the bare area of the liver; the upper half of the left adrenal is covered by peritoneum of the lesser sac and the lower half is covered by the pancreas and splenic vessels (Fig. 3-2).

BLOOD SUPPLY

The arterial blood supply to the adrenal comprises many small and medium-size twigs that enter the gland in a radiating spokelike manner along its entire margin and over its anterior surface. These vessels arise from the inferior phrenic artery above, via a small direct branch from the abdominal aorta medially, and from the renal artery inferiorly (Fig. 3-3).

The arrangement of the adrenal veins is much simpler. Almost all of the smaller veins channel into one large central vein that lies in the substance of the gland. On the right side, this vein emerges for about 1 cm before emptying directly into the inferior vena cava. At this point, the cava is vulnerable to injury during the course of an adrenalectomy, and disastrous hemorrhage can occur unless the right adrenal vein is dissected and ligated with great care. The left adrenal vein is somewhat larger; it leaves the gland and descends obliquely to enter the left renal vein. Occasionally, the left adrenal vein empties into the left inferior phrenic vein or, less commonly, it crosses over the aorta to enter the inferior vena cava.

ACCESSORY ADRENAL TISSUE

The adrenals are really compound glands derived by the union of two types of tissue: the cortex is derived from the urogenital portion of the coelomic mesoderm and produces various adrenal steroid hormones; the medulla is derived from the ectoderm of the neural crest and secretes the catecholamines, epinephrine, and norepinephrine.

True accessory adrenal glands, containing both cortical and medullary components, are exceedingly rare. However, it is not uncommon to find nodules of accessory cortical tissue in the periadrenal fat, and ectopic cortical tissue has also been described in the substance of the spleen, below the kidneys, and associated with the testes or ovaries.

Chromaffin tissue resembles the tissue of the adrenal medulla and is derived from the same source. It is found in sites close to autonomic ganglia (paraganglion bodies) and along the aorta. Chromaffin tissue at any site may give rise to a pheochromocytoma; one of the most common locations for an extraadrenal pheochromocytoma is the organ of Zuckerkandl, which is a chromaffin deposit on the ventral surface of the aorta close to its bifurcation.

The distribution of chromaffin tissue is maximal at birth, after which it involutes progressively until puberty. This may explain, in part, why extraadrenal and multiple pheochromocytomas are more common in children (1).

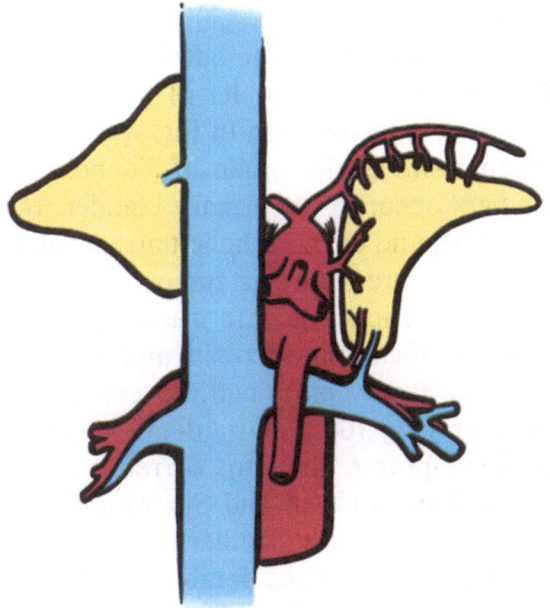

Blood supply of the adrenal glands. For clarity, only the arterial blood supply to the left adrenal gland is depicted (the arrangement is essentially duplicated on the right). Small arterial twigs are derived from three main vessels, all branches of the aorta, and form a striking arborization at the periphery of the gland. The adrenal vein on the right is short and makes a 45° angle as it passes superiorly to enter the inferior vena cava. The vein on the left is longer and descends obliquely to enter the left renal vein. Note the anterior position of the adrenal veins as they leave the glands.

Fig. 3-3.

Pheochromocytoma

Pheochromocytomas are rare: the estimated incidence in the hypertensive population is 0.1%–1.0% (2–5). Approximately 400 new cases of pheochromocytoma, 40 of which are malignant, probably occur each year in the United States. Diagnosis is critical, as curative resection is possible in 90% of cases (6–8) and failure to recognize it is often lethal (9,10). Since the first successful resection of a pheochromocytoma in the United States was performed by Mayo in 1927 (11), considerable progress has been made in understanding the physiology and designing the management of these tumors, particularly in the multidisciplinary approach to preoperative, intraoperative, and postoperative management.

PATHOLOGY

Pheochromocytoma has been called the "10% tumor" because approximately 10% are bilateral, malignant, extraadrenal, multiple, familial, and occur in children—although bilaterality and extraadrenal tumors in children occur in 25% (4,6,7,10,12–15) (Table 3-1). Extraadrenal tumors

Table 3-1. Pheochromocytoma, the "10% Tumor"

Bilateral
Malignant
Extraadrenal
Multiple
Familial
Occurs in children

have a higher malignancy rate of 25%–40% (7,16,17). While 80%–90% of pheochromocytomas arise from the adrenal medulla, they may also be found anywhere along the remainder of the paraganglionic system extending from the pelvis to the base of the skull (Fig. 3-4). The most common extraadrenal site is the organ of Zuckerkandl at the aortic bifurcation, but others occur in the urinary bladder, renal hilum, chest and neck (less than 1%), and even in the left atrial wall of the heart (18).

Pheochromocytomas are vascular tumors with a thin connective tissue capsule. On cut section, they are usually pink-tan in color, with foci of hemorrhage, calcification, necrosis, and gelatinous change (Fig. 3-5). They vary in size from very small (several grams) to very large (1000 g or more), averaging 100 g and a diameter of 2–4 cm (15). The severity of clinical symptoms does not correlate with the size of the tumor. In fact, according to Crout and Sjoerdoma (19), larger tumors are metabolically less active than smaller lesions; hence, they escape detection longer and grow to a considerable size before discovery.

Microscopically, the tumor cells are arranged in a cordlike or alveolar pattern, with a very vascular stroma (Fig. 3-6). The cytoplasm is finely granular and basophilic, corresponding on ultrastructural study to dense-core neurosecretory granules that are believed to contain packets of catecholamine (Fig. 3-7).

DIAGNOSIS

CLINICAL FEATURES

There is no significant sex bias and all ages may be affected. The peak age of onset is about 40 years. The protean clinical features of patients with pheochromocytoma have often caused delayed diagnosis; some patients have been labeled as functional or as having a psychoneurotic disorder until a medical catastrophe signaled the true pathology. Perhaps cases recognized clinically actually represent only the tip of an

Fig. 3-4. **Sites of extraadrenal pheochromocytomas.** Most extraadrenal pheochromocytomas are found within the abdomen, usually in lumbar and aortic paraganglia.

Fig. 3-5. **Well-circumscribed pheochromocytoma of the adrenal gland.** Areas of hemorrhage, necrosis, and gelatinous change on the cut surface are characteristic.

Fig. 3-6. **Microscopic appearance of pheochromocytoma.**

Fig. 3-7. **Electron microscopic appearance of two adjacent cells from a pheochromocytoma.** The dense-core intracytoplasmic granules are believed to represent packets of catecholamine. ×40,000.

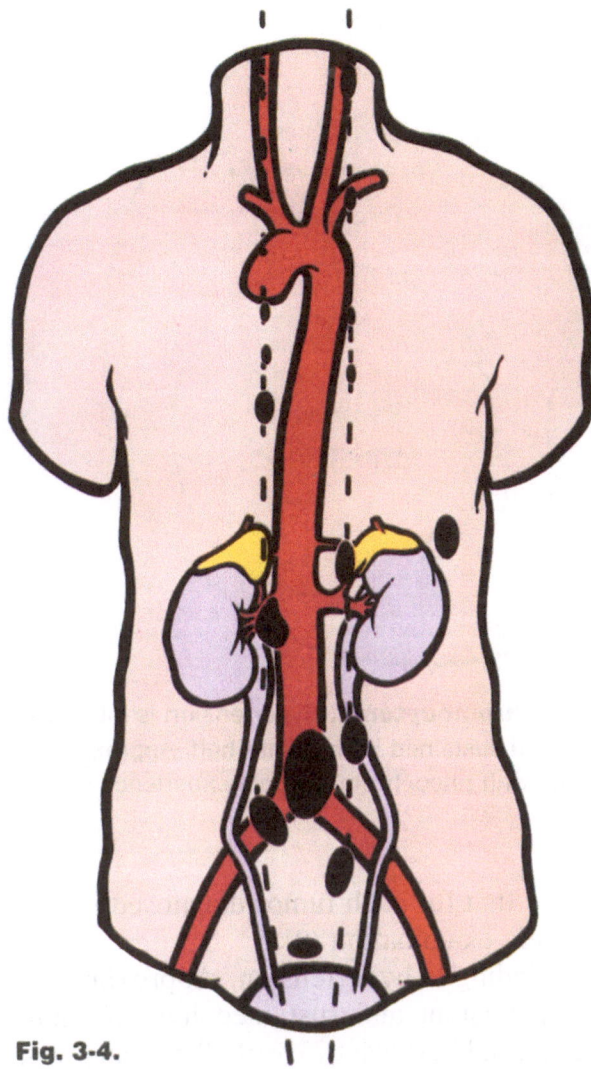

Fig. 3-4.

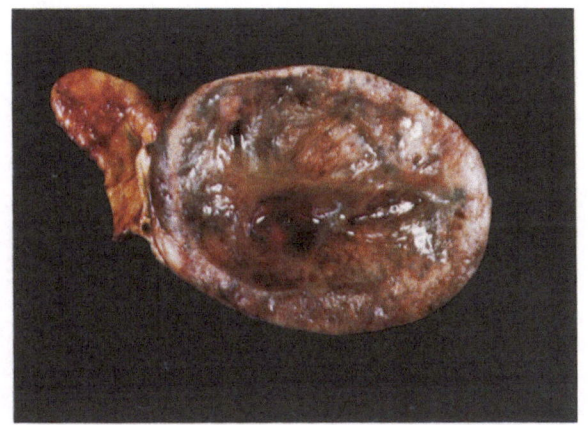

⊢——⊣ 1 cm

Fig. 3-5.

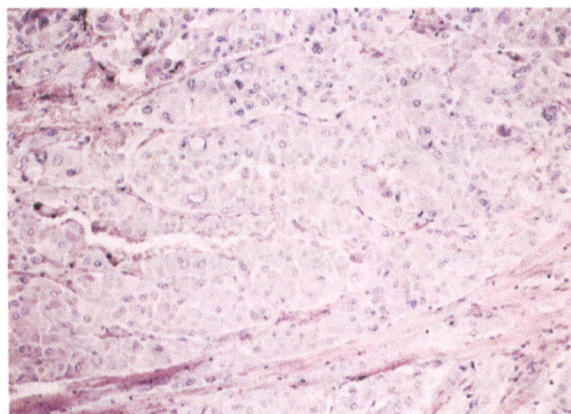

Fig. 3-6.

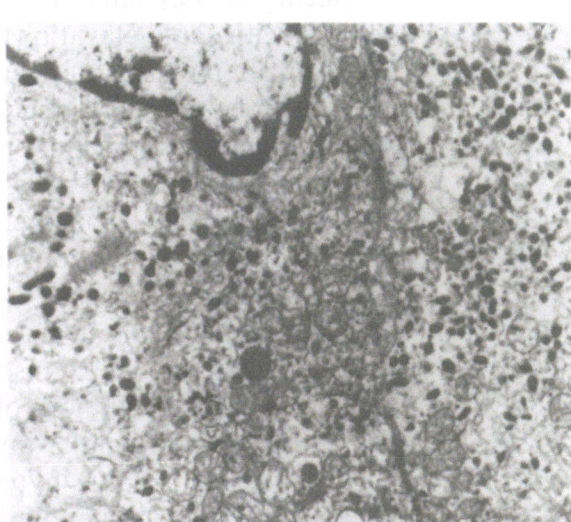

Fig. 3-7.

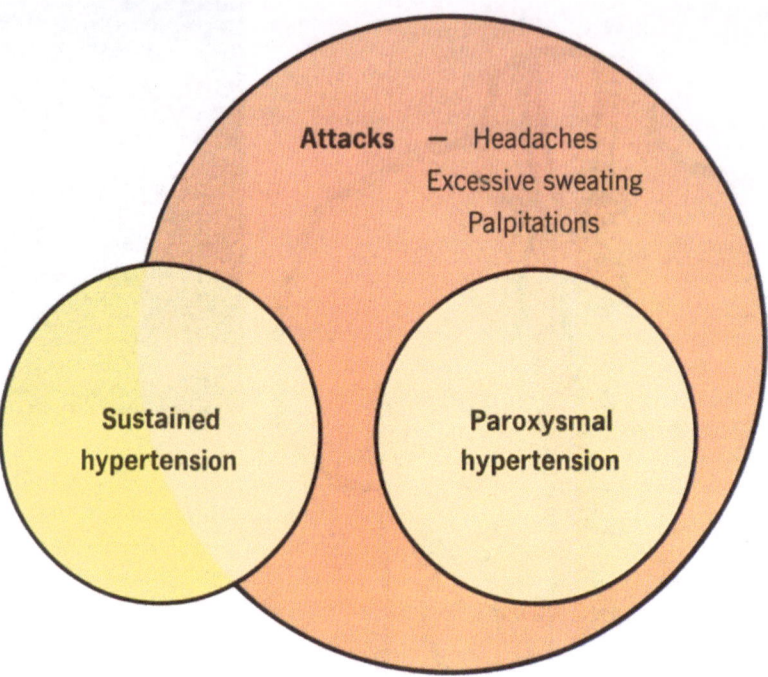

Fig. 3-8. **Salient clinical features of pheochromocytoma.** Hypertension is intermittent in about one-half of the cases and sustained in the other half. Approximately three-quarters of the patients with pheochromocytoma experience paroxysmal symptomatic attacks.

iceberg, as it has been suggested that for each tumor diagnosed in life, two are discovered at postmortem examination (9).

The most common clinical finding is hypertension. Approximately one-half of the patients have persistent and sustained hypertension, while it is intermittent in the other half. At least 75% of all patients with pheochromocytoma suffer paroxysmal symptomatic episodes associated with acute elevations in blood pressure (6) (Fig. 3-8). Such paroxysms often consist of headache, palpitations, perspiration, angina, and tachyarrhythmias related to the unpredictable secretory release of catecholamines by the tumor (6,20,21). They typically last less than 15 minutes but become more frequent as time goes on. During the attack, the patient may also experience flushing or pallor, vomiting, abdominal pain, and acute nervousness or anxiety. Death from cerebrovascular attacks and myocardial infarction have occurred (9,10). Symptomatic paroxysms usually occur spontaneously, but in some patients they can be precipitated by exercise, overeating, local pressure, defecation, micturition (seen in tumors of the bladder), sexual intercourse, and, perhaps most importantly, invasive diagnostic procedures and general anesthesia. Orthostatic hypotension (i.e., a decrease in blood pressure when the patient stands) is a frequent finding in pheochromocytoma, and in the absence of antihypertensive medications it is virtually unique to this form of hypertension; it is probably the result of a marked attenu-

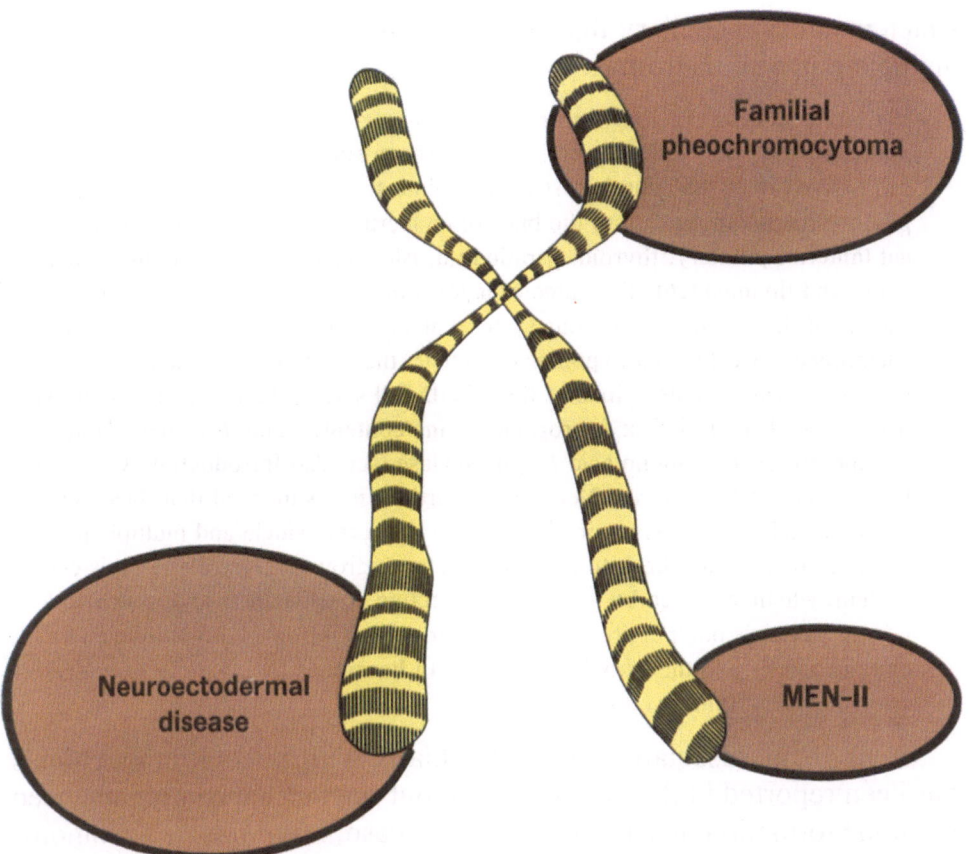

Genetically associated diseases in pheochromocytoma. Familial **Fig. 3-9.**
pheochromocytoma (often bilateral) may occur alone or associated with neuroectodermal disorders, such as von Recklinghausen's neurofibromatosis, and
with MEN-II.

ation of normal sympathetic reflexes secondary to the excess levels of
circulating catecholamine.

Glucose intolerance is found in some patients with pheochromocytoma and frank hyperglycemia may be present, particularly during a
symptomatic attack or immediately following operative resection.
Much of the altered carbohydrate metabolism is thought to be caused by
the alpha-adrenergic effect of norepinephrine and epinephrine, which
inhibits the release of insulin from pancreatic islet cells and is a stimulus
for glycolysis.

Pheochromocytoma is genetically associated with other endocrine
and nonendocrine conditions in about 10% of cases (Fig. 3-9). The first
recognized associations were in families with neuroectodermal tissue
diseases, such as von Recklinghausen's neurofibromatosis, Lindau-von
Hippel disease, and tuberous sclerosis (22). It also assumes a prominent
role in the multiple endocrine neoplasia type II syndromes: MEN-IIa
(Sipple's syndrome), which is composed of medullary thyroid carcinoma, pheochromocytoma, and hyperparathyroidism; and MEN-IIb,

which includes medullary thyroid carcinoma, pheochromocytoma, and multiple mucosal neuromas.

> Various workers have sought to explain the association of these synchronous abnormalities in many different organs. It has been suggested that a common stem cell derived from the neural crest migrates into the primitive alimentary and respiratory tracts, and then into the buds of endocrine glands derived from the foregut (anterior pituitary, thyroid, parathyroid, islets of Langerhans, ultimobrachial body, and thymus) (26). The same cells form the adrenal medulla and paraganglia of the autonomic nervous system, melanin-producing cells in the skin, chemoreceptor cells, and hypothalamic nuclei that give rise to posterior pituitary hormones. They are described as the APUD cell series, the initials being derived from three characteristics: fluorogenic *Amine* content, amine *Precursor Uptake*, and the presence of amino acid *Decarboxylase* (see also Introduction, Common Denominators of Endocrine Neoplasia). Further, it is supposed that these multipotential endocrine cells retain the capacity to secrete single and multiple peptide hormones under the autonomy of neoplastic growth. Dysplasia of this cell system, whether caused by genetically defective or spontaneously occurring mutant genes, is one possible explanation for the syndromes of multiple endocrine neoplasia and the ectopic production of hormones by a variety of nonendocrine malignant tumors (26).

A frequent association of cholelithiasis with pheochromocytomas has been reported in the literature (20), but the mechanism of enhanced gallstone formation, if such is actually the case, is unknown. Vasomotor instability, manifested by livedo reticularis, Raynaud's phenomenon, or both, is also seen. Accelerated malignant hypertension, severe congestive heart failure secondary to so-called catecholamine myocardopathy (15), ischemic enterocolitis (24), and peripheral vasoconstriction producing intermittent claudication (25) are some of the less common but dangerous clinical syndromes that may be associated with these tumors.

LABORATORY STUDIES

A hypertensive patient who complains of episodic headaches, excessive sweating, palpitations, or "nervous attacks" should be evaluated for pheochromocytoma. Likewise, those patients with paroxysmal hypertension—especially following trauma, surgery, or childbirth—or with a neurocutaneous syndrome, medullary carcinoma of the thyroid, or a family history of pheochromocytoma should be tested (Fig. 3-10).

Urine Studies. The principal biochemical diagnostic modalities confirming the diagnosis of pheochromocytoma have been the 24-hour urine levels of metanephrines (TMN) and vanillylmandelic acid (VMA) (5–8, 15) (Fig. 3-11).

Under normal circumstances, VMA comprises more than 75% of the total urinary catecholamine metabolites, TMN adds 10%, and the free urinary catecholamines (UCA) about 1%. The pattern of urinary metabolites in patients with pheochromocytoma varies. In small tumors

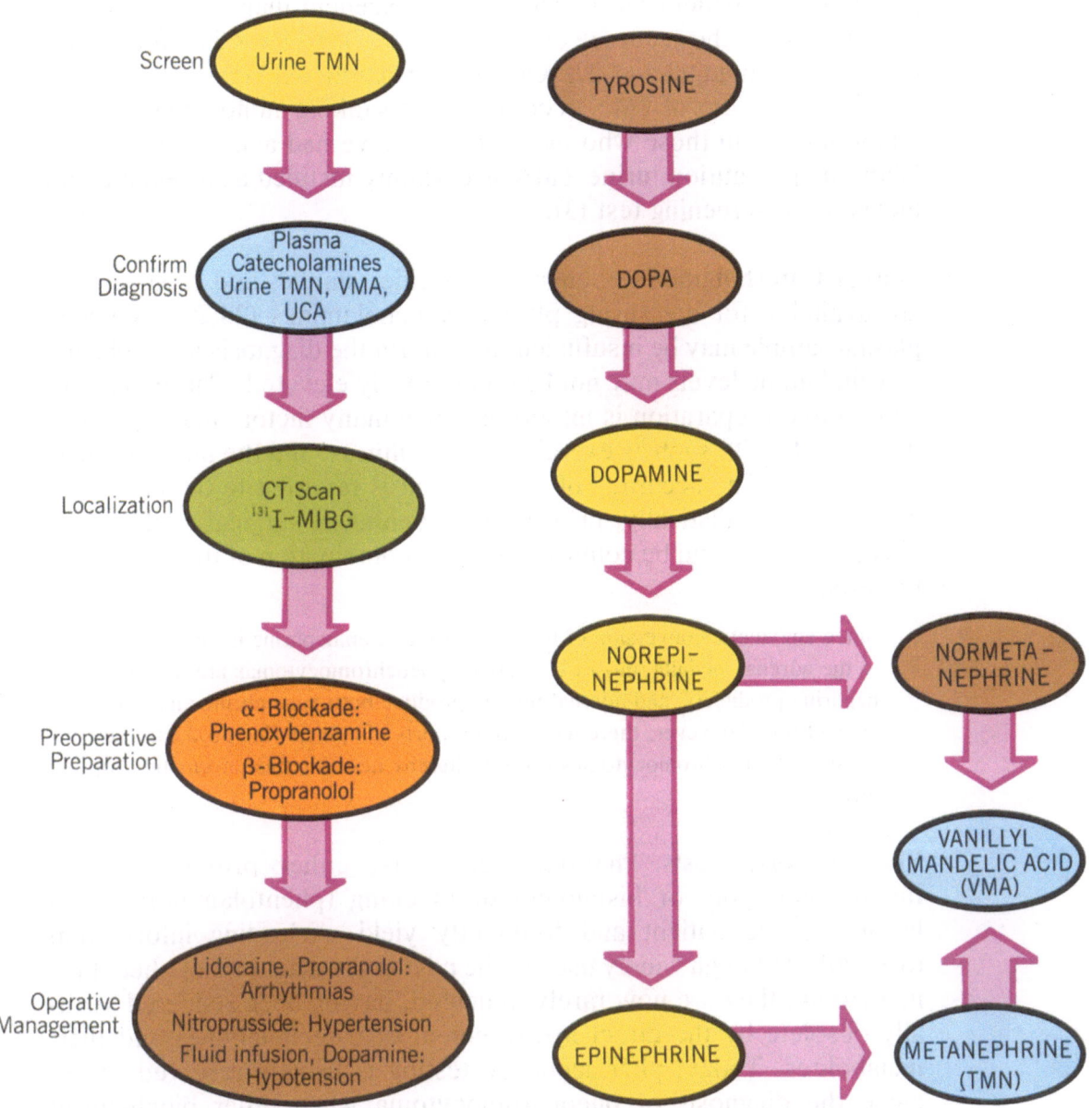

Fig. 3-10. Preoperative evaluation of pheochromocytoma.

Fig. 3-11. Catecholamine metabolism.

(less than 50 g) there is rapid synthesis of catecholamines and preferential excretion of free UCA in the urine. In contrast, in large tumors (more than 50 g) there is a slow turnover and most of the norepinephrine and epinephrine produced is degraded within the tumor itself, resulting in a relatively high excretion rate of VMA and TMN and a low rate of excretion of UCA (19). Strikingly elevated levels of UCA may be found in patients following a symptomatic paroxysmal attack. Although in the past colorimetric assays for VMA were unreliable due to the influence of certain foods and medications (5), high-pressure liquid chromatography and electrochemical detection yield excellent diagnostic accuracy (2). At present, the accuracy of TMN is 95% (7), VMA is 89–96% (7,26), and UCA is about 90% (7,27). One must be cautious, however, as false-positive elevations of TMN occur in patients taking monoamine oxidase inhibitors and in those who may recently have had angiographic dyes. With this precaution, urine TMN is certainly justified as a reliable and inexpensive screening test (3).

Plasma Catecholamines. Sensitive, specific, simple, and rapid assays are available for measuring plasma catecholamines (28,29). A single plasma sample may be insufficient to confirm the diagnosis since plasma catecholamine levels may not be continuously elevated. Careful patient and sample preparation is important since many factors may influence these levels (30), such as exercise, severe illness, and the medication α-methyldopa. The accuracy of this method is reported to be more than 90% (7,29). Realistically, prior to the planning of surgical exploration, the diagnosis should be confirmed using a combination of these diagnostic tests.

> Since enzymatic conversion of norepinephrine to epinephrine is virtually unique to the adrenal medulla, most extraadrenal pheochromocytomas are norepinephrine producers, and adrenal tumors produce both epinephrine and norepinephrine. However, there have been reports of epinephrine production by extraadrenal pheochromocytomas (31,32), thereby negating this information for any localizing value.

Pharmacologic Tests. Pharmacologic tests, either provocative (tyramine, glucagon, or histamine) or blocking (phentolamine) pose a hazard to the patient and frequently yield misleading information (6,15,26). Although widely used in the past in the diagnosis of pheochromocytoma, they are now rarely indicated, having been rendered virtually obsolete by the direct measurement of catecholamines and their metabolites. Today, pharmacologic testing is usually reserved to exclude the diagnosis of pheochromocytoma when other biochemical results are equivocal. No patient should undergo surgery on the basis of a positive blood pressure response alone—confirmation with appropriate urine and blood studies is mandatory.

PREOPERATIVE

At this stage a definitive diagnosis of pheochromocytoma has been confirmed. This can be primary, recurrent, or metastatic disease. Localization is the next step in the evaluation of these patients (Fig. 3-10).

COMPUTERIZED TOMOGRAPHY

CT has emerged as the localizing modality of choice for this disease as well as all adrenal tumors (7,33). Utilizing present-day, state-of-the-art

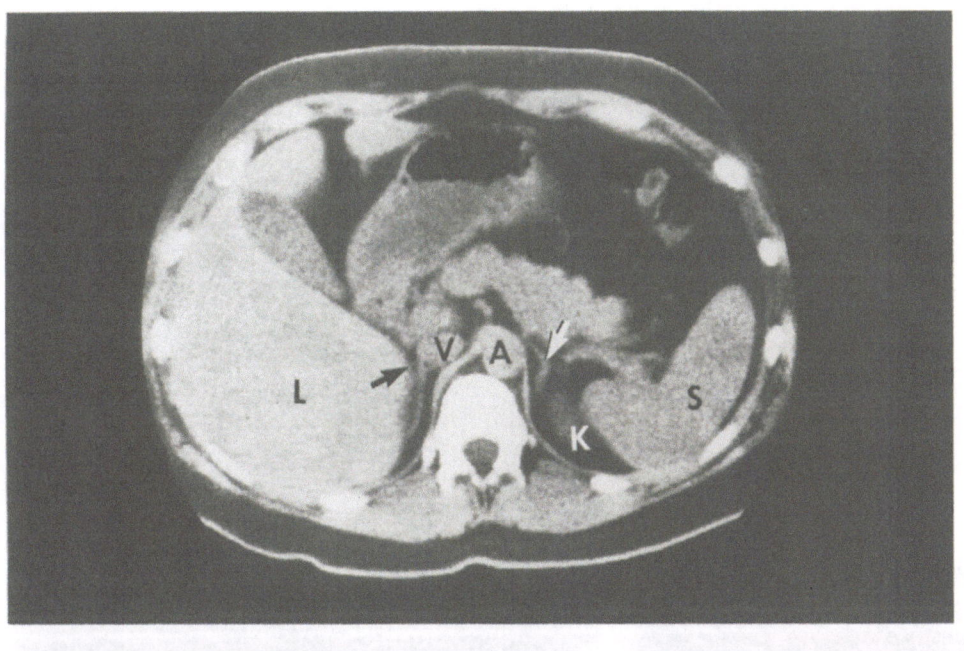

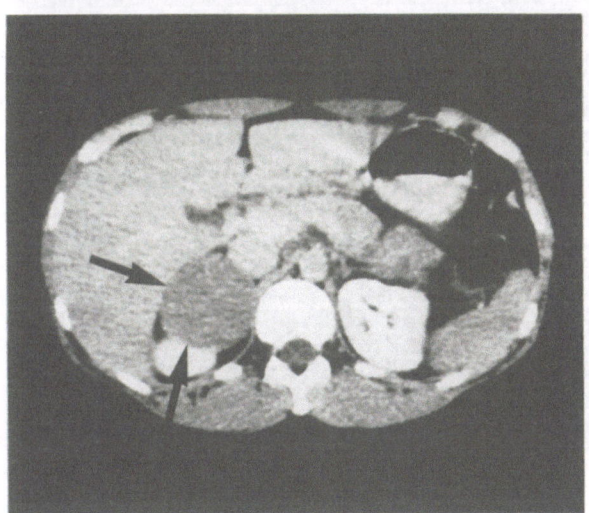

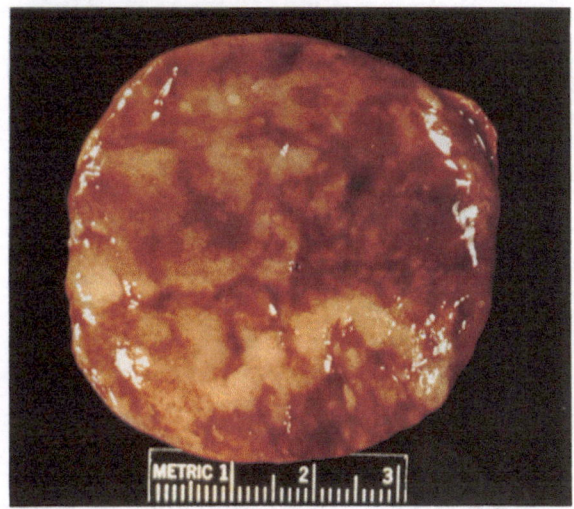

CT scans. **A.** Normal adrenal glands (*arrows*). The liver (*L*), vena cava (*V*), aorta (*A*), spleen (*S*), and kidney (*K*) are identified. **B.** Right adrenal pheochromocytoma. **C.** Corresponding gross specimen.

Fig. 3-12.

scanners, diagnostic accuracy should approach 90%–95% (7,34,35). Except in very large and vascular tumors, CT scanning will no doubt replace arteriography, which is both more invasive and more hazardous. Of major importance, however, is the knowledge that glucagon, which is frequently administered by radiologists to quell bowel peristalsis during examination with CT, should never be given to a patient with a pheochromocytoma as it is a potent stimulus for catecholamine release. The CT scan includes the liver in order to detect metastases, and may also be extended to encompass the remainder of the abdomen, pelvis, and thorax if the screening chest x-ray is normal (Fig. 3-12).

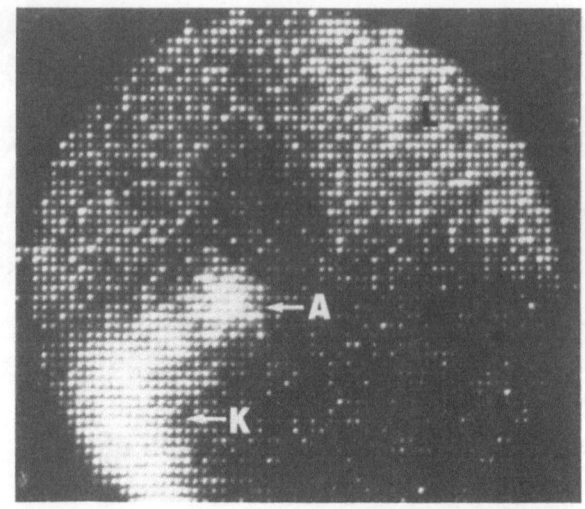

A

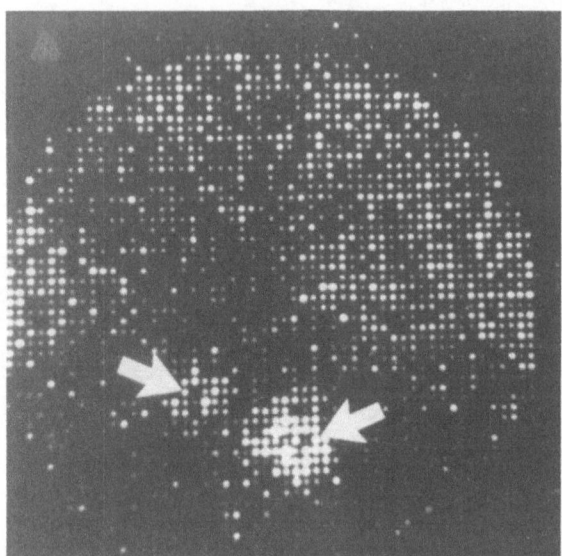

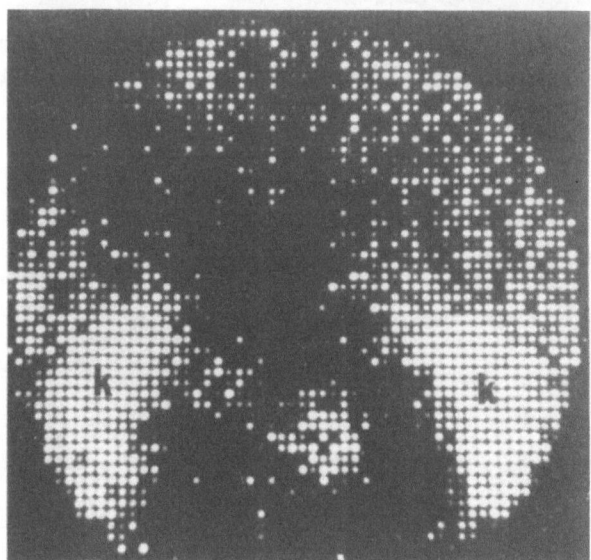

B

Fig. 3-13. **¹³¹I-MIBG scans.** **A.** Posterior abdominal view, with a superimposed renal scan, demonstrates a solitary left kidney (*K*), an intraadrenal pheochromocytoma (*A*), and the usual liver uptake (*L*). **B.** Left: midline, extraadrenal pheochromocytomas (*arrows*). Right: renal scan shows relationship of kidneys (*K*). **C.** Symmetric abnormal adrenal uptake (*arrows*), which proved to be adrenal medullary hyperplasia. **D.** Cystic pheochromocytoma with metastases in the spine and rib. Left: anterior abdominal view. Right: posterior view. (Courtesy of Drs.

ADRENAL RADIONUCLIDE IMAGING

A recent and exciting technologic development has been the introduction of the radiopharmaceutical agent ¹³¹I-metaiodobenzylguanidine (¹³¹I-MIBG), which is specifically taken up and concentrated in adrenergic vesicles (36,37). Only abnormal sites of adrenergic tissue—pheochromocytomas, metastases, paragangliomas—show uptake of the

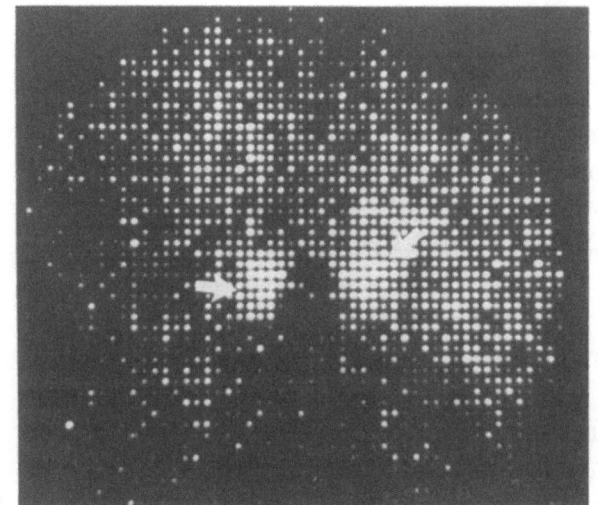

C

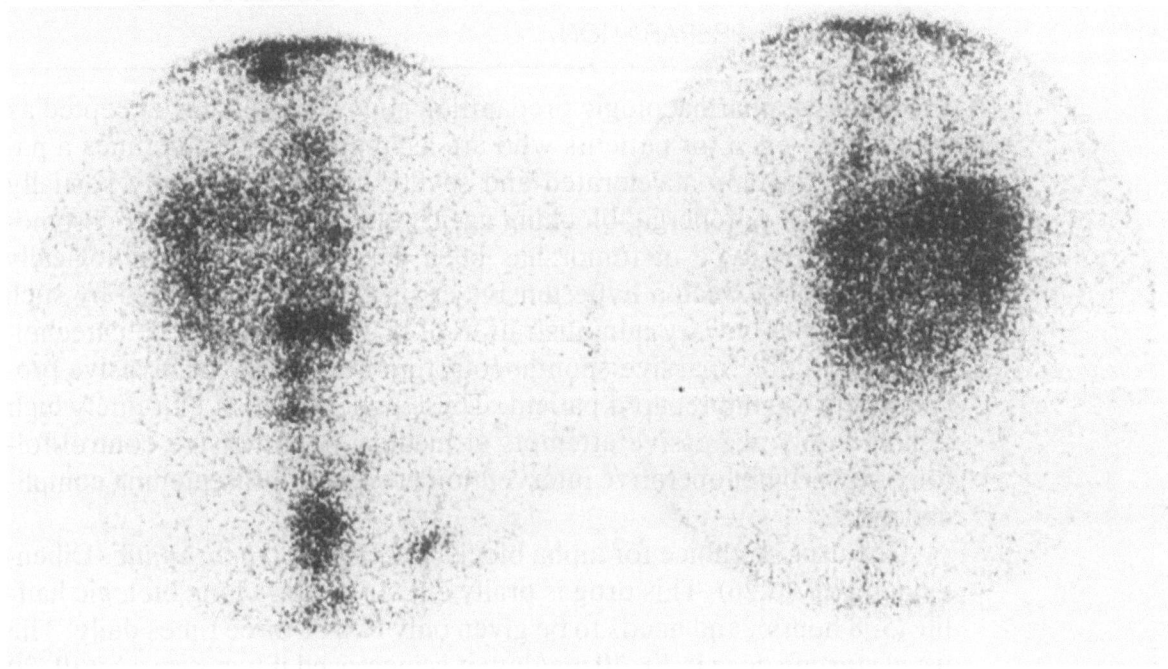

D

James Sisson and Norman Thompson, Ann Arbor, Michigan. Fig. 3-13.A from
Surgery 91(4):374, 1982; Fig. 3-13.B reprinted by permission of The New En-
gland Journal of Medicine 305:12, 1981; Fig. 3-13.C from Ann Intern Med
94(6):762, 1982.)

^{131}I-MIBG, whereas normal adrenals fail to visualize (Fig. 3-13). Since
its first human application in August 1980, numerous patients with adrenal, ectopic (including intracardiac), recurrent, and metastatic pheochromocytomas have been scanned using this agent in the United States
(18) and Europe (38). Only rare false-negative scans occur. The possible
therapeutic implications for managing metastatic pheochromocytomas
(analogous to ^{131}I treatment for metastatic differentiated thyroid carcinoma) seem appealing but have yet to be delineated.

VENA CAVAL CATHETERIZATION AND BLOOD CATECHOLAMINE ASSAY

Only following the exceedingly rare failure to localize with CT scan or ^{131}I-MIBG should vena caval sampling be necessary. As in the case of arteriography, full pharmacologic preparation should be instituted prior to caval catheterization.

TREATMENT

The only satisfactory treatment for pheochromocytoma is surgical removal. In recent years, the use of specific alpha- and beta-adrenergic blocking agents, both to prepare patients preoperatively and for intraoperative control of paroxysmal hypertension and cardiac arrhythmias, has greatly improved the safety of operation.

PREOPERATIVE PREPARATION

Preoperative pharmacologic preparation is now universally accepted as mandatory, even for patients who are asymptomatic. Sometimes a patient may develop accelerated and severe hypertension only partially controlled by adrenergic blocking agents (so-called acute pheochromocytoma). This type of tumor has been described as "physiologically malignant" (1). Such a hypertensive crisis can be precipitated by such factors as the unwary administration of drugs that stimulate catecholamine secretion, massive spontaneous tumor necrosis, or invasive procedures in the unprepared patient. These patients are at extremely high risk and only aggressive attempts at medical hypertensive control followed by prompt operative intervention prevent life-threatening complications.

The drug of choice for alpha blockade is *phenoxybenzamine* (Dibenzyline) (7,8,15,26). This drug is orally effective, has a long biologic half-life (5–8 hours), and needs to be given only two or three times daily. The usual starting dose is 20–40 mg/day; it is increased if necessary by 10–20 mg/day until hypertension and other symptoms are controlled, with a desired end point of moderately symptomatic orthostatic hypotension. Treatment is usually continued for 7–14 days preoperatively (Fig. 3-14). Phenoxybenzamine may cause gastrointestinal distress, nasal stuffiness, excessive sedation, and lassitude, but it is tolerated fairly well by most patients. Occasionally it produces an exaggerated antihypertensive effect and tachycardia. This occurs when the pheochromocytoma secretes large amounts of epinephrine; alpha blockade unmasks the beta-adrenergic vasodilatation and positive chronotropic effect of epinephrine to cause hypotension and tachycardia. This problem is averted by using combined alpha and beta blockade.

Although not uniformly accepted, *propranolol* (Inderal) is usually

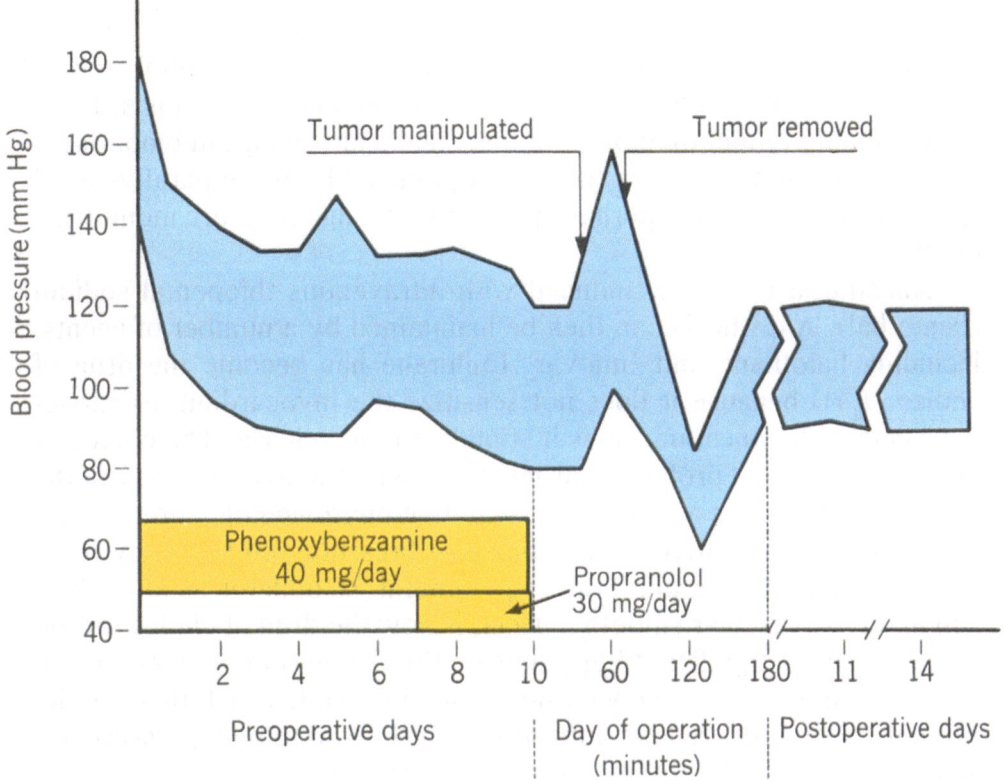

Blood pressure recordings before, during, and after operation for Fig. 3-14.
pheochromocytoma. Preoperative treatment with phenoxybenzamine brings
the blood pressure down to normal levels over a period of several days. Although the patient is protected by alpha-adrenergic blockade from violent paroxysms of hypertension during manipulation of the tumor, some fluctuations of
blood pressure may occur, as shown in this case.

added to the regimen for 3–7 days before surgery to control and prevent
tachyarrhythmias (7,15). Patients with pheochromocytoma appear to be
quite sensitive to propranolol, so the starting dose is usually 30–40 mg/
day (given in three or four divided doses) (Fig. 3-14). Cautious incre-
ments in dosage are added every 3–4 days until cardiac rhythm and rate
are controlled. Administration should be continued through the morning
of operation, and should be started after alpha blockade is established to
avoid unopposed intense vasoconstriction, severe hypertension, and
precipitate congestive heart failure.

Other drugs, such as α-methylparatyrosine, have been used to decrease catecholamine synthesis (14). While catecholamine synthesis can
be significantly reduced, alpha and beta blockade are still necessary to
avoid significant hypertensive episodes and tachycardia (39).

INTRAOPERATIVE DRUG MANAGEMENT

A narcotic analgesic or powerful tranquilizer has been favored for pre-anesthetic medication. Atropine should be avoided because it causes tachycardia. Successful anesthetic management requires skillful control of acute and severe hypertension, hypotension, and arrhythmias. Even with optimal preoperative preparation, significant swings in blood pressure are common. Safety is therefore optimized by intraoperative arterial, central venous, and perhaps pulmonary wedge pressure monitoring (7,40).

Anesthesia is usually induced with intravenous thiopental sodium (Pentothal). Anesthesia can then be maintained by a number of agents, including halothane and Innovar. Enflurane has become the drug of choice (7,41) because it does not sensitize the myocardium to exogenous catecholamines, nor does it stimulate their release. The choice of an anesthetic agent probably has less to do with the overall safety of the procedure than does adequate preoperative pharmacologic preparation and adept intraoperative control of blood pressure and heart rhythm.

Sodium nitroprusside, a direct peripheral vasodilator as a result of action on the vascular smooth muscle, is now the drug of choice for the management of significant hypertension (7). A solution of 50 mg in 250 ml 5% dextrose gives a concentration of 100 μg/ml, which then can be titrated as an intravenous infusion according to blood pressure response. It is a highly potent hypotensive agent with an almost immediate effect that ends abruptly when the infusion is stopped (Fig. 3-15A). These properties are ideally suited for this intraoperative use, and this technique has replaced the use of bolus injections of phentolamine (Regitine).

Hypotension may occur shortly after the main adrenal vein has been ligated or following control of the numerous small peripheral tributaries as the tumor is completely resected. Contracted blood volume was originally blamed for the marked hypotension (42), but it is now thought that three different factors are responsible: (a) there is a sudden decrease in circulating catecholamines (which intraoperatively may reach 600 times the preoperative levels (29)); (b) the alpha-adrenergic blockade medication is still effective; and (c) there appears to be a relative refractoriness to normal tone following the relief from chronic catecholamine stimulation of the vascular bed. Seemingly excessive *fluid administration* is still commonly necessary despite careful preoperative blockade. On occasion, the use of a pressor agent such as *dopamine* (200 mg in 250 ml 5% dextrose) may be helpful.

Intraoperatively, the onset of premature contractions or marked sinus tachycardia, the most commonly encountered *cardiac arrhythmias,* usually signals an increase in blood pressure. Treatment of the hypertension alone is often enough to cause resolution of the cardiac irregularity. Repeated intravenous administrations of lidocaine (50–100

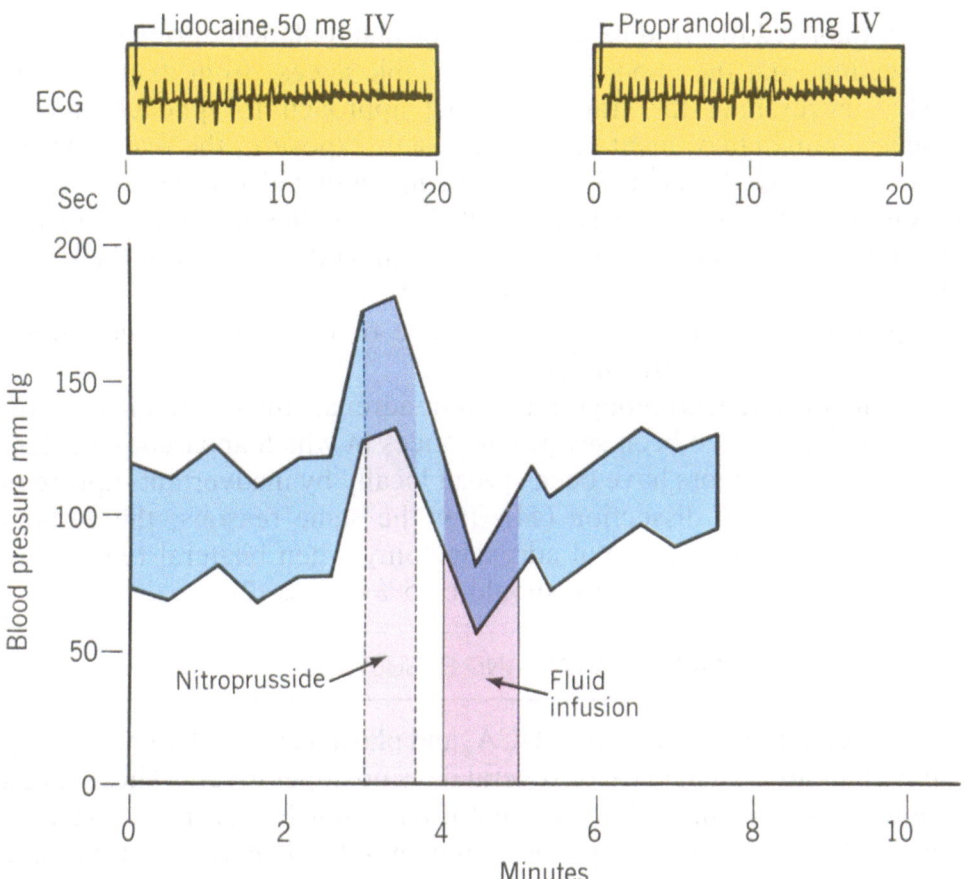

Intraoperative drug treatment. Blood pressure recording during operation. Paroxysm of hypertension controlled by intravenous nitroprusside. This is usually not necessary with adequate preoperative alpha-adrenergic blockade. The decrease in blood pressure following removal of the tumor is best treated by volume infusion. Ventricular bigeminy converted to normal sinus rhythm by lidocaine and by propranolol.

Fig. 3-15.

mg bolus, or intravenous infusion of 1 g in 250 ml 5% dextrose then 1–4 mg/min) or propranolol (0.5–1 mg IV) may be required to abolish significant ventricular arrhythmias (Fig. 3-15). The bolus effect of lidocaine is very transient, whereas propranolol is usually effective for 15–30 minutes or longer. Equipment for cardioversion should be available.

If bilateral total adrenalectomy is anticipated, preoperative steroid preparation is instituted. If no preparation has been used, any suitable intravenous corticosteroid preparation should be started intraoperatively, be continued in adequate doses to cover perioperative stress, then be reduced to standard steroid replacement therapy.

OPERATIVE STRATEGY

Even though preoperative localization is highly reliable, the possible multiplicity of tumors (i.e., intraadrenal and unsuspected extraadrenal

(43)), the need to avoid excessive tumor manipulation during operative dissection, and the importance of available access from diaphragm to pelvis necessitate the transabdominal approach for pheochromocytoma. Upon achievement of excellent safe exposure, the main adrenal vein is controlled. The tumor should be manipulated as little as possible, even after the hilar vein is controlled, as smaller tributaries are frequently present and hypertensive crises can still occur. After the tumor has been removed, the abdominal cavity is systematically explored; particular note is taken of any evidence of metastases, contralateral adrenal tumor, or extraadrenal tumors.

When a pheochromocytoma is intraadrenal, the entire gland is removed. There have been several instances in which apparently benign, encapsulated tumors have been spread locally by inadvertant rupture of the tumor during dissection (44). For the same reasons, the authors usually prefer bilateral total adrenalectomy when bilateral tumors are present. Operative mortality should be 5% or less (7).

POSTOPERATIVE MANAGEMENT AND RESULTS

Measurement of TMN, VMA, UCA, and plasma catecholamines is very important after an interval of several days postoperatively. These levels should return completely to normal if all tumor has been removed. In this way, residual or metastatic tumor may be detected, and baseline values are recorded for future comparisons. Levels of UCA, VMA, and TMN excretion should be checked at 6-month intervals for about 2 years and yearly thereafter for an indefinite period. The possibility of future tumor recurrence can never be entirely discounted.

Following resection of benign pheochromocytomas, 95% of patients with paroxysmal and 67% of those with sustained hypertension become normotensive; the others are managed with conventional antihypertensive programs (7). The actuarial survival curve for those with benign pheochromocytoma is comparable to the expected survival in age- and sex-matched controls.

MALIGNANT PHEOCHROMOCYTOMA

Malignant pheochromocytoma is a rare and challenging tumor to accurately diagnose, localize, and treat. The clinical presentation of a primary, recurrent, or metastatic pheochromocytoma is virtually indistinguishable from its benign counterpart. Paroxysmal attacks of hypertension and concomitant symptoms of catecholamine bursts as well as sustained hypertension have been recorded (43). Metastatic or recurrent tumor is usually functional and the urinary biochemical diagnostic tests often presage tumor recurrence. The median time lapse between initial operation and recurrence was 5.6 years in one study (6); thus long-term follow-up is advisable.

Even on retrospective review, the distinction between a malignant and benign primary adrenal tumor is often impossible. Mitotic figures and vascular and capsular invasion can be readily identified in both benign and malignant neoplasms. Malignancy can be positively diagnosed only when metastases to non-chromaffin-bearing tissue, such as liver, lung, nodes, or bone (most commonly as lytic bone metastases) have been confirmed (6,14,18). In the past, invasive localization utilizing "vena caval search" was necessary; CT and ^{131}I-MIBG have revolutionized this task (18,37,45).

Radical en bloc resection of the tumor and lymph nodes (6,7,14), re-resection of recurrences, and palliative debulking of functioning metastases presently constitute the best accepted, although sometimes suboptimal, treatment. Alpha and beta blockade together with the synthesis inhibitor α-methylparatyrosine offer palliative symptomatic relief. Chemotherapy has been disappointing, but radiotherapy may effect significant palliation, especially from painful osseus metastases (43,46).

Five-year survival of patients with adrenal malignancies averages 40% (6,7,14), whereas the prognosis for those with malignancies of extraadrenal origin is much less favorable (14).

PHEOCHROMOCYTOMA DURING PREGNANCY

Pregnancy complicated by pheochromocytoma is extremely dangerous for both mother and fetus. Unfortunately, the diagnosis of pheochromocytoma is established antepartum in only one-third of these patients (47). Even when the diagnosis is established during pregnancy, maternal and fetal mortalities are 17% and 40%, respectively, whereas these rates soar to 58% and 50% when the disease remains unsuspected (48). Urinary catecholamines are normal during pregnancy. Even though rare, the disastrous complications of pheochromocytoma during pregnancy seem to warrant urinary TMN screening of hypertensive patients.

When this problem is encountered during the first or second trimester, the first priority is maternal safety. Prompt surgical excision after appropriate preoperative blockade is usually undertaken (21,49). In the third trimester, adrenergic blockade is instituted and full-term cesarean section and synchronous tumor excision are recommended. These are general guidelines; each case must be individually considered with close collaboration of the obstetrician, pediatrician, radiologist, endocrinologist, anesthesiologist, and surgeon.

PHEOCHROMOCYTOMA IN MEN-II SYNDROMES

Pheochromocytomas that develop in patients with MEN-II syndromes follow a capricious course: sometimes they remain subtle, yet they may unpredictably evolve into a malignancy or present as a lethal, hypertensive crisis (50,51). Once unequivocally positive biochemical tests document the presence of pheochromocytoma, bilateral adrenal medullary disease is invariably present (36,52). One finds either pheochromocytomas or bilateral adrenal medullary hyperplasia—analogous to the precursor, C-cell hyperplasia of medullary thyroid carcinoma. Bilateral total adrenalectomy is recommended in these circumstances (36,53,54).

Primary Aldoste-ronism

Primary aldosteronism is a surgically correctable type of hypertension found in 1%–2% of all hypertensive patients (55–57). It is characterized by autonomous, excessive aldosterone secretion, which causes sodium retention, potassium wasting, hypertension, and suppression of plasma renin activity (PRA). Five subgroups of the syndrome have emerged:

1. Aldosterone-producing adenoma (APA)
2. Idiopathic hyperaldosteronism due to bilateral adrenocortical hyperplasia (IHA)
3. Aldosterone-producing adenocarcinoma
4. Glucocorticoid-remediable hyperaldosteronism (58,59)
5. "Indeterminate" hyperaldosteronism.

Only APA and IHA are of practical significance. Aldosterone-producing adenocarcinoma is very rare, as is the glucocorticoid-remediable form; the latter is most often seen in young males or a few kindreds, and it is curable with oral corticosteroids.

Secondary aldosteronism, or hyperreninemic hyperaldosteronism, typified by renal artery stenosis, is characterized by a decreased renal artery perfusion pressure and flow, which stimulates renin secretion by the juxtaglomerular apparatus and leads to increased angiotensin and, ultimately, elevated aldosterone. Thus, the two forms of hyperaldosteronism can be clearly differentiated by determining the PRA: renin is low in primary and high in secondary aldosteronism.

PATHOLOGY

Controversy abounds in endocrine surgery surrounding the vague distinctions between adenoma and hyperplasia. Primary aldosteronism is no exception. A clear separation of IHA and APA is sometimes difficult, and even categories of multiple adenomas and macronodular hyperplasia have been introduced, raising the possibility that the clinical syndrome is produced by an entire spectrum of pathology. To add confusion, it is well known that an APA and definite hyperplasia of the zona glomerulosa can coexist in the same adrenal gland (60–62). "Nonfunctioning" nodules may also accompany an APA and share similar gross, light, and electron microscopic features (63). To provide unequivocal identification, in vitro studies to determine if the nodule can produce aldosterone are necessary. Only an APA produces aldosterone; non-

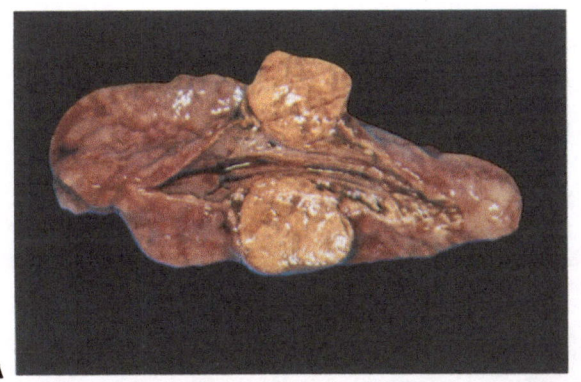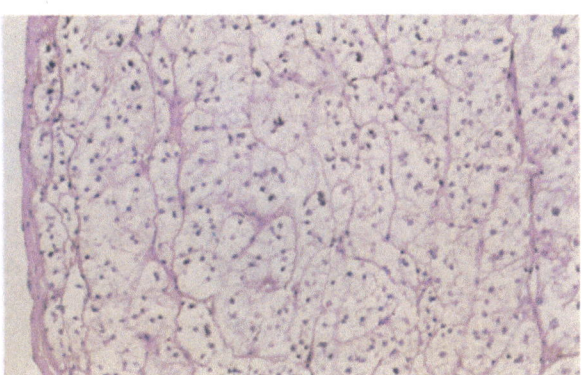

A   ⊢———⊣ 1 cm   B

Aldosteronoma. **A.** Gross appearance. The color is distinctive. Most of these   **Fig. 3-16.**
tumors are less than 2 cm in diameter. **B.** Large lipid-laden clear cells of an
APA on histologic section.

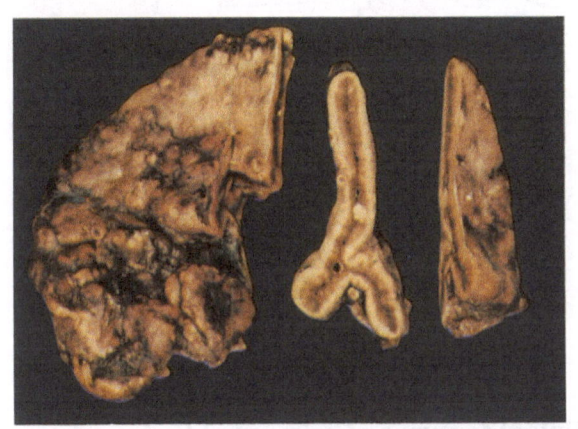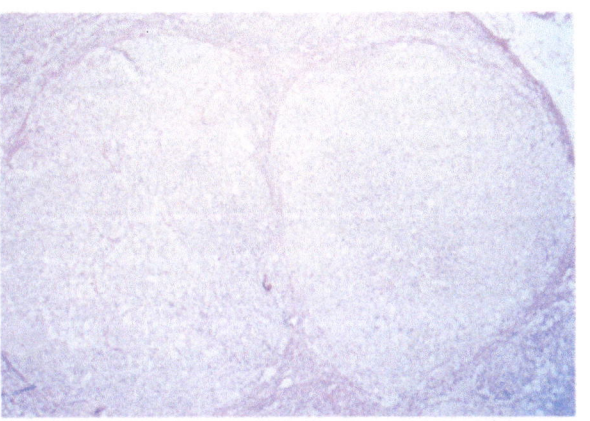

A   ⊢———⊣ 1 cm   B

Bilateral nodular hyperplasia causing primary aldosteronism. **A.** Adre-   **Fig. 3-17.**
nal from a patient with IAH. Several macronodules are easily visible. **B.** Histologic appearance of a nodule.

functioning nodules cannot (63,64). Given the inexact pathology, APAs
seem to represent 50%–75% of the cases of primary aldosteronism; IHA
constitutes the other 25%–50%. Carcinoma is extremely rare.

A typical APA is small (three-quarters measure 8–20 mm in diameter), solitary, well demarcated, and distinctively golden yellow (Fig.
3-16A). It may project from the surface of the adrenal or be wholly
intraglandular and visible only after the gland has been removed and
sectioned. Several different histologic cell patterns exist, but the most
frequent consists of large lipid-laden cells arranged in small cords or
acini and separated by fine connective tissue trabeculae (Fig. 3-16B).

With IHA, both adrenal glands show diffuse or nodular hyperplasia
of the zona glomerulosa (Fig. 3-17). When a macronodule is present
within a hyperplastic gland and is visible to the naked eye it may be
extremely difficult to distinguish from a small APA.

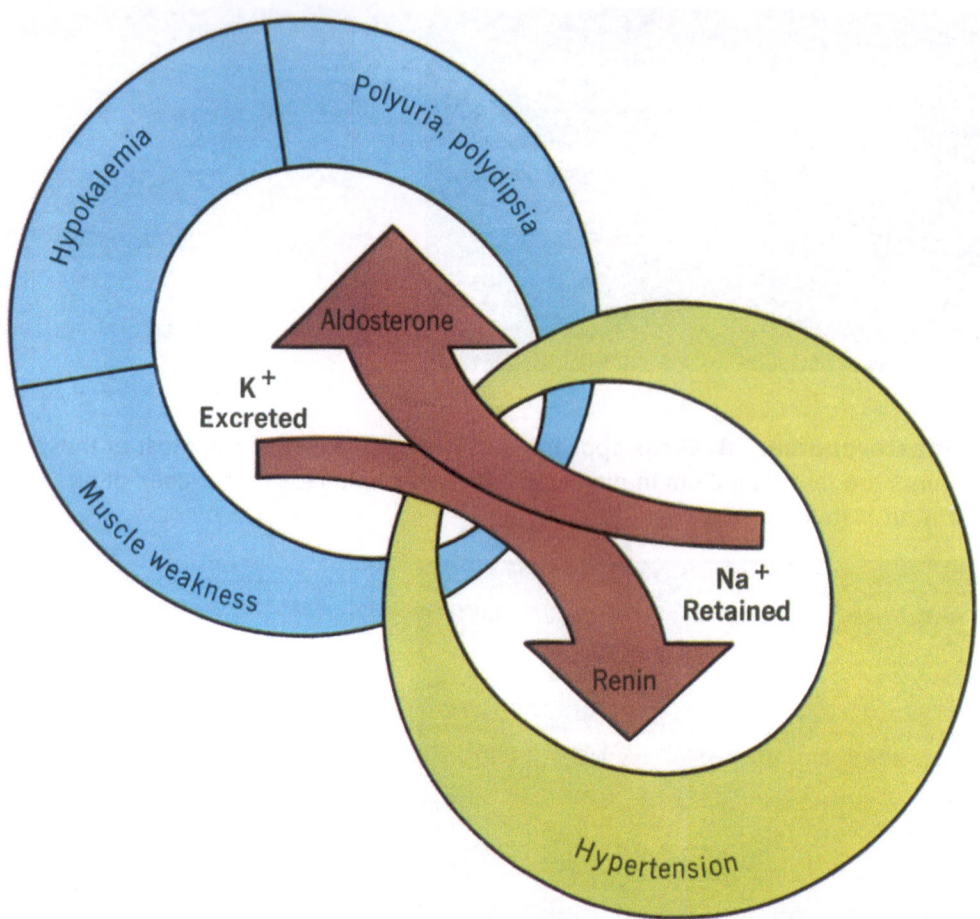

Fig. 3-18. **Pathophysiology and major clinical features of primary aldosteronism.**

DIAGNOSIS

CLINICAL FEATURES

Malignant hypertension is rarely present (65), but moderate to severe hypertension is common (60,61,66), and cardiac (61,65), vascular (61,67), and renal (60,65) complications provide impetus for early diagnosis and treatment. Conn (68) first recognized the associated constellation of symptoms, including muscle weakness, polydipsia, polyuria, nocturia, muscle cramps, and headache attributable to the hypokalemia and hypertension (Fig. 3-18). Primary aldosteronism is more common in women, and the mean age at diagnosis is 40–50 years (61,66,69).

LABORATORY STUDIES

The diagnosis of primary aldosteronism can be subdivided into three stages: screening; confirming the diagnosis; and differentiating APA from IHA (Fig. 3-19).

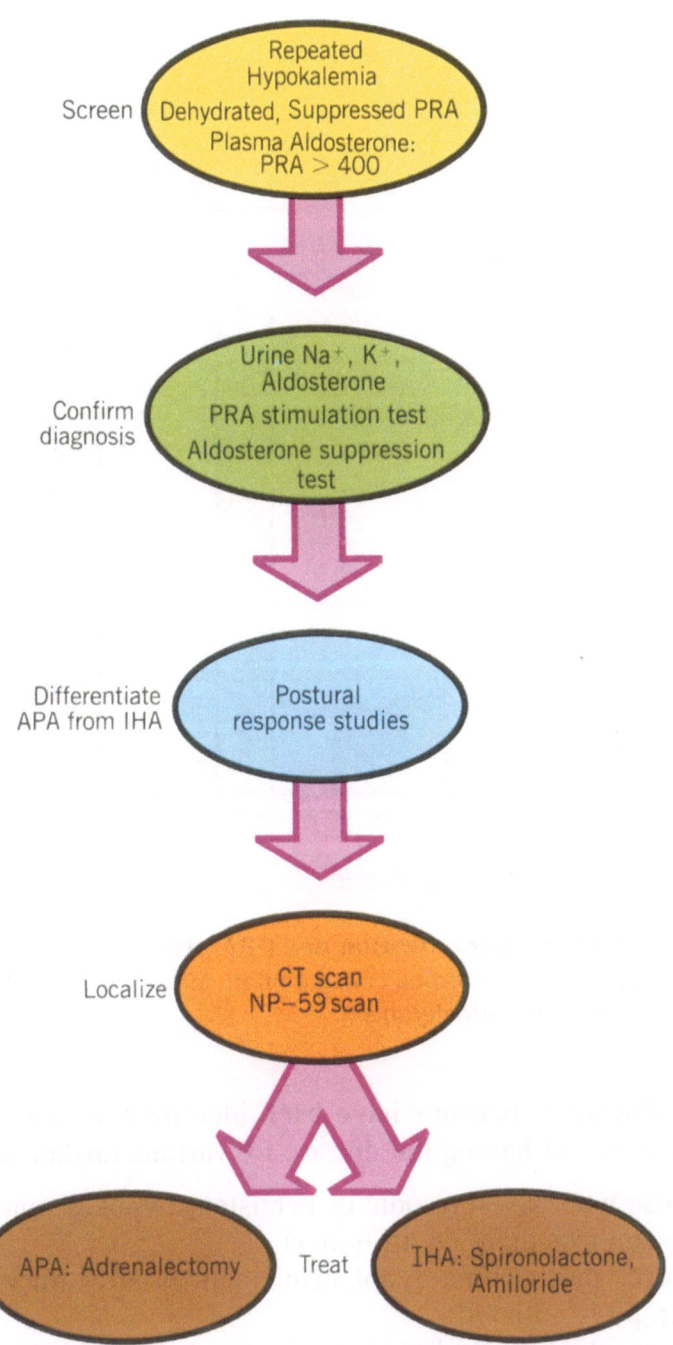

Screen — Repeated Hypokalemia / Dehydrated, Suppressed PRA / Plasma Aldosterone: PRA > 400

Confirm diagnosis — Urine Na⁺, K⁺, Aldosterone / PRA stimulation test / Aldosterone suppression test

Differentiate APA from IHA — Postural response studies

Localize — CT scan / NP–59 scan

Treat — APA: Adrenalectomy / IHA: Spironolactone, Amiloride

Evaluation and treatment of patients with primary aldosteronism. **Fig. 3-19.**

Screening. Unprovoked hypokalemia in hypertensive patients is the usual trigger to further investigation. Used as the sole screening test, however, it may miss 20% of patients with primary aldosteronism (57,70). A convenient, sensitive, reliable, and cost-effective screening test has yet to be developed. A plasma aldosterone to PRA ratio of greater than 400 has been reported as highly accurate in identifying patients with APA (71). Its widespread use awaits further confirmation.

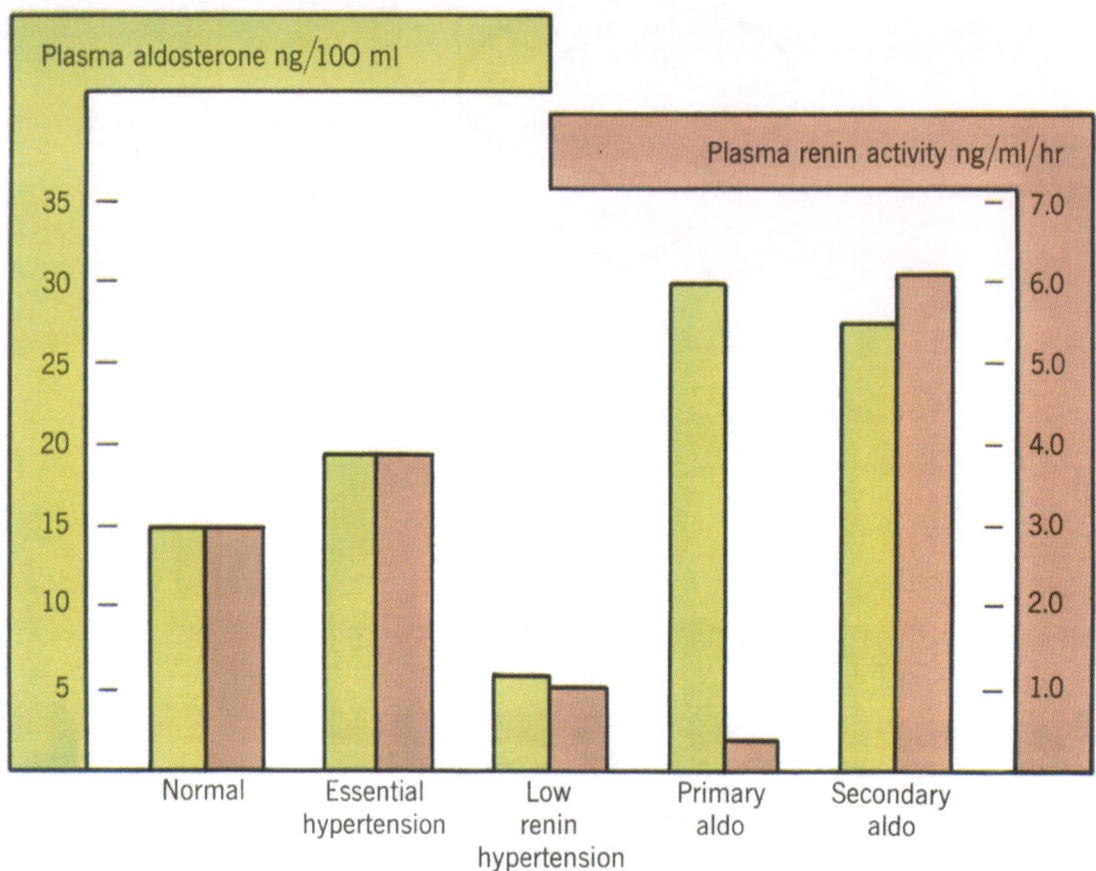

Fig. 3-20. **Plasma aldosterone concentration and PRA after 2 hours of erect position.** A high plasma aldosterone concentration combined with a low PRA is characteristic of primary aldosteronism.

The following subgroups have been identified as possessing sufficient probability of having the disease to warrant further workup (72):

1. Those who have episodic or persistent hypokalemia (serum potassium less than 3.6 mEq/liter)
2. Those who become hypokalemic shortly after thiazide diuretic therapy is initiated
3. Those who become hypokalemic after ingesting large amounts of sodium chloride.

Confirming the Diagnosis. Primary aldosteronism is the only recognized condition that produces high secretory rates of aldosterone and low serum renin levels in a patient who is hypertensive. Thus, the diagnostic aim is to prove unsuppressible hyperaldosteronism and PRA that cannot be stimulated (Fig. 3-20).

Low serum potassium reflects the renal effects of excess aldosterone—namely, elevated urinary potassium excretion. Initial tests, therefore, should include 24-hour urine collections for sodium, potassium,

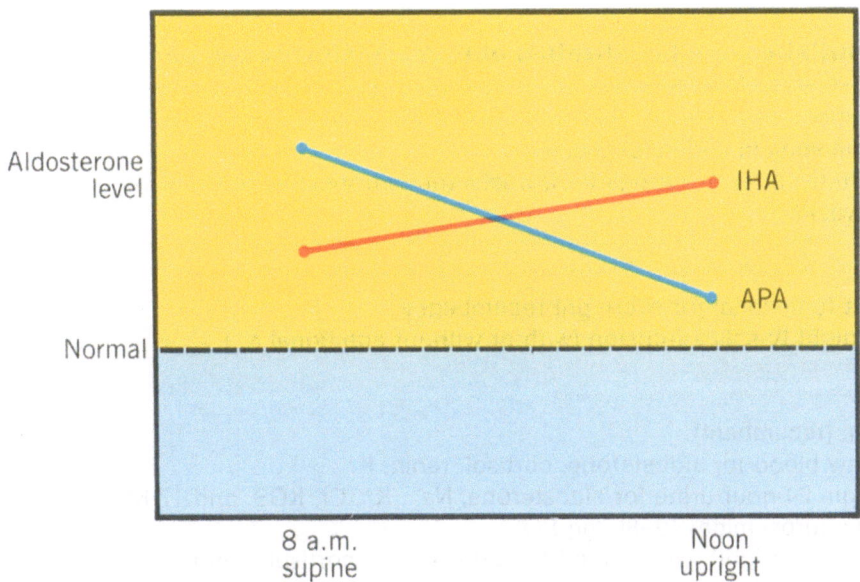

Differentiating APA from IHA by postural response studies. Levels of aldosterone *decrease* in patients with APA when upright from 8 a.m. until noon. Aldosterone levels *increase* in patients with IHA in a similar setting.

Fig. 3-21.

and aldosterone. A serum potassium less than 3 mEq/liter with a concomitant urinary potassium excretion exceeding 40 mEq/liter is highly suspect for primary aldosteronism (73). An elevated urinary aldosterone level lends further support to the diagnosis.

A *subnormal PRA* in the face of an acute diuresis, induced by 80 mg of furosemide orally and the assumption of an upright posture for 4 hours, is strong evidence in support of primary aldosteronism (74,75).

Failure to suppress aldosterone secretion by intravascular volume expansion is the fundamental basis for establishing the diagnosis.

This test is best carried out by administering the following:

1. High sodium chloride diet (9 g) for 3 days
2. Fludrohydrocortisone (Florinef), 0.5 mg/day for 3 consecutive days (deoxycorticosterone, 10 mg IM in two doses administered 12 hours apart, may be substituted for Florinef).

Plasma aldosterone and 24-hour urine aldosterone levels are then determined.

If the results of the PRA stimulation test and aldosterone suppression tests demonstrate that the aldosterone levels remain elevated in the face of volume expansion, and that the PRA is not stimulated by acute diuresis, the diagnosis is confirmed.

Differentiation of APA and IHA. The development of a highly reliable and accurate radioimmunoassay for plasma aldosterone (76) and advances in our understanding of the renin–angiotensin–aldosterone axis have laid the foundation for a quick, reliable, and relatively inexpensive method to differentiate APA from IHA. Ganguly et al. (77) introduced

Table 3-2. **Differentiation and Localization of Primary Aldosteronism**

Preparation
  Liberal sodium intake for 5 days
  No antihypertensive drugs for 2 weeks (no spironolactone for 6
    weeks)

Day 1
  Admit to hospital for overnight recumbency
  Overnight IV saline infusion (with or without additional K$^+$)

Day 2
  8 a.m. (recumbent):
    Draw blood for aldosterone, cortisol, renin, K$^+$
    Begin 24-hour urine for aldosterone, Na$^+$, K$^+$, Cr, KGS, and 17-KS
    Give furosemide, 40–80 mg PO
  12 noon (upright): Draw blood for aldosterone, cortisol, renin, K$^+$
  Afternoon: CT scan of adrenal glands

Day 3
  Complete 24-hour urine collection
  Discharge in morning

the concept and others (61,78,79) confirmed that postural response studies tend to distinguish APA from IHA.

> Levels of plasma aldosterone decrease in patients with APA when they are upright between the hours of 8:00 a.m. and 12 noon, reflecting their responsiveness to the inherent circadian rhythm of plasma adrenocorticotropic hormone (ACTH). In contrast, aldosterone levels increase in patients with IHA under similar conditions, owing to their hypersensitivity to angiotensin II. Even a slight increase in angiotensin II, reflected by PRA, seen with upright posture causes a significant increase in plasma aldosterone (80) (Fig. 3-21).

APA and IHA can thus be clearly differentiated in approximately 75%–85% of patients within as little as 36 hours of hospitalization (61) (Table 3-2).

PREOPERATIVE LOCALIZATION STUDIES

CT scanning and adrenal scintigraphy using ^{131}I-6β-iodomethylnorcholesterol (NP-59) with dexamethasone suppression have almost completely superseded other localizing modalities. Current, state-of-the-art CT scanners are able to detect adenomas less than 1 cm in diameter (81,82), require low radiation doses, are widely available, and are well accepted by the patient because they are noninvasive. The normal adrenal can be visualized in up to 95% of patients (83) and an APA can be localized in 75%–90% (61,82,84). This technique has thus become the localizing technique of choice.

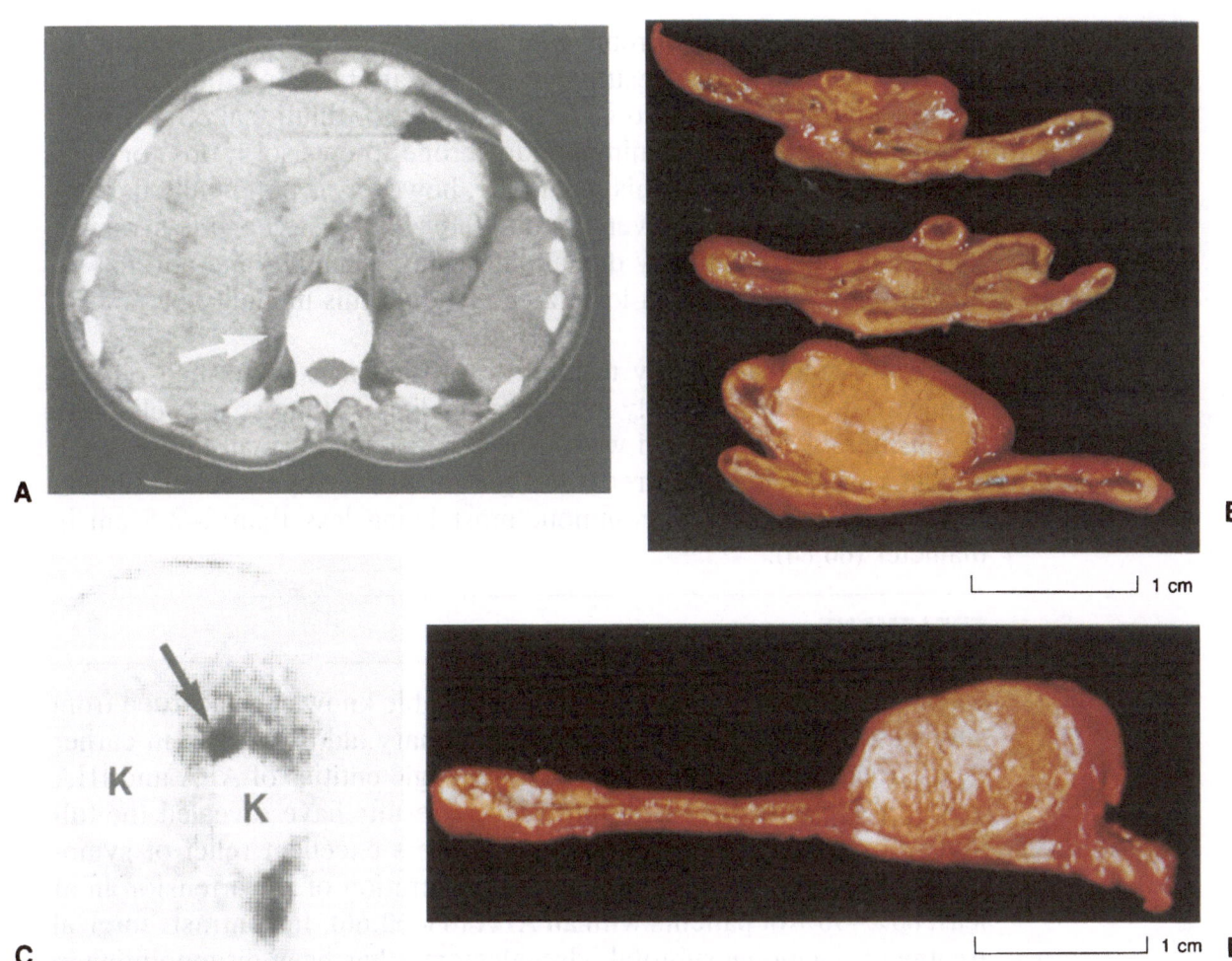

Noninvasive localization studies in primary aldosteronism. **A.** CT scan of right adrenal aldosteronoma. **B.** Corresponding gross specimen. **C.** NP-59 scan (posterior view) with renal scan subtraction (*K*), which shows a right adrenal aldosteronoma (*arrow*). **D.** Corresponding gross specimen. (Scale is in centimeters.)

Fig. 3-22.

Of nearly equal accuracy but encumbered by higher radiation doses, more extensive patient preparation, and less convenience, NP-59 with dexamethasone suppression (61,85,86) is the second choice. This noninvasive technique employs radioactively labeled cholesterol, which is detected by gamma camera tomography. The NP-59 is injected intravenously and subsequently incorporated by the adrenal cortex for use in the synthesis of the various steroid hormones. Photoscans after injection of the radioiodine reveal a hot spot at the site of an APA. Patients with IHA ideally exhibit diffuse bilateral uptake, ranging from minimally to moderately intense imaging. Dexamethasone inhibits the uptake of labeled cholesterol by hyperplastic glands but does not interfere with the uptake by an APA. CT scan and NP-59 scintigraphy should be regarded as complementary, not exclusive tests (Fig. 3-22).

Although bilateral adrenal venous sampling is quite accurate in some hands (60,87), the results are highly variable. Variations in aldosterone levels secondary to catheter slippage or dilutional effects have been minimized by determining aldosterone to cortisol ratios for each adrenal venous sample. This technique, however, is potentially dangerous when combined with venography (88) (Fig. 3-23A) and is invasive, expensive, and technically demanding. Only when CT and adrenal radioisotope scanning fail in localization should this modality be considered (Fig. 3-23B).

Arteriography is rarely needed; at present it is performed only to delineate the arterial supply in large or malignant tumors. Its reliability is considerably diminished when it is used to detect small tumors (61). Aldosterone-producing adrenal malignancies are very rare, and tumors larger than 3 cm are uncommon, most being less than 2–2.5 cm in diameter (66,84).

TREATMENT

Current treatments in part reflect considerable knowledge accrued from surgical treatment of all patients with primary aldosteronism in earlier years. Recognition of the separate pathologic entities of APA and IHA and correlation of their different clinical results have revealed the following: unilateral total adrenalectomy offers excellent relief of symptoms, and either cure or significant amelioration of hypertension in at least 80%–90% of patients with an APA (60–62,66). In contrast, surgical treatment, including subtotal adrenalectomy, has been disappointing in patients with IHA (61,62,70,89) with response rates ranging from 22% (60) to 54% (61). Therefore, spironolactone and Amiloride have become the first-line treatments in this subset of patients (60,61,90). Spironolactone, either alone (in doses of 100–400 mg/day) or in combination with other antihypertensives, has usually been quite effective in both symptomatic and hypertensive control. However, side effects, in particular gynecomastia and impotence in males, may make the drug unacceptable. A suitable alternative is Amiloride, a potassium-sparing diuretic with a different mechanism of action, whose use alone or with other antihypertensives has been described clinically (91) at a dosage of 40 mg/day.

For *preoperative preparation,* spironolactone may be given for 1–2 weeks prior to operation. It facilitates potassium repletion (oral supplements of about 50 mEq/day) and substantially corrects the hypertension. The incidence of operative and postoperative complications, such as cardiac irregularities and paralytic ileus, are thought to be thereby reduced.

In patients with an APA, a unilateral total adrenalectomy is the preferred surgical management. The posterior approach has been shown to be superior to the anterior, transperitoneal option as it is

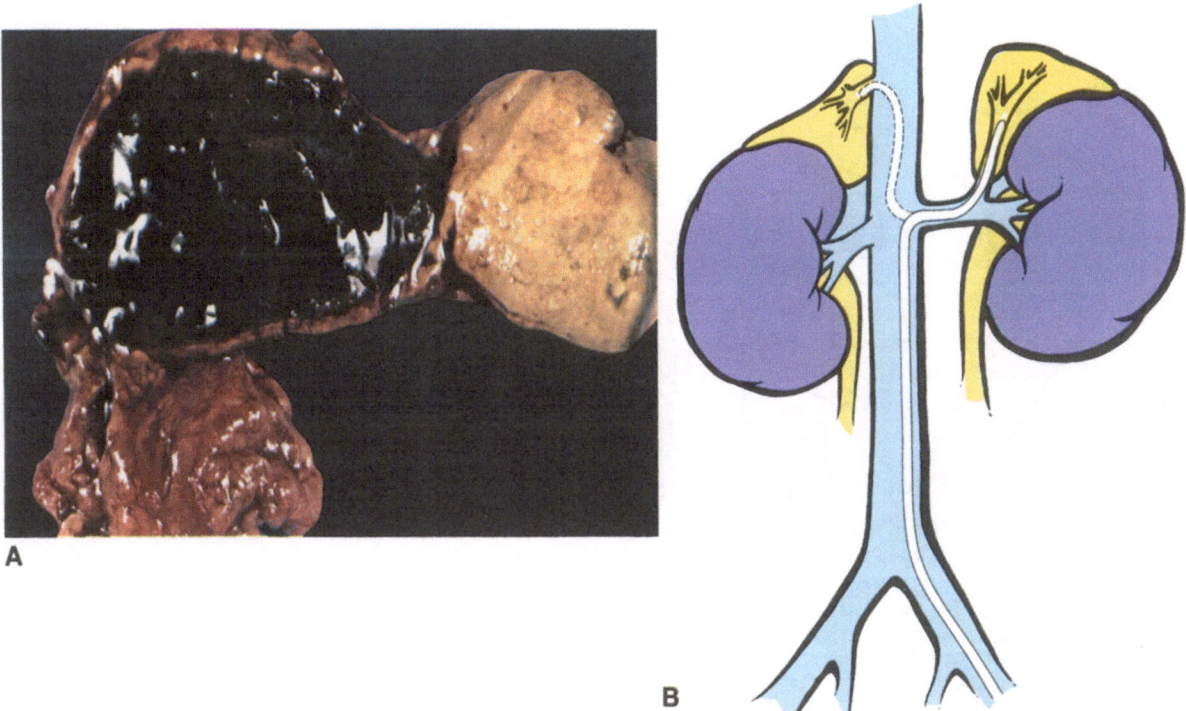

A

B

Invasive localization studies in primary aldosteronism. **A.** Intraadrenal   **Fig. 3-23.**
hemorrhage caused by dye extravasation during the course of adrenal venography.   **B.** Bilateral adrenal vein catheterization technique for sequential sampling of the left and right adrenal venous effluent and plasma aldosterone assay.
The technique lateralizes hyperfunction to one side in the case of an APA, and
to both sides in IHA. (Adapted from Melby JC et al: Diagnosis and localization of
aldosterone-producing adenomas by adrenal-vein catheterization. N Engl J Med
277:1051, 1967.)

accompanied by shorter hospitalization and decreased morbidity and
mortality (92). Among patients with IHA, surgical intervention is indicated only in those rare patients who have failed or cannot tolerate
medical therapy.

Postoperatively, serum electrolytes usually return to normal within
a day or so, and blood pressure reverts to normal within a matter of
weeks. The theoretical suppression of the contralateral zona glomerulosa has not been appreciated as a clinical problem.

Cushing's syndrome refers to the constellation of symptoms and signs   **Cushing's**
resulting from persistent elevation of plasma glucocorticoid. The most   **Syndrome**
common present cause is the excessive exogenous administration of
glucocorticoid medications. Cushing's disease, first described in 1932
(93), is this syndrome when caused by excess pituitary ACTH secretion
("pituitary Cushing's"). Up to 50% of patients with untreated Cushing's syndrome may die within 5 years (94); however, if the underlying
cause is treated, there is no malignancy, and plasma cortisol is carefully

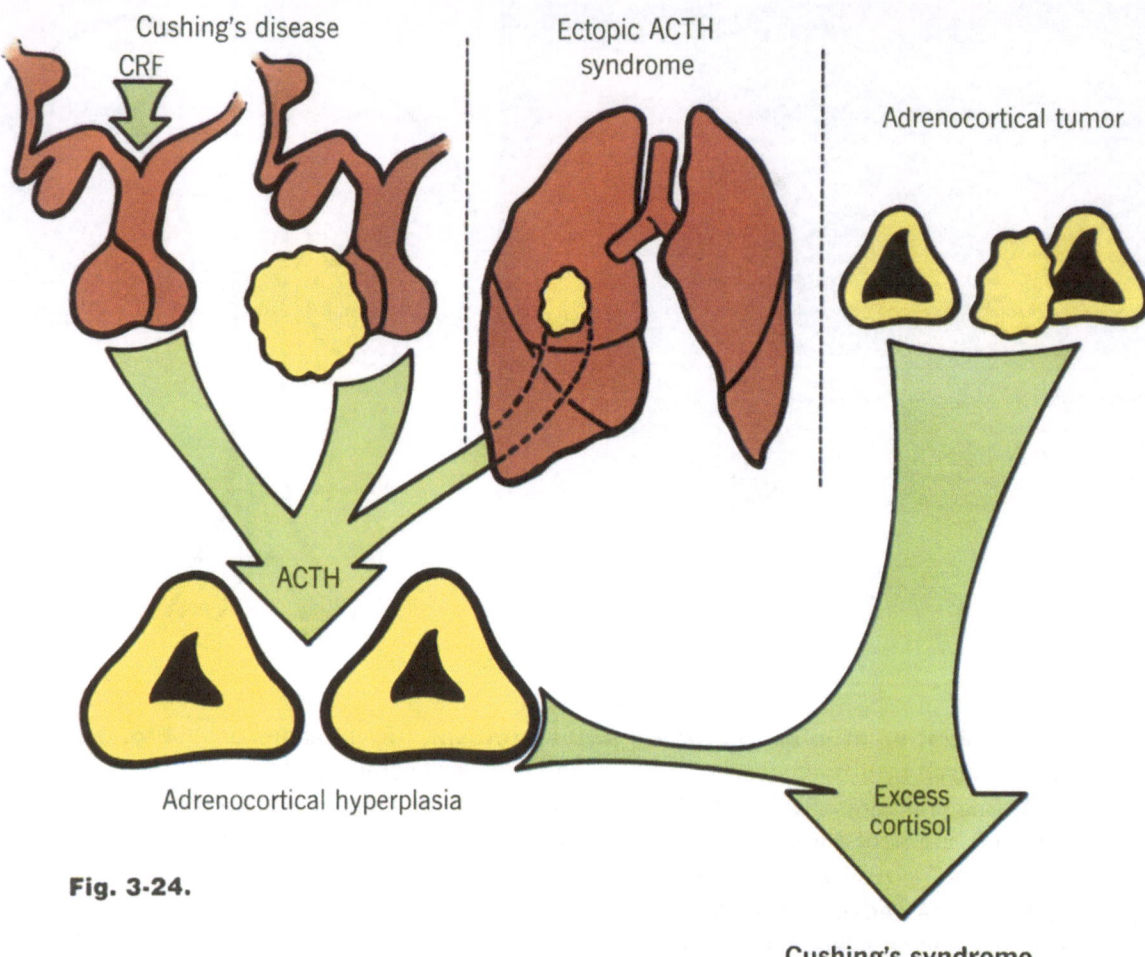

Fig. 3-24.

controlled, these patients probably may expect a normal life span (95). The clinical presentation alone may frequently solidify the diagnosis, but more subtle or atypical cases demand extensive investigation. Such factors as depression or stress can elevate serum cortisol. "Pseudo-Cushing's" syndrome has been described in alcoholic patients: the clinical features and biochemical tests unequivocally support the diagnosis of Cushing's syndrome, but the syndrome completely resolves with abstinence from alcohol (96,97). In addition to a confirmed diagnosis, identification of the specific etiologic source of Cushing's syndrome is critical in planning appropriate therapy.

CLASSIFICATION

There are three main causes of Cushing's syndrome (Fig. 3-24): pituitary-dependent Cushing's disease accounts for 65%–70% of cases, adrenal adenomas or carcinoma cause approximately 20%, and ectopic ACTH production by nonadrenal, nonpituitary tumors leads to 5%–10% (98). To these should be added the rare condition of non-ACTH-dependent bilateral adrenal hyperplasia (14).

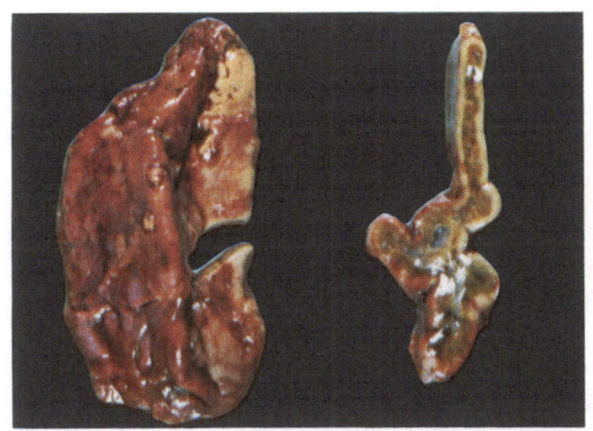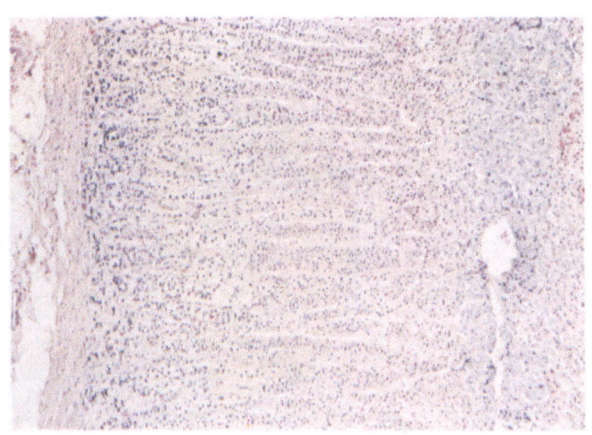

A   B

⊢_____⊣ 1 cm

Bilateral adrenal hyperplasia causing Cushing's syndrome. **A.** Gross
specimen. Glands are enlarged and rounded. **B.** Microscopic specimen. The
cortex is broadened with compact cell zona reticularis forming the inner one-
half and clear cell zona fasciculata forming the outer zone.

Fig. 3-25.

◀ **Causes of Cushing's syndrome.** Bilateral adrenocortical hyperplasia is produced by the increased secretion of ACTH either by the pituitary (Cushing's disease) or by an ectopic tumor (ectopic ACTH syndrome). Adrenocortical adenomas and carcinomas can both lead to the secretion of excess cortisol. CRF:
corticotropin-releasing factor.

Fig. 3-24.

PITUITARY

Our understanding of the pathology, localization, and appropriate treatment has evolved considerably since the discovery and clinical introduction of cortisone by Kendall and Hench allowed successful management of patients treated for Cushing's disease. While the pituitary was
recognized as the source of the problem, the standard, most effective,
and widely accepted form of treatment was bilateral total adrenalectomy (99) (Fig. 3-25) after which the patient was totally dependent on
glucocorticoid and mineralocorticoid replacement therapy. In an attempt to avert this problem, subtotal adrenalectomy was tried (100).
Unpredictable remnant function with high recurrence rates of Cushing's
syndrome led to the abandonment of this procedure. Radiotherapy to
the pituitary reflected efforts to redirect treatment at the etiologic
source and avert Nelson's syndrome (hyperpigmentation and pituitary
tumors that ''develop'' following total adrenalectomy for bilateral adrenocortical hyperplasia) (101). This was effective in only about 20% of
cases (99), in part due to techniques that are now outmoded. With the
introduction and refinement of transsphenoidal *selective* resection of
*micro*adenomas (102), the focus has been sharpened on the pituitary
(Fig. 3-26).

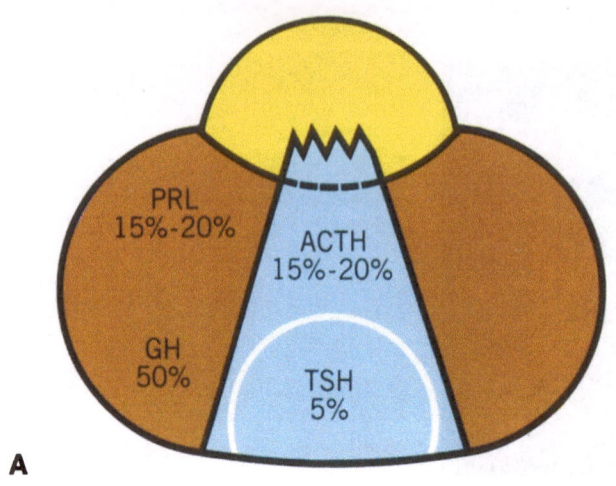

A

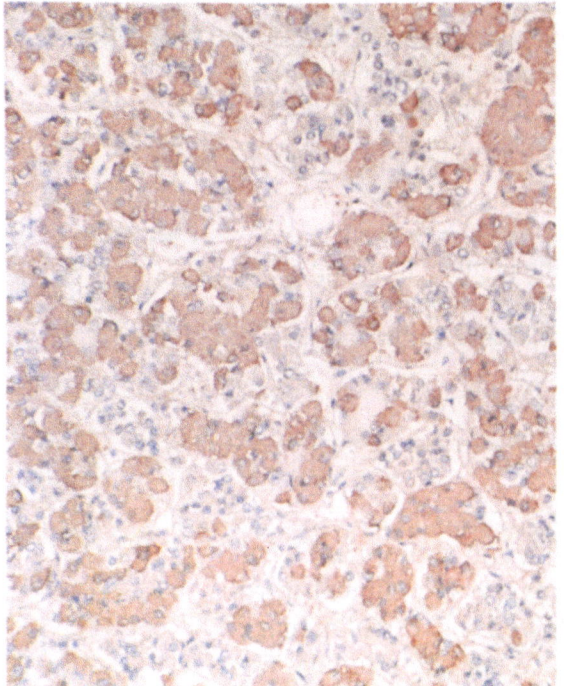

B

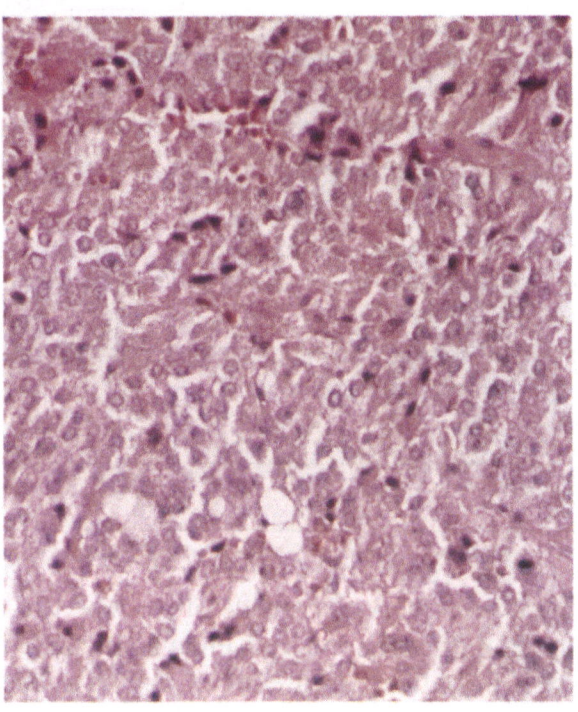

C

Fig. 3-26.   Pituitary: Normal and Cushing's Disease.   A. Typical cell distribution of the normal pituitary gland. Yellow, neurohypophysis; *PRL,* prolactin; *GH,* growth hormone; *TSH,* thyroid-stimulating hormone; *ACTH,* adrenocorticotropic hormone located in the midline "mucoid wedge" of the adenohypophysis.   **B.** Immunoperoxidase staining (for ACTH) of the normal pituitary "mucoid wedge."   **C.** Hematoxylin and eosin staining of Cushing's adenoma: mildly basophilic cytoplasmic staining.   **D.** Periodic acid–Schiff staining of Cushing's adenoma: characteristic positive cytoplasmic staining.   **E.** Immunoperoxidase staining of Cushing's adenoma: characteristic positive cytoplasmic staining.   **F.** Electron micrograph of Cushing's adenoma cell. Note modest variation in granule size, shape, and electron density as well as presence of cytoplasmic type 1 microfilaments (*arrows*).

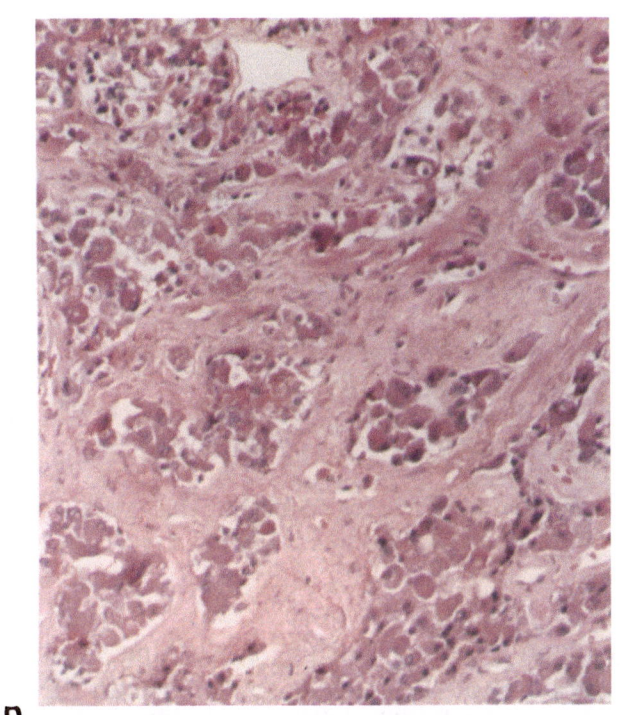

D

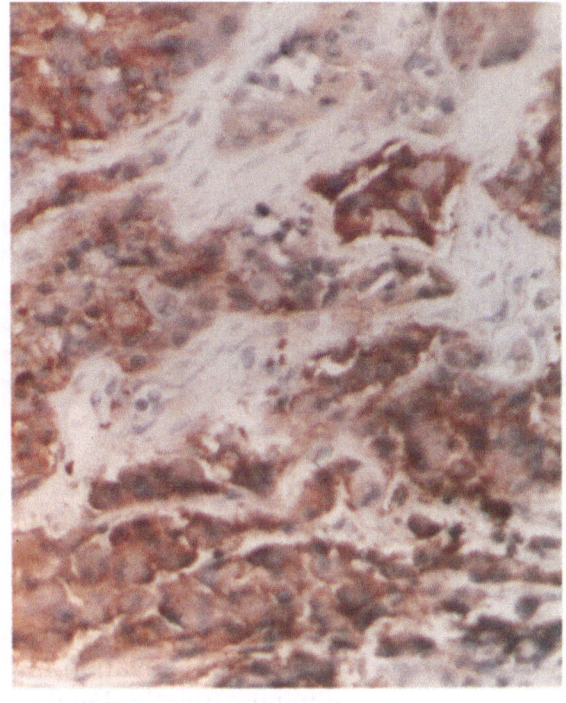

E

F

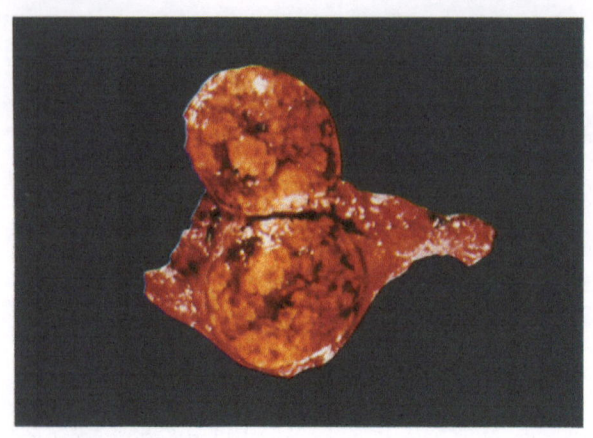
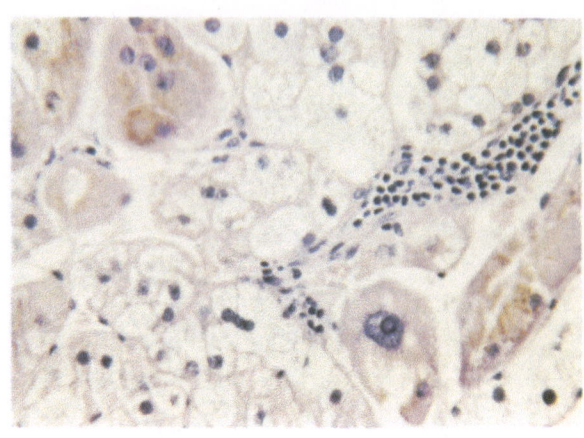

A

B

⌊___⌋ 1 cm

Fig. 3-27. Adenoma causing Cushing's syndrome. A. Gross specimen. This is a typical yellow, encapsulated tumor. **B.** Microscopic specimen. The adenoma consists of large clear cells.

Physiologically, one may regard pituitary Cushing's (Cushing's disease) as an elevation in the set point of ACTH release rather than the pituitary functioning totally autonomously. The pituitary is still responsive to steroid suppression (albeit in high doses) and metyrapone stimulation—perhaps implicating hypothalamic corticotropin-releasing factor (CRF) in the genesis of the disease. At least in part, the hypothesis implicating CRF forms the basis for the use of central nervous system–active treatment medications such as bromocriptine and cyproheptadine. Studies with the recently isolated and synthesized mammalian CRF may clarify the role of CRF in Cushing's disease (103).

ADRENAL

Cushing's syndrome produced by benign adrenal adenomas (Fig. 3-27) is more common than that caused by carcinomas in adults (Fig. 3-28). In contrast, carcinoma is by far the more common cause in children. As in many endocrine tumors, the pathologic distinction of adenoma versus carcinoma is sometimes quite difficult, the only definitive characteristic of malignancy being the presence of metastases.

ECTOPIC ACTH SYNDROME

In 1962, Liddle et al. (104) coined the term ''ectopic ACTH syndrome'' which referred to adrenocortical hyperplasia caused by ectopic ACTH production by nonadrenal, nonpituitary tumors. The overall incidence is commonly noted as 5%–10% (98,105), but this is probably a gross underestimation. In one series of patients with oat cell bronchial carcinomas, one-half demonstrated unsuppressible, elevated evening plasma cortisol levels (106). The tumors most commonly associated with ec-

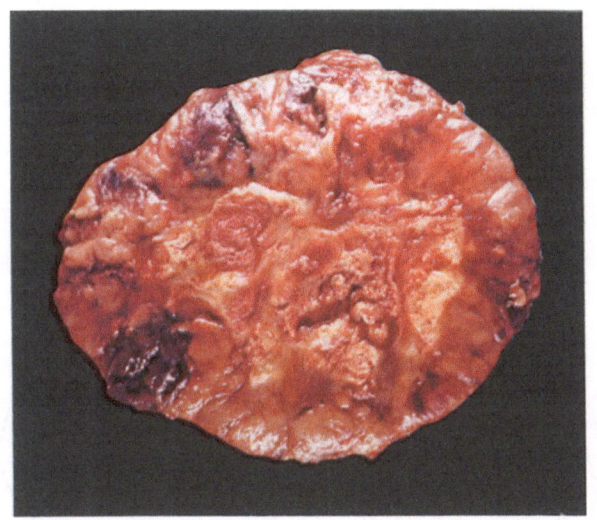
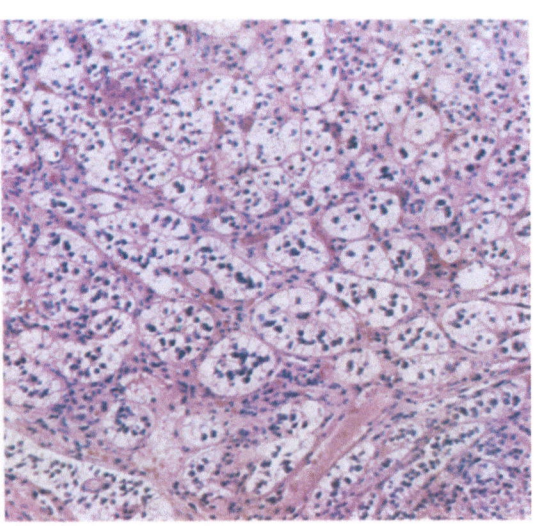

A

B

└─┘ 1 cm

Adrenal carcinoma causing Cushing's syndrome. **A.** Gross specimen. **Fig. 3-28.** These tumors are usually large; the cut surface shows broad areas of hemorrhage and necrosis. **B.** Microscopic specimen. Most carcinomas are a mixture of compact and clear cells.

topic ACTH secretion are part of the APUD cell system, including the following: thymoma; islet cell tumors of the pancreas; carcinoid tumors of the lung, pancreas, stomach, and ovary; medullary thyroid carcinoma; pheochromocytoma; and the principal one, oat cell bronchial carcinoma (107,108). If the tumor is benign (e.g., a bronchial carcinoid), removal is curative. However, most of these tumors are malignant, and the patient may die of the primary disease before becoming overtly cushingoid. Cushing's syndrome has also been reported in patients whose tumors presumably elaborate CRF (109).

NON-ACTH-DEPENDENT BILATERAL ADRENAL HYPERPLASIA

This disease entity is quite rare but is noteworthy in that it sometimes affects children and teenagers and may be associated with severe osteoporosis (110). Pathologically, the diagnostic features include bilateral non-ACTH-dependent nodular hyperplasia with intervening atrophic adrenal cortex in normal-sized adrenal glands. This suggests primary adrenal pathology, and bilateral total adrenalectomy is the recommended curative procedure (14).

DIAGNOSIS

Definitive diagnosis and precise localization utilizing both biochemical and radiologic techniques are pivotal in selecting the appropriate surgical approach.

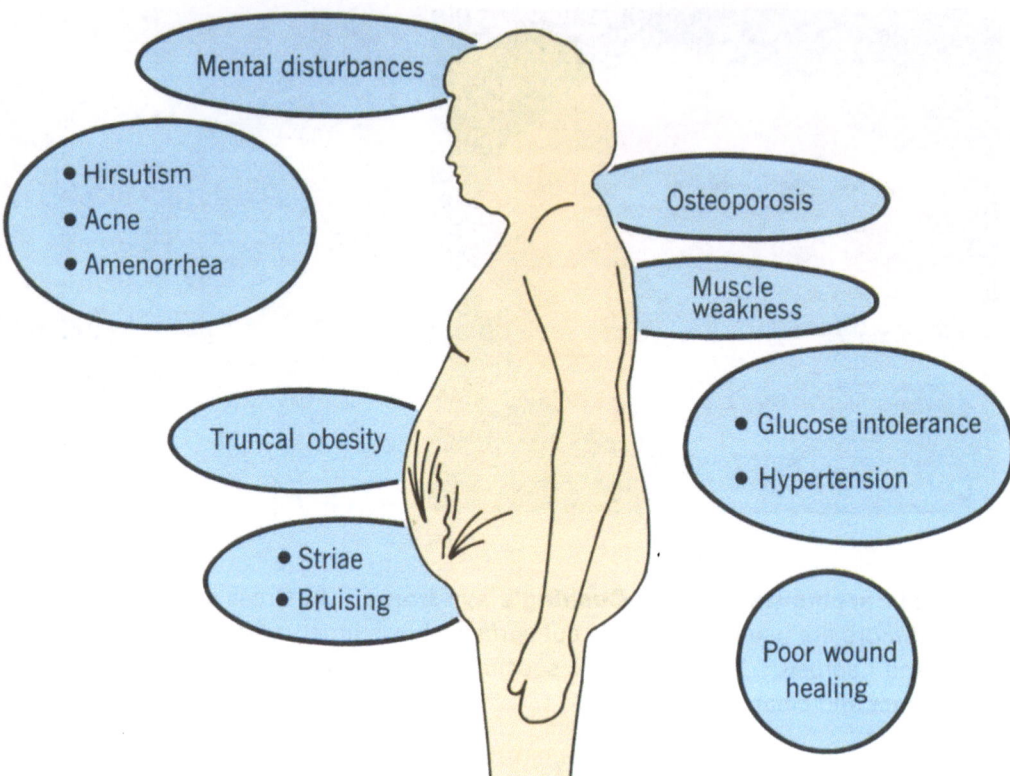

Fig. 3-29.   **Major clinical features of Cushing's syndrome.**

CLINICAL FEATURES

The major clinical features of Cushing's syndrome are shown in Figure 3-29. Cushing's disease affects women four times more often than men; it usually presents between the ages of 30 and 40 years (109,111,112). The most common clinical manifestation—obesity—is characteristically limited to the head, neck, and trunk, in sharp contrast to the thin, muscle-wasted arms, legs, and buttocks (14). This peculiar centripetal truncal fat distribution ordinarily distinguishes the patient with Cushing's syndrome from the one with simple, generalized obesity.

The skin may be atrophic and the face plethoric with prominent vessels, and there may be purplish striae on the abdomen, hips, flanks, breasts, and across the axillae. Capillary fragility is increased in Cushing's syndrome, and most patients describe skin bruising after minimal or unnoticed trauma. Not unexpectedly, wound healing is notoriously poor in these individuals (113,114). Acne of the face and trunk, hirsutism, and oligomenorrhea are helpful diagnostic signs in women; if virilism is pronounced, an adrenal carcinoma should be suspected. Males may manifest decreased libido and some have testicular softening and gynecomastia. Some degree of proximal muscle weakness and wasting is present in most patients with Cushing's syndrome. Os-

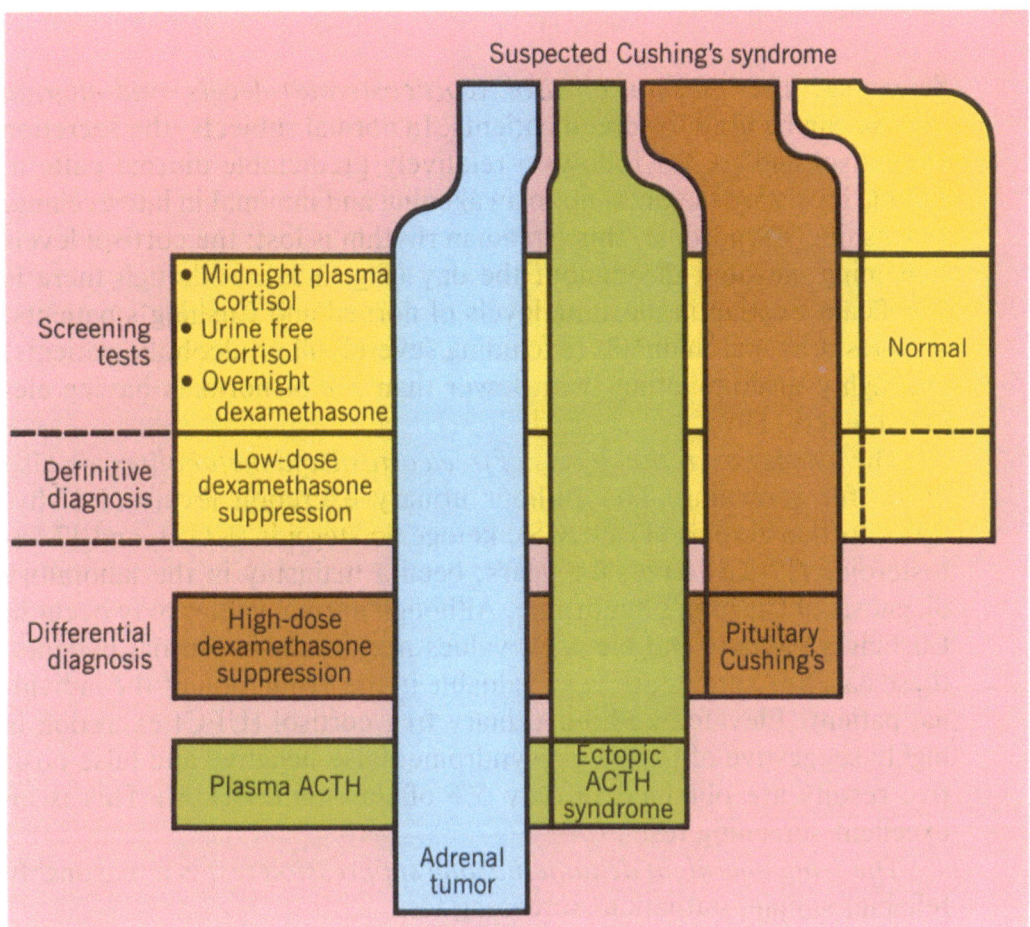

Suspected Cushing's syndrome

| Screening tests | • Midnight plasma cortisol • Urine free cortisol • Overnight dexamethasone | | | | Normal |

Low-dose dexamethasone suppression — Definitive diagnosis

Differential diagnosis — High-dose dexamethasone suppression — Pituitary Cushing's

Plasma ACTH — Ectopic ACTH syndrome

Adrenal tumor

Laboratory tests to determine the etiology of Cushing's syndrome.   **Fig. 3-30.**

teoporosis also is very common, and patients may present with pathologic fractures of the ribs or long bones, and especially vertebral body collapse.

A high incidence of hypertension has been noted, but it is rarely severe. Similarly, most patients have some degree of glucose intolerance, but frank diabetes with ketosis is distinctly uncommon. A complete spectrum of psychiatric illness, ranging from mild depression to major psychosis may be seen; mental disturbances are probably more common than is generally recognized. In patients with ectopic ACTH production, the typical clinical manifestations often are overshadowed by the weight loss and generalized tissue wasting secondary to advanced malignancy.

LABORATORY STUDIES

General plasma biochemical studies are not diagnostically helpful, although severe hypokalemia is a clue to the diagnosis of ectopic ACTH syndrome (115). Laboratory studies specific for Cushing's syndrome may be categorized as tests for screening, definitive diagnosis, and differential diagnosis (Fig. 3-30).

Screening. The *plasma cortisol (corticosteroid) levels and diurnal rhythm* can be used to screen patients. In normal subjects, the secretion of cortisol and ACTH follows a relatively predictable diurnal pattern: plasma levels are maximal upon awakening and minimal in late evening. In Cushing's syndrome, this circadian rhythm is lost: the cortisol levels remaining elevated throughout the day (Fig. 3-31). Although there is significant overlap in morning levels of normal and Cushing's patients, samples drawn at midnight (excluding severely ill or alcoholic patients) are highly discriminating, with fewer than 5% of normals having elevated levels (116).

The *urinary excretion levels of free cortisol and metabolites* are also useful for screening. The 24-hour urinary excretion levels of 17-hydroxycorticosteroids (17-OHCS), ketogenic steroids (KGS), and 17-ketosteroids (17-KS) have, for years, been a mainstay in the laboratory diagnosis of Cushing's syndrome. Although normal values may occur in Cushing's patients and elevated values may occur in normal patients, these baseline studies are very valuable in the evaluation of the individual patient. Elevated 24-hour urinary free cortisol (UFC) excretion is highly suggestive of Cushing's syndrome; false-negative and false-positive results are obtained in only 5% of the studies (116). This is an excellent screening test.

The *1-mg overnight dexamethasone suppression test* is a reasonably reliable, simple, outpatient screening test.

> The patient is given 1 of dexamethasone by mouth at 11 p.m. The following morning, at 8 a.m., the plasma cortisol level is drawn.

In normal patients, the clearly low cortisol level reflects the suppressed pituitary–adrenal axis. Fewer than 2% of Cushing's patients are suppressed normally (116); however, a significant number of obese, depressed, alcoholic, or chronically ill patients fail to show suppression.

Definitive Diagnosis. When Cushing's syndrome is suspected either clinically or by biochemical screening tests, appropriate confirmation employing the *low-dose dexamethasone suppression test* becomes necessary.

> The patient receives 0.5 mg dexamethasone orally every 6 hours for 2 consecutive days. On the second day, the 24-hour urine collection is sent for 17-OHCS, 17-KS, KGS, and UFC determinations.

With rare exceptions, normal subjects demonstrate suppressed urinary levels (as defined by each laboratory), but levels from patients with Cushing's syndrome are not suppressed normally (117). This test is highly reliable in making a definitive diagnosis of Cushing's syndrome.

Differential Diagnosis. As has been stated, establishing the etiology of Cushing's syndrome is critical to subsequent therapy. These tests are based on the fact that, in general, adrenal tumors and ectopic ACTH-

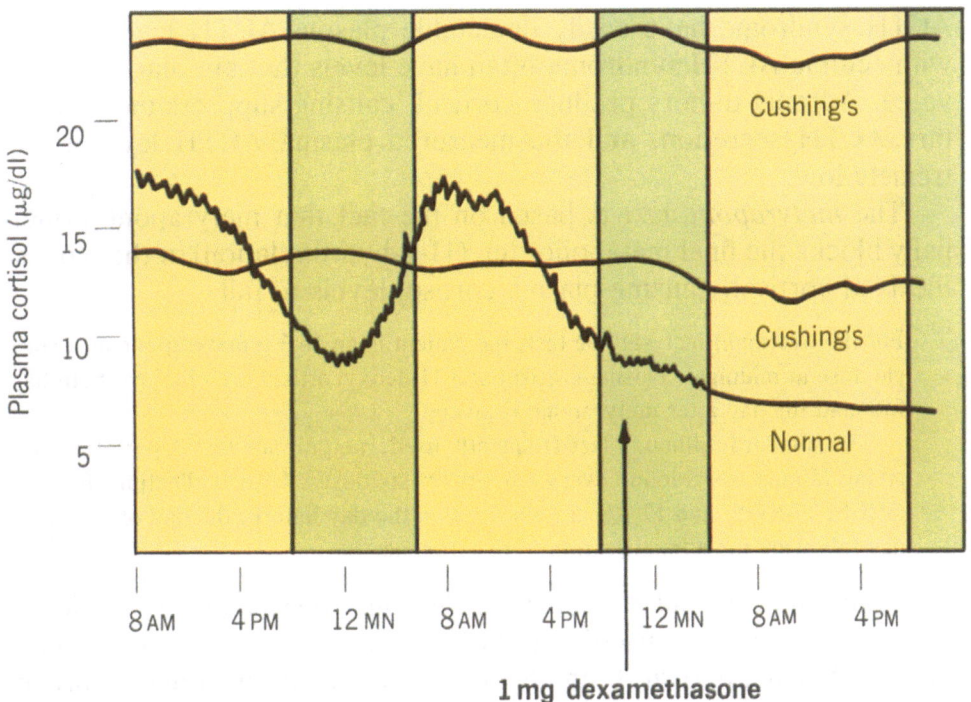

1 mg dexamethasone

Plasma cortisol rhythms. Plasma cortisol rhythms in normal subject and in two patients with Cushing's syndrome. The normal diurnal variation in plasma cortisol concentration is lost in Cushing's syndrome. One milligram of dexamethasone given at 11 p.m. suppresses the 8 a.m. plasma cortisol level in normal subjects but not in patients with Cushing's syndrome.

Fig. 3-31.

secreting tumors function autonomously and are virtually unaffected by hormonal manipulation. In contrast, the feedback mechanism in pituitary Cushing's is functioning, although it is abnormal.

The *high-dose dexamethasone suppression test* is conducted as follows:

> The patient is given 2 mg dexamethasone orally every 6 hours for 2 consecutive days (rarely extended to 3 days). On the second day, the 24-hour urine collection is sent for 17-OHCS, 17-KS, KGS, and UFC determinations. Results are compared to baseline urinary studies obtained prior to any dexamethasone administration.

When pre- and postsuppression urinary values are compared, nearly all patients with *adrenal* tumors fail to suppress to 40% of baseline; however, most patients with pituitary Cushing's suppress to at least 40% of baseline (117). As many as 15% of patients with Cushing's disease may require higher (16 or 24 mg/day) doses of dexamethasone to suppress. (Some patients with presumed ectopic CRF production show substantial suppression of steroid production with a high dose of dexamethasone.)

The keystone to the valuable *plasma ACTH assay* is a sensitive and reliable assay technique. Patients with Cushing's disease or ectopic

ACTH syndrome have easily detectable plasma ACTH levels, those with ectopic ACTH syndrome often have levels that are markedly elevated. Adrenal tumors produce cortisol, causing suppression of pituitary ACTH secretion, and the measured plasma ACTH level is extremely low.

The *metyrapone test* is based on the fact that metyrapone principally blocks the final metabolic step (11-β-hydroxylation) in the biosynthesis of cortisol, causing plasma cortisol levels to fall.

> For the overnight metyrapone test, the patient is given 3 g metyrapone as a single dose at midnight. Plasma cortisol and 11-deoxycortisol are obtained both before and the day after metyrapone is given.
>
> The standard, although less frequently used, metyrapone test is performed by giving 750 mg metyrapone every 4 hours for six doses. Urine collections for 17-OHCS, 17-KGS, and 17-KS are obtained on the day before, the day of, and the day following the administration of metyrapone.

In normal subjects and patients with Cushing's disease, the reduction in plasma cortisol is "sensed" by the pituitary, and ACTH secretion is increased. This, in turn, promotes increased synthesis of deoxycortisol (compound S, which has no suppressive action on pituitary ACTH secretion)—the immediate precursor of cortisol. Increased compound S production is reflected in either increased serum levels or increased urinary excretion of 17-OHCS or KGS. If urinary values or serum compound S levels fail to rise in a properly administered metyrapone test, the diagnosis of Cushing's disease is virtually excluded. In contrast, patients with Cushing's syndrome due to adrenal neoplasm or ectopic ACTH syndrome usually do not show an increase in 17-OHCS excretion with metyrapone.

PREOPERATIVE LOCALIZATION STUDIES

Localization studies are frequently delayed until biochemical results offer an appropriate direction, but they may facilitate an earlier, definitive diagnosis (118). Nephrotomography, selective angiography, and adrenal venography are very rarely used since the advent of high-resolution CT scanners.

COMPUTERIZED TOMOGRAPHY

CT scanning provides a rapid, accurate, and reliable method for identifying virtually all adrenal tumors in patients with Cushing's syndrome (33,118,119) and it is the localizing modality of choice (Fig. 3-32). This is also the technique of choice in detecting nodules in the lungs, mediastinum, and pancreas (120,121), all of which are potential tumor sites for ectopic ACTH syndrome (115,118).

Pituitary CT scanning has superseded skull x-rays, angiography, and even multidirectional sellar tomography for the evaluation of Cush-

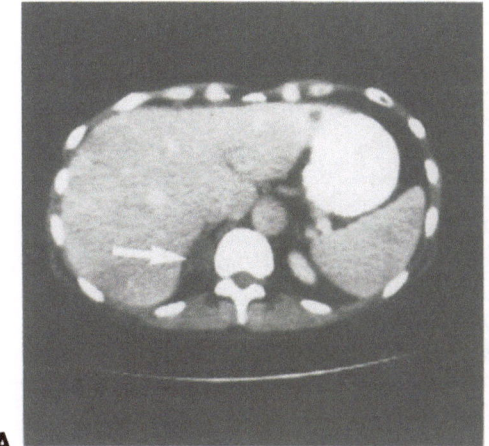

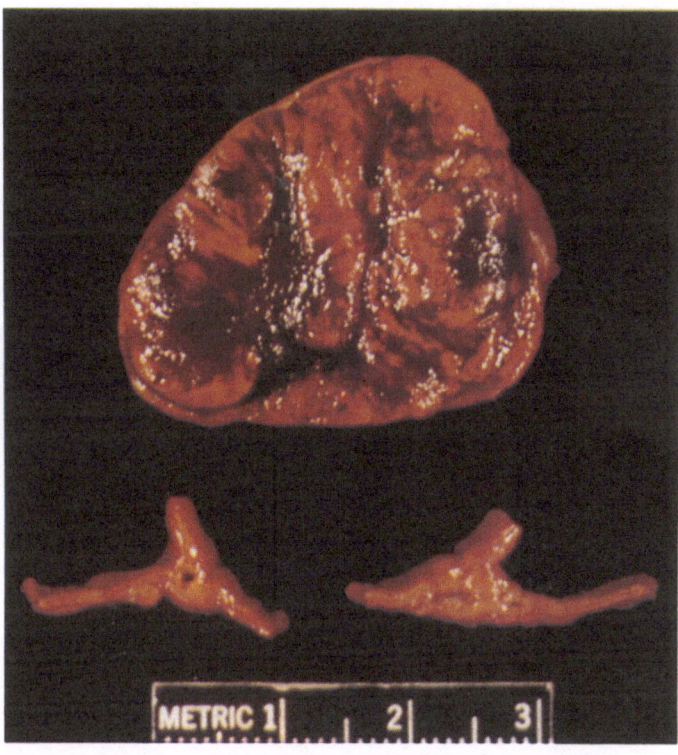

Cushing's adenoma. **A.** CT scan of right adrenal Cushing's adenoma (*arrow*). **B.** Corresponding gross specimen.   **Fig. 3-32.**

ing's disease. However, even with state-of-the-art CT scanners, only about 50% of surgically proven pituitary microadenomas are preoperatively identified (122).

ADRENAL SCINTIGRAPHY

Radionuclide adrenal scintigraphy with NP-59 (using gamma camera tomography) is a useful, reasonably accurate, and noninvasive adrenal imaging technique that provides both physiologic and anatomic information (86). A functioning, benign tumor shows up as a unilateral hot spot (usually with no uptake by the contralateral, suppressed gland); hyperplasia is characterized by a bilaterally increased uptake of radioactivity, the appearance of which is described as "headlights burning through a fog." An adrenocortical carcinoma generally does not show uptake; however, due to contralateral suppression, the other adrenal does not visualize either.

Several important drawbacks detract from the use of the NP-59 scan. Pre- and postscan thyroid blocking is important, since a potentially thyroid-ablative dose of ^{131}I is given. Poor storage properties, moderate expense, time delay, and significant radiation exposure make restricted and thoughtful patient selection for this examination important.

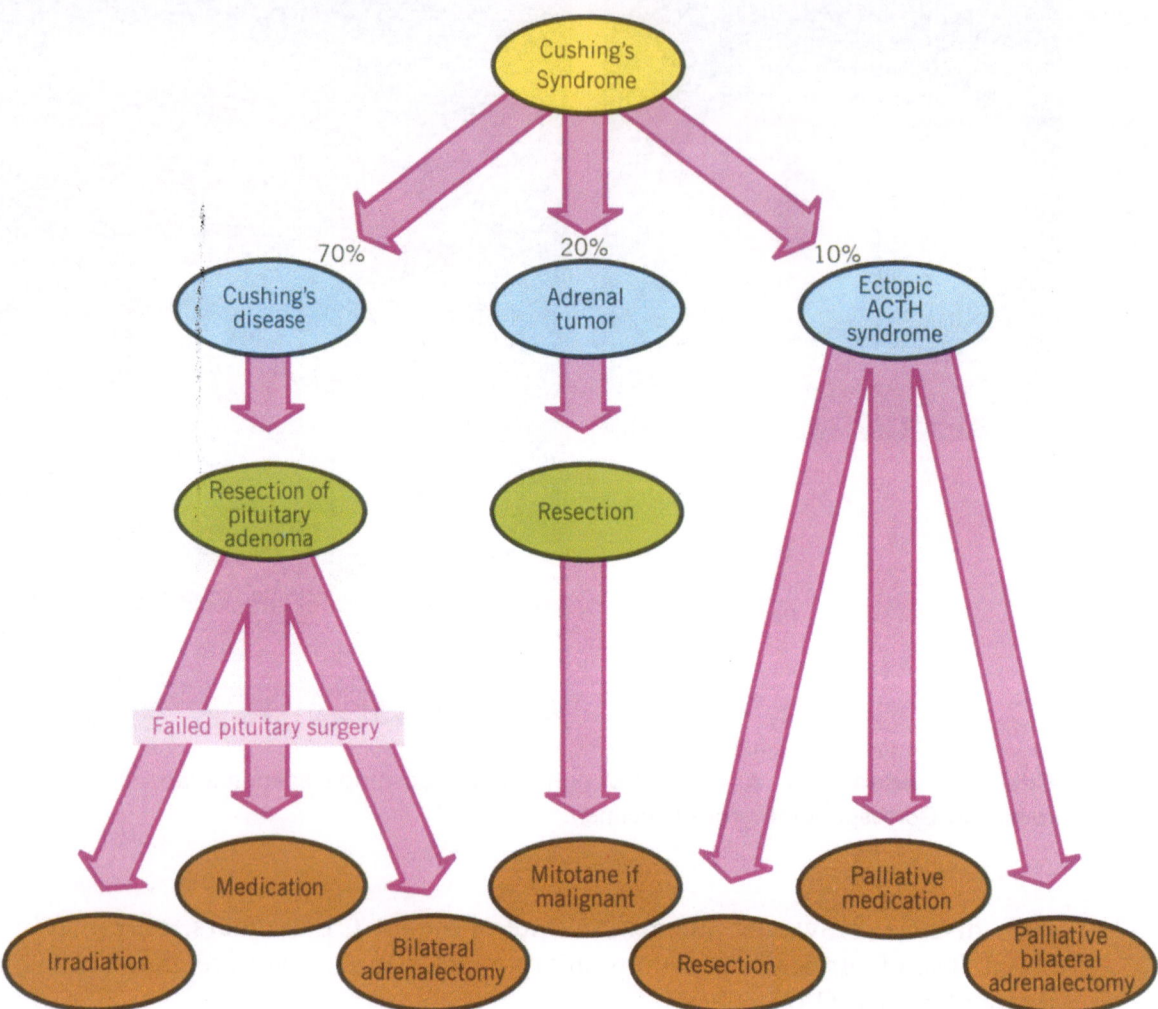

Fig. 3-33.   **Therapeutic alternatives in Cushing's syndrome.**

TREATMENT

CUSHING'S DISEASE

A number of both medical and surgical options are available for the treatment of Cushing's disease (Fig. 3-33). Surgically, the primary choices are (a) transsphenoidal excision of a micro- or macroadenoma or (b) bilateral total adrenalectomy followed by prophylactic pituitary irradiation to prevent Nelson's syndrome. Medically, one may choose among (a) pituitary irradiation, (b) medications "inhibiting" the CRF–ACTH axis, (c) cortisol synthesis blockers, and (d) adrenolytic drugs.

Surgical. The recent dramatic neurosurgical advances, which have been substantiated by excellent results (123,126), qualify surgery as the

Steroid Replacement Therapy After Bilateral Adrenalectomy for Hyperplasia (Cushing's Syndrome) Table 3-3.

Perioperative steroid preparation (Table 3-5)
Postoperative days 1–3
  Prednisolone sodium phosphate (Hydeltrasol), 40 mg IM or IV every 12 hours
After day 3 (oral intake)
  Hydrocortisone, 20 mg in a.m., 10 mg in p.m. + fludrocortisone acetatate
    (Florinef), 0.1 mg daily
  Medialert bracelet
  Provide dexamethasone 4-mg syringe for emergency self-injection

---

current treatment of choice for Cushing's disease. Among over 100 patients so treated, the 80% overall cure rate, 95% remission rate of noninvasive tumors, 6% recurrence rate, and minimal morbidity and mortality attest to this choice (123). Cure of the hypercortisolism is immediate, and experienced surgeons can safely perform this operation on these high-risk patients. Bilateral total adrenalectomy remains a reliable, acceptable form of therapy for pituitary-treatment failures (126,127) (Table 3-3).

Nonsurgical. Present-day external pituitary radiation as primary treatment of Cushing's disease has had variable success. It may be the treatment of choice in children (80% success rate), but only 50%–60% of adults sustain remissions (128). These results, along with the delay of 6–18 months for response, dampen enthusiasm for this approach. The implantation of yttrium-90 has not been well evaluated in the United States.

Cyproheptadine, which acts as a serotonin antagonist, is thought to inhibit CRF. Some successful remissions have been reported (129), but the many cases in which it has been ineffective relegate it to secondary importance. Bromocriptine, a dopamine agonist, has been effective in only sparse reports (130), presumably by an inhibitory effect on pituitary ACTH secretion. Its clinical utility awaits further investigation. Metyrapone has enjoyed popularity in Europe both as chronic therapy and for preoperative preparation (131). Its use in the United States, however, has been principally restricted to adjunctive therapy for pituitary irradiation, or to palliation of either ectopic ACTH syndrome or adrenocortical carcinoma (115,132).

Aminoglutethimide, an inhibitor of the conversion of cholesterol to pregnenolone, also has been given for palliation, similar to metyrapone. There has been much greater interest and more investigations regarding its effectiveness in metastatic breast carcinoma (see the next section). Mitotane (*O,p'*-DDD) causes necrosis of the zona fasciculata and zona reticularis. Long-term results have been poor, with only a 17% sustained, 2-year remission following an 8-month course of medication (133).

ADRENAL TUMOR

There is little disagreement concerning the need for surgical resection in patients with an adrenal tumor (111,127). If the tumor is greater than 10–15 cm in diameter it may necessitate a thoracoabdominal approach for necessary exposure to proceed safely with en bloc resection. For smaller benign tumors the posterior retroperitoneal approach is preferred. (134) Adrenalectomy for Cushing's syndrome may be followed by significant complications. Increased susceptibility to wound infections, delayed wound healing, thromboembolism, and atelectasis and pneumonitis require special attention. Of particular note, despite perioperative exogenous steroid support, during the early postoperative period prominent symptoms of malaise, myalgias, arthralgias, and even gastrointestinal upset may occur, reflecting the acute decline in endogenous cortisol. This period is followed by an interval of variable length during which the contralateral adrenal assumes fully supportive adrenocortical capacity. The patient may again suffer similar symptoms, presumably indicative of a relative hypocortisolism stimulating pituitary ACTH, and resumption of the normal servo mechanism. The weaning of exogenous cortisol can best be titrated by an intelligent, informed patient who expects these symptoms yet avoids serious adrenocortical insufficiency (Table 3-4).

ECTOPIC ACTH SYNDROME

If the tumor is benign (e.g., a bronchial carcinoid), removal is curative. Many ectopic ACTH-secreting tumors, however, are malignant and widely metastatic at the time Cushing's syndrome becomes clinically apparent. Palliation using the aforementioned medications may offer metabolic control. Rarely, bilateral total adrenalectomy becomes justified in less aggressive but unresectable primary tumors.

Table 3-4.   Steroid Replacement Therapy After Unilateral Adrenalectomy for Tumor (Cushing's Syndrome)

Perioperative steroid preparation (Table 3-5)

Postoperative days 1–3
Prednisolone sodium phosphate (Hydeltrasol), 40 mg IM every 12 hours or IV every 8 hours

After day 3 (oral intake)*
1 month prednisone, 5 mg in a.m., 2.5–5 mg in p.m.
1 month prednisone, 5 mg in a.m.
1 month prednisone, 2.5 mg in a.m.

* Titrate dose according to withdrawal symptoms, i.e., myalgia, arthralgia, anorexia, nausea (increase dose before vomiting, hypotension).

PERIOPERATIVE STEROID PREPARATION

Many patients undergoing operation are, or have recently taken, cortisone or one of its analogues. The predictable suppressed endogenous adrenocortical secretion following unilateral or bilateral adrenalectomy for Cushing's syndrome, or potential suppression in the face of exogenous corticosteroid administration must be borne in mind (Table 3-5). Physiologic stress such as serious infection or general anesthetic can be extremely hazardous in the unprepared patient, leading to circulatory shock or even death due to adrenal insufficiency.

As a general guideline, the quantity of adrenal steroids taken by a patient must equal or exceed the normal physiologic output (assume the equivalent of 25 mg cortisone per day, Table 3-6) of the adrenal for 1

Perioperative Steroid Preparation* Table 3-5.

*Intramuscular**
  Dexamethasone (Decadron), 4 mg IM at least 1 hour preoperatively and every 12 hours on day of surgery
or
  Prednisolone sodium phosphate (Hydeltrasol), 40 mg IM at least 1 hour preoperatively and 40 mg every 8 hours on day of surgery

*Intravenous**
  Dexamethasone (Decadron), 4 mg IV on call to the operating room and every 6 hours on day of surgery
or
  Prednisolone sodium phosphate (Hydeltrasol), 40 mg IV on call to the operating room and every 6 hours on day of surgery
or
  Methylprednisolone (e.g., Solu Medrol), 40 mg IV on call to the operating room and every 6 hours on the day of surgery

* Adequate steroid preparation can be administered by either the intramuscular or intravenous route.

Relative Potencies and Sodium Retention of Various Glucocorticoids Table 3-6.

Medication	Equivalent Dose (mg)	Salt Retention
Hydrocortisone (cortisol)	20	1.0
Cortisone	25	0.8
Prednisone	5	0.8
Prednisolone	5	
Methylprednisolone	4	0
Dexamethasone	0.75	0
Betamethasone	0.6	0

week or more. After steroid medication is discontinued, a variable interval is required for normalization of the pituitary–adrenal axis and for normal adrenal responsiveness to occur. The exact chronologic relationship cannot be stated precisely. In order to provide a sufficient margin of safety, one should assume inadequate adrenal responsiveness persists for 6 months after physiologic doses have been stopped, and for 1 year if large doses have been taken.

Appropriate tapering of corticosteroids is also critical for safe patient management and must be individualized, precluding a standard recommendation. Following bilateral adrenalectomy, one cannot accurately judge the adequacy of cortisone replacement by ACTH levels. The reason for this is that in normal individuals, while ACTH follows a diurnal pattern, its actual secretion is continuous. Replacement is in effect "bolus" therapy. If the measured fasting morning ACTH is "normal," most patients will be receiving excessive cortisone replacement.

Adrenal Gland and Metastatic Breast Carcinoma

Breast cancer is a clinical disease of immense proportions. A prevalence of over 500,000, an estimated 110,000 newly diagnosed cases per year (135), and the grim fact that only about one-half of these will be cured by primary therapy (136) attest to its serious nature. Only 2 years after Halsted's publication (137) of surgical therapy for patients with extensive breast cancer in 1894, Beatson demonstrated favorable effects of oophorectomy in these patients (138). Huggins and Bergenstal, in 1952, were the first to demonstrate striking remission of advanced breast carcinoma after bilateral total adrenalectomy (139). Until recently, adrenalectomy (with previous or concomitant oophorectomy) remained the "supercastration" procedure of choice, with objective response rates of 25%–50% in selected patients (140).

Numerous reports suggest that estrogen is the major hormonal stimulus for growth in hormone-dependent breast carcinoma. The distinction between hormone-dependent and hormone-independent tumors is of major importance because their biologic behavior and treatment responsiveness are quite different. The measurement of estrogen receptors (ER) and progesterone receptors (PgR) facilitates categorizing these subtypes. Estrogen-receptor negative (ER−) tumors grow faster, recur earlier, and cause shortened patient survival compared to ER+ tumors (141). While fewer than 5% of ER− tumors respond to hormonal therapy, 50%–60% of ER+, and 80% of ER+, PgR+ tumors respond to endocrine treatment (136).

The initial endocrine treatment of choice is the nonsteroidal competitive binder, antiestrogen tamoxifen. It has emerged as a highly effective, nontoxic medication that appears equivalent to surgical oophorectomy in rate and duration of tumor remission (142,143).

In postmenopausal women, however, direct secretion of estrogen

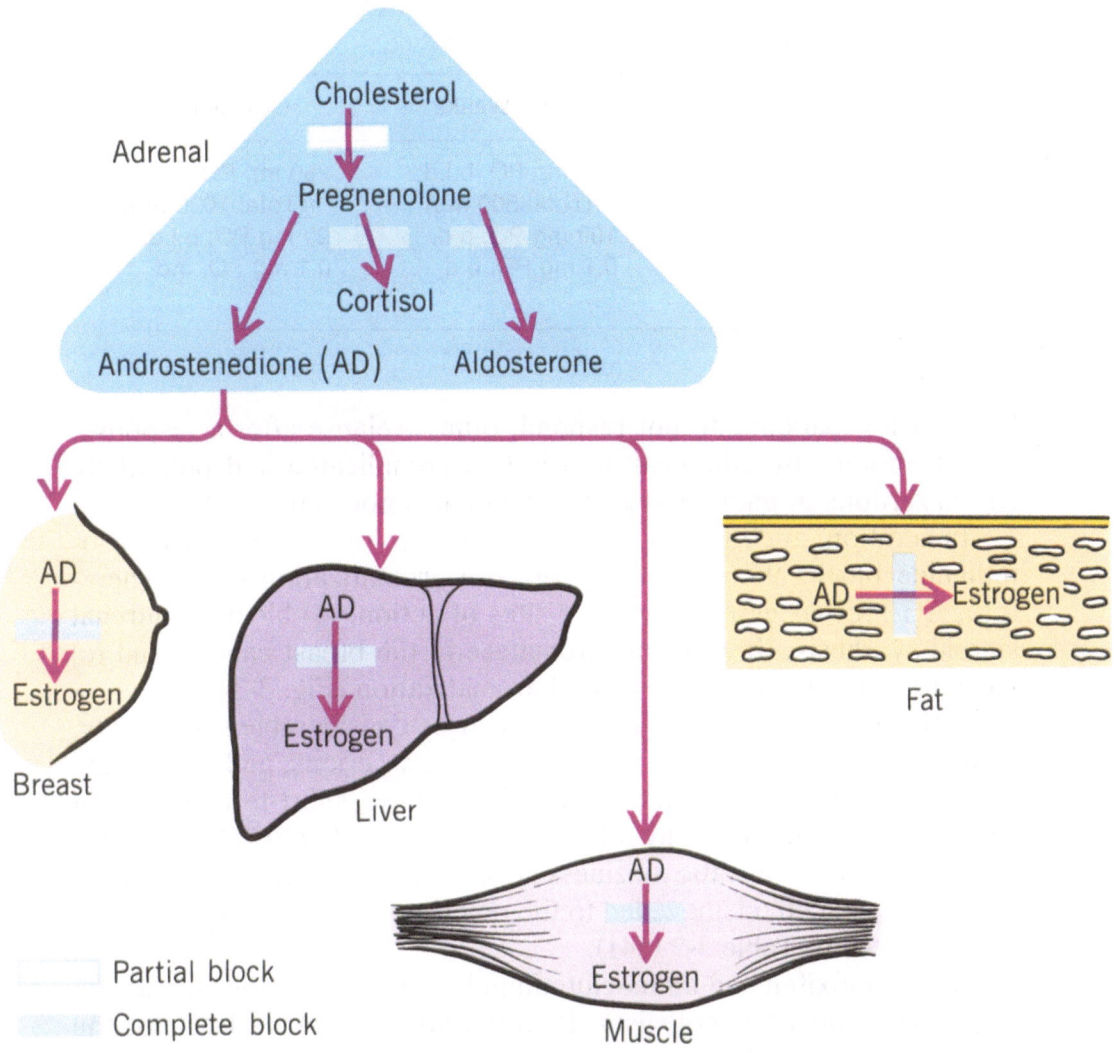

Sites of action of aminoglutethimide.   **Fig. 3-34.**

by the ovaries is minimal (144). Adrenalectomy has been used as further ablation of estrogen production. However, direct adrenal secretion of estrogen is also low (144). It is now known that the major source of estrogen in postmenopausal women with metastatic breast cancer is through the conversion of adrenally derived estrogen precursors (catalyzed by the enzyme *aromatase*) by *peripheral* sources such as fat, muscle, liver, and the breast cancer itself (145). "Medical adrenalectomy," employing the steroid biosynthesis blocker aminoglutethimide together with hydrocortisone (AG-HC), has been shown to be equally as effective as surgical adrenalectomy (146,147). Drug therapy (AG-HC) has the advantages that it (a) avoids surgical morbidity and rare mortality, (b) can be used in nonsurgical candidates, and (c) is totally reversible. It is fully reversible in that full adrenal function returns within days of stopping the medication (141). This is very important because one-

Table 3-7. **Recommended Regimen for "Medical Adrenalectomy" in the Treatment of Metastatic Breast Cancer**

Medication	First 2 Weeks	Chronic
Aminoglutethimide	250 mg PO, b.i.d. (Total 500 mg)	250 mg PO, q.i.d. (Total 1000 mg)
Hydrocortisone	100 mg PO, q.d.	20 mg PO, b.i.d.
Fludrocortisone acetate (Florinef)	0.1 mg PO, q.d.	0.1 mg PO, q.d.

half of ER+ patients do not respond, others relapse after a response, and chemotherapy administration is less complicated and potentially less hazardous in patients with normal endogenous adrenal function.

In addition, and of even greater therapeutic significance, aminoglutethimide blocks 95%–98% of peripheral aromatization (148). Therefore, AG-HC has essentially three sites of action: (a) blocking adrenal steroid synthesis, (b) blocking aromatase in the breast cancer, and (c) blocking extraglandular, peripheral aromatization (Fig. 3-34).

Unfortunately, aminoglutethimide causes considerable side effects, although they are usually temporary and rarely serious, and they rarely cause total cessation of the medication. These short-term/long-term symptoms include lethargy (42%/15%), skin rash (30%/1%), ataxia (11%/3%), and orthostatic dizziness (16%/10%) (141). Attempts to minimize these side effects have led to the recommended medication schedule presented in Table 3-7 (141).

Both tamoxifen and aminoglutethimide have gained widespread acceptance by breast oncologists. It would appear that, at least for the present, medical endocrine manipulation has virtually replaced surgical ablation in the treatment of women with metastatic breast carcinoma.

Adrenocortical Carcinoma

Adrenocortical carcinoma is a rare, often highly malignant neoplasm that is usually diagnosed late in its course, resulting in short life expectancy (149–152). The reported incidence is 2 per million population per year (153); it accounts for only 0.2% of all deaths from cancer (154). The tumor may excessively secrete one or more cortical steroids to produce a clinical syndrome, thereby being classified as "functioning." The majority of functioning carcinomas occur *before* the age of 40 years (151) and have a *female:male* ratio of 4:1 (150). Those cancers that do not produce hormones causing a clinical syndrome are considered "nonfunctioning" (155); 75% are found in patients *over* the age of 40, with the *reverse* sex ratio of *male:female*, 2:1 (156). Functioning adrenal cancers may produce Cushing's syndrome (hypercortisolism), virilizing or feminizing syndromes, Conn's syndrome (hyperaldosteronism), or mixed syndromes.

DIAGNOSIS

CLINICAL FEATURES

Mixed syndromes such as Cushing's and virilization strongly suggest adrenal carcinoma. The combination of hirsutism, acne, amenorrhea, and rapidly progressing Cushing's syndrome in a young female is a classic example (157). When Cushing's syndrome occurs in a child, adrenal carcinoma is a common cause (153).

In infancy, the "adrenogenital syndrome" is usually caused by an enzyme deficiency leading to congenital adrenal hyperplasia. However, in prepubertal females, virilization is most commonly caused by adrenal carcinoma. In a child normal at birth who later develops precocious virilization, adrenal carcinoma should be suspected. Feminization in the adult male is very rare (158) and highly suspect for adrenal carcinoma; it is heralded by gynecomastia, testicular atrophy, and impotency.

Nonfunctioning cancers are usually discovered late because the lack of an endocrine syndrome allows marked growth until a mass or flank pain leads to the diagnosis (156).

LABORATORY STUDIES

When an adrenal carcinoma is functioning the patient almost invariably excretes inordinately large amounts of 17-KS, irrespective of the clinical syndrome (150). Adrenal carcinoma is characteristically inefficient in producing normal steroid hormones. This is reflected in the fact that only when the mass of cancer attains large size does it produce the syndrome. This is also the reason the urine has markedly elevated levels of steroid precursor metabolites. Adrenal cancers fail to become suppressed with high-dose dexamethasone (Fig. 3-30). Such tumors can form pregnenolone or other early precursors in steroid synthesis (rather than the typical steroid products), which can be used as markers to gauge the clinical status of the patient (156).

PREOPERATIVE LOCALIZATION STUDIES AND STAGING

The tumor is reliably localized by CT scanning, which may also demonstrate signs of malignancy, including an irregular, poorly defined margin, inhomogeneous density from necrosis, local invasion, and distant metastases (33) (Fig. 3-35). Vena caval studies may be indicated to define local invasion, extrinsic compression, or tumor thrombus (159,160). Arteriography is occasionally used to define the vascular anatomy to aid in planning surgical excision.

Staging is important from both therapeutic and prognostic standpoints. The most widely accepted system is. that proposed by Macfarlane and modified by Sullivan (155) (Table 3-8).

Table 3-8.

Staging of Adrenocortical Cancers

Stage	Size (cm)	Nodes*	Local Invasion*	Metastases*
I	≤5	–	–	–
II	>5	–	–	–
III	Any size	+	+	–
IV	Any size	+	+	+

* –, absent; +, present.

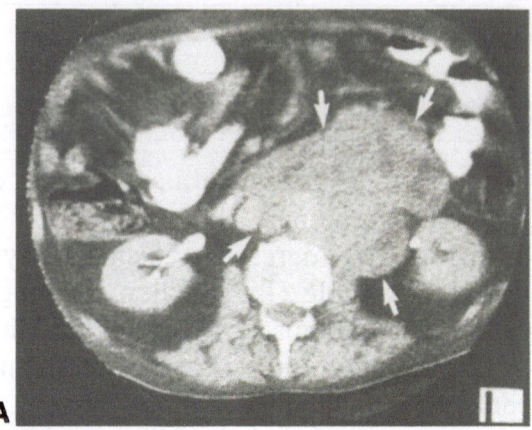

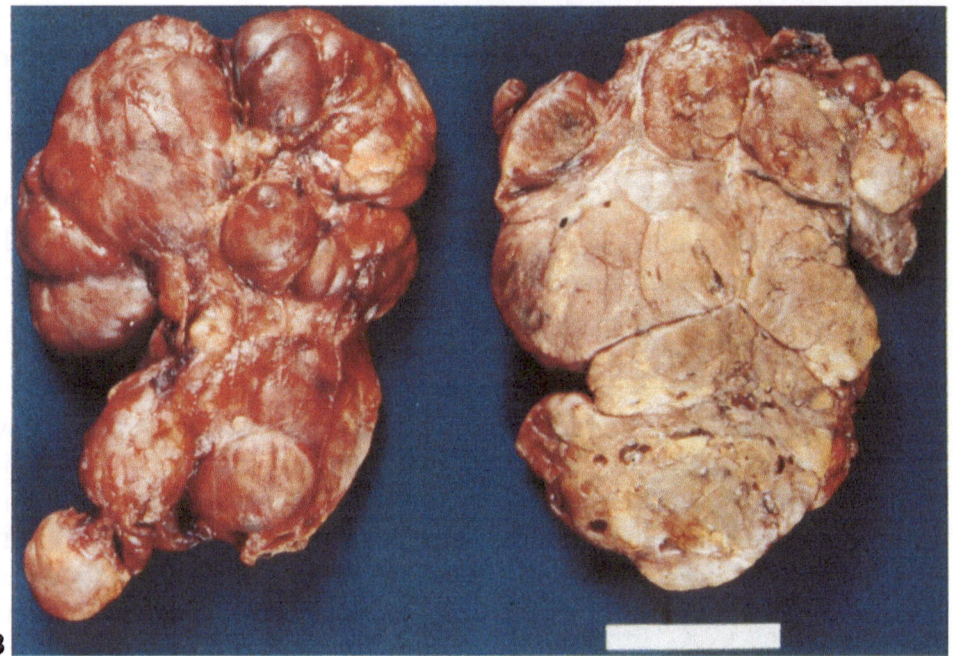

Fig. 3-35. **Adrenocortical carcinoma.** **A.** CT scan of massive adrenocortical carcinoma (*arrows*). **B.** Corresponding gross specimen. Scale = 4 cm.

TREATMENT

SURGICAL

Most adrenal carcinomas are unresectable for cure due to local invasion, lymph node metastases, or distant metastases, most commonly to liver or lung (150,151,158,161). Radical excision remains the primary treatment (152,153,162). Since these tumors are almost uniformly large, transabdominal or thoracoabdominal incisions may be necessary for adequate, safe exposure.

Nephrectomy, splenectomy, partial pancreatectomy, and partial colectomy may all be necessary to excise the mass en bloc. This implies that preoperative assessment of renal function and bowel preparation are advisable. Perioperative steroid administration is critical to avoid intra- or postoperative adrenal insufficiency as a result of the suppression and atrophy of the contralateral adrenal in cases with Cushing's syndrome. Aggressive debulking of the primary tumor (163) and even repeated resections of recurrent tumor may be justified (164).

CHEMOTHERAPY AND RADIOTHERAPY

Results of conventional chemotherapy have been discouraging. Several investigators have reported significant tumor regression (165,166) using adrenolytic drug mitotane; and even a cure of metastatic disease has been reported (167). However, the mean survival of these patients was only 8.4 months, somewhat better than the previously reported mean survival of 2.9 months in untreated patients (151).

When mitotane has been used as adjuvant therapy (6-g dose) and continued indefinitely as low-dose therapy (1–2 g/day), a significantly longer mean survival of 74 months has been reported (168). These lower doses are far better tolerated than 8–20 g/day, which leads to significant gastrointestinal and neuromuscular toxicity in up to 90% of patients (169). It should be noted that the need for both glucocorticoid and mineralocorticoid replacement should be anticipated.

For palliative relief of Cushing's syndrome, aminoglutethimide and metyrapone have been employed. By blocking the enzymatic conversion of cholesterol to 5-pregnenolone (170) or 11-deoxycortisol to cortisol, respectively, they may cause rapid and sustained suppression of steroid synthesis (171). The usual dose is 1–2 g/day for aminoglutethimide or 2–6 g/day for metyrapone, which is increased until plasma or urinary free cortisol falls and symptomatic relief is achieved or toxicity is intolerable.

The effectiveness of radiotherapy has been disputed. Some investigators have stated that it was ineffective for inoperable lesions (165), whereas others have reported useful palliation (170) for painful osseus metastases and significant tumor regression (161).

PROGNOSIS

Of those patients with stage I and II disease, 5-year survivals of 35% (152) to 63% (161) have been reported. In contrast, the majority of patients with stage III and IV disease generally do not survive beyond 12–18 months.

Nonfunctioning Adrenal Tumors

Until recently, small, nonfunctioning adrenocortical nodules had rarely been detected clinically. The advent of CT with its extreme sensitivity in imaging the adrenal (33) has in essence produced a new clinical phenomenon: the small, nonfunctioning adrenal tumor.

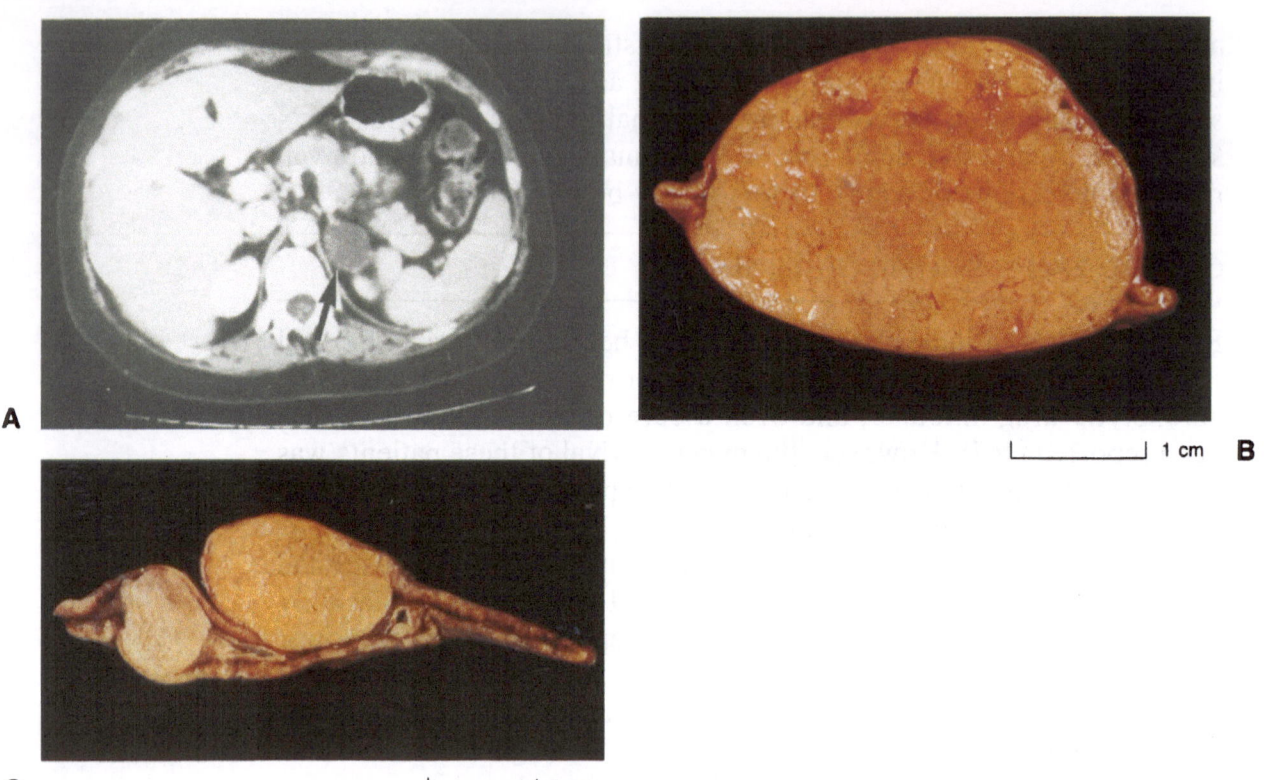

Fig. 3-36. **Nonfunctioning adrenal adenoma.** **A.** CT scan of nonfunctioning left adrenal adenoma (*arrow*). **B.** Corresponding gross specimen. **C.** An adrenal gland with a pale, nonfunctioning adenoma and a typically yellow aldosterone-producing adenoma.

This radiologic "discovery" clinically highlights the known pathologic incidence of nonfunctioning adrenal nodules, which occur in 1.45% (172) to 15% (173) of autopsies. These tumors actually represent localized overgrowth of adrenocortical cells; they may be considered a normal part of the aging process and are more common in patients with hypertension, cardiovascular disease, and diabetes (63). The exact stimulus remains unknown, but they are theorized to represent reactive hyperplasia to localized, ischemic, cortical atrophy (173). They are therefore a *result* of hypertensive changes, not the cause. Despite attaining a size in excess of 3 cm, they have never demonstrated any specific abnormal hormone imbalance. In contrast to the gross appearance of a typically golden-yellow aldosterone-producing adenoma, or the mottled yellow-brown Cushing's adenoma, nonfunctioning nodules are pale yellow (Fig. 3-36).

When such a nodule is discovered, one should first obtain appropriate tests to exclude the presence of a functioning adrenal tumor, since an unsuspected pheochromocytoma has been diagnosed in this manner (174). The non-functioning nodule presents a therapeutic dilemma. The risk of failing to excise a cancer before it reaches the all-too-common incurable stage must be balanced against recommending adrenalectomy for numerous asymptomatic patients. No present biochemical or radio-

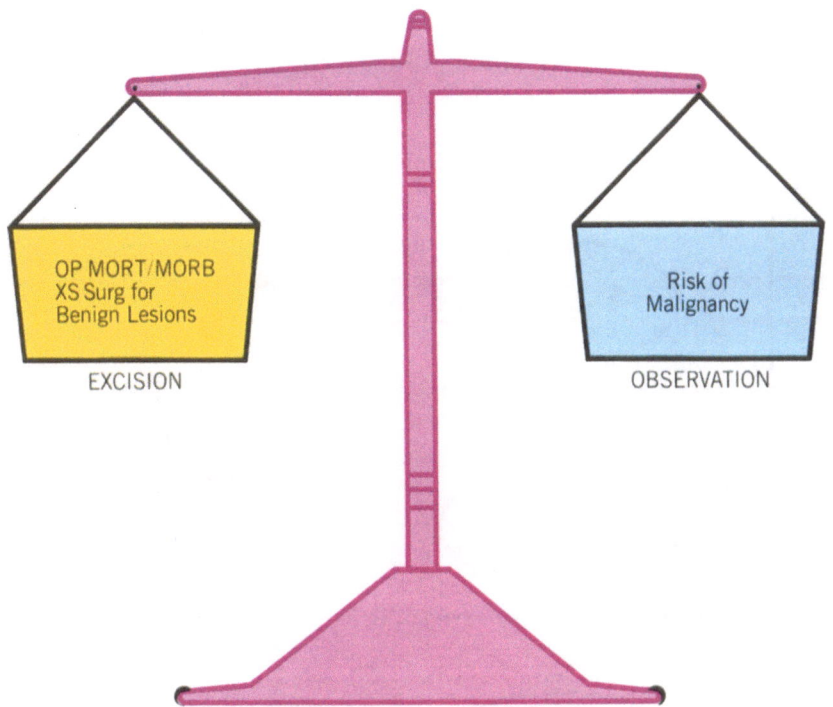

Small, nonfunctioning adrenal tumors. Weighing the risks and advantages of excision versus observation.

Fig. 3-37.

logic test can definitely distinguish these tumors as benign or malignant. Even needle biopsy is unreliable since there are no histologic criteria that can reliably differentiate benign from malignant tumors (156). Even more disconcerting, malignant change in a previously benign lesion has been reported (151), although most cancers are presumed to start de novo. Despite the fact that 75%–80% of nonfunctioning cancers occur after the age of 40 years, they have developed in both men and women in their late twenties and early thirties (175). These facts have prompted some investigators (156,176) to consider all nonfunctioning tumors malignant, although this conclusion predated CT scanning and was based only on large masses.

At present, therapeutic recommendations must be individualized and are somewhat arbitrary (Fig. 3-37). Adrenalectomy is generally advised for any one of the following: tumors in patients who are under age 50; lesions greater than 3 cm; or nodules that enlarge on CT scan. Otherwise, serial follow-up CT scans are indicated.

Congenital adrenal hyperplasia is almost always caused by an inherited deficiency of one of the enzymes involved in the five metabolic steps leading to the synthesis of cortisol (most commonly C-21 hydroxylase). Synthesis of cortisol and/or aldosterone are impaired and precursor compounds, metabolites, or alternate pathway end products are produced (Fig. 3-38). The overproduction of adrenal androgens in utero produces a pseudohermaphrodite, with ambiguous genitalia in females

Congenital Adrenal Hyperplasia (Adrenogenital Syndrome)

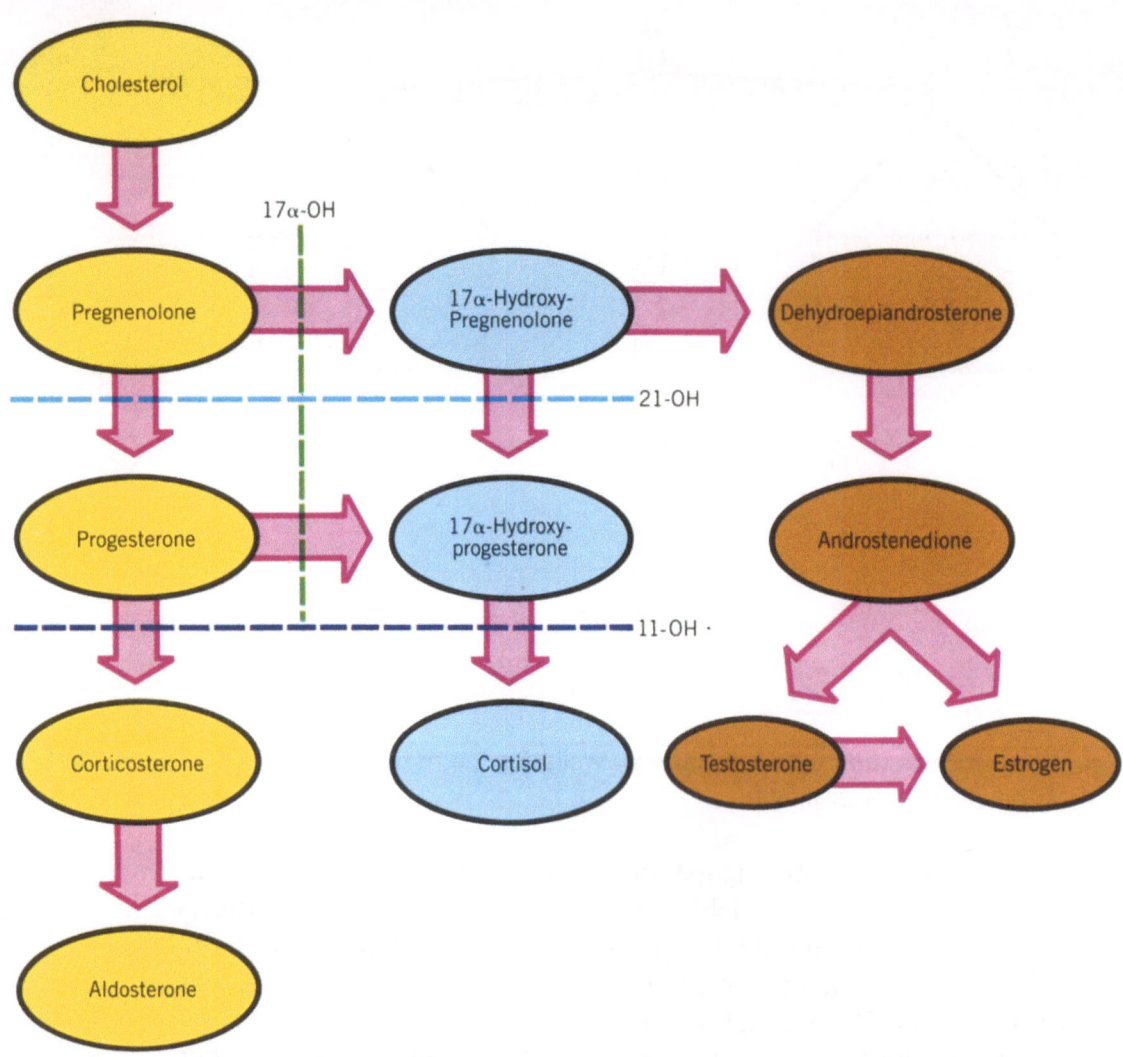

Fig. 3-38. **Congenital adrenal hyperplasia: major steps in the steroid synthesis metabolic pathways.** The three most commonly encountered enzyme deficiencies producing congenital adrenal hyperplasia are demonstrated.

and various degrees of macrogenitosomia in the male. Salt-losing crisis, hypertension, or addisonian crisis precipitated by stress in the newborn are also strong clues to this diagnosis.

The metabolic treatment of congenital adrenal hyperplasia is nonoperative and requires indefinite ACTH-*suppressive* doses of glucocorticoids together with replacement doses of mineralocorticoids. The prospects for normal childhood growth and development and normal adult life expectancy, fertility, and childbearing are quite good.

Operative Technique

POSTERIOR APPROACH TO ADRENALECTOMY

The posterior approach to adrenalectomy, as popularized by Young (177), is associated with a lower morbidity and mortality than the anterior route. The approach should be considered when operating on pa-

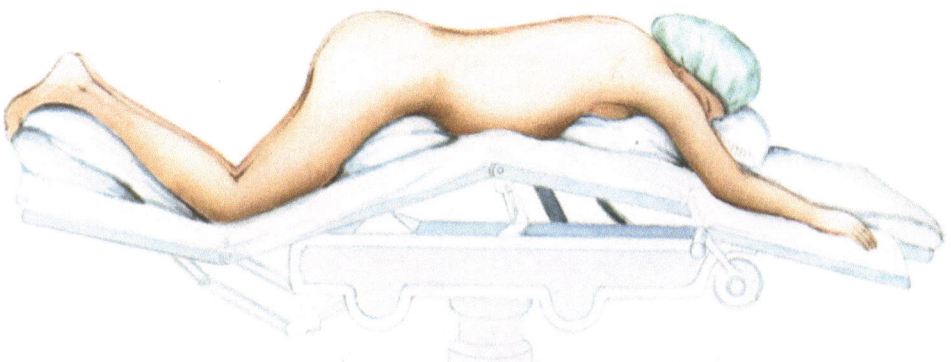

Position. Following induction of anesthesia and insertion of an endotracheal tube, the patient is turned gently to the prone position. Rolled blankets or firm pillows are placed beneath the chest and pelvis, allowing the abdomen to sag and the peritoneal contents to fall away from the retroperitoneal area. The table is flexed into the jackknife position to eliminate lumbar lordosis. The knees are flexed and the legs supported on pillows to reduce venous pooling in the lower extremities during the operative procedure.

Fig. 3-39.

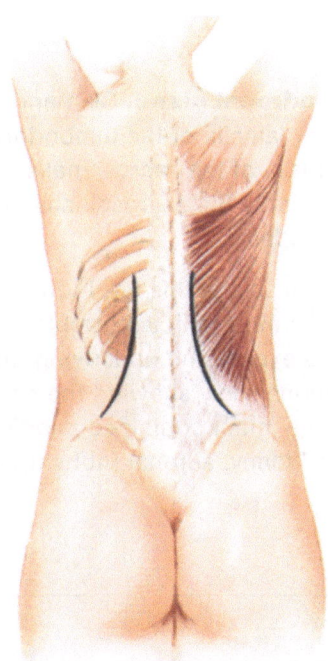

Incision. A curvilinear incision is made through the skin, subcutaneous fat, and latissimus dorsi muscle down to the posterior lamella of the lumbodorsal fascia. The upper end of the incision is about three fingerbreadths from the midvertebral line at the level of the 10th rib; the lower end is at the iliac crest about four fingerbreadths from the midline. Bilateral incisions are shown marked in relation to underlying bony landmarks, muscles, and viscera.

Fig. 3-40.

tients with primary aldosterone-producing adenomas, bilateral hyperplasia of Cushing's syndrome, and nonfunctioning adrenal tumors. The positioning of the patient and incision placement are shown in Figures 3-39 and 3-40.

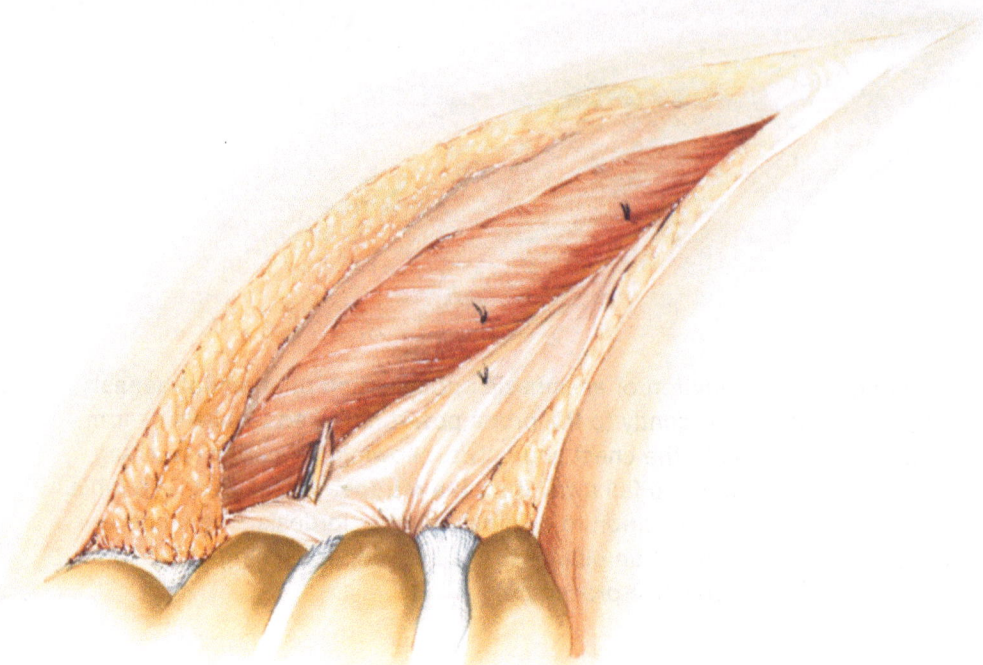

Fig. 3-41. **Incision to expose right adrenal gland.** Skin and subcutaneous bleeders are secured and the posterior lamella of the lumbodorsal fascia is incised to expose the underlying fleshy mass of the sacrospinalis muscle. Several lumbar cutaneous vessels and nerves pierce the sacrospinalis muscle and tether it laterally; these are ligated and divided.

Fig. 3-42. **A.** Because the lumbodorsal fascia at this level forms a smooth, nonadherent investment for the sacrospinalis muscle, it is possible to retract the muscle belly medially against the spine to expose the underlying middle lamella of fascia and the 12th rib. **B.** Cross-sectional view showing the sacrospinalis muscle retracted medially to expose the intact conjoined middle and anterior lamellae of the lumbodorsal fascia. The kidney, adrenal (not shown), and retroperitoneal fat are directly subjacent.

RIGHT ADRENALECTOMY

The posterior approach to the adrenal gland is a direct one (Figs. 3-41 and 3-42), and ligation of the right adrenal vein, a delicate step in adrenal surgery, is facilitated. The key to operative exposure is resection of the 12th rib (Figs. 3-43 to 3-45). The pleura is then reflected upward out of the way, and the diaphragm is divided to give an excellent view of the retroperitoneal space and adrenal area (Figs. 3-46 to 3-48). After the gland is mobilized (Figs. 3-49 and 3-50), the vein can be ligated (Fig. 3-51). If the inferior vena cava is accidentally torn at this point, bleeding is best controlled by a pack and firm pressure for 5–10 minutes. Large tears require 5–0 vascular suture.

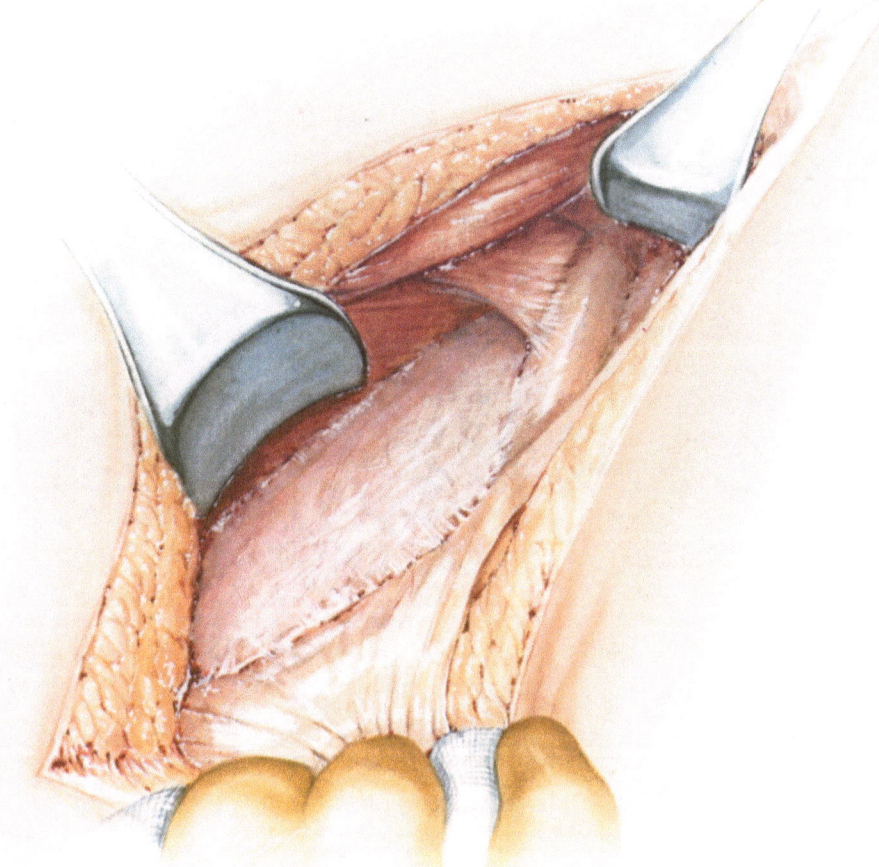

Fig. 3-42.

A

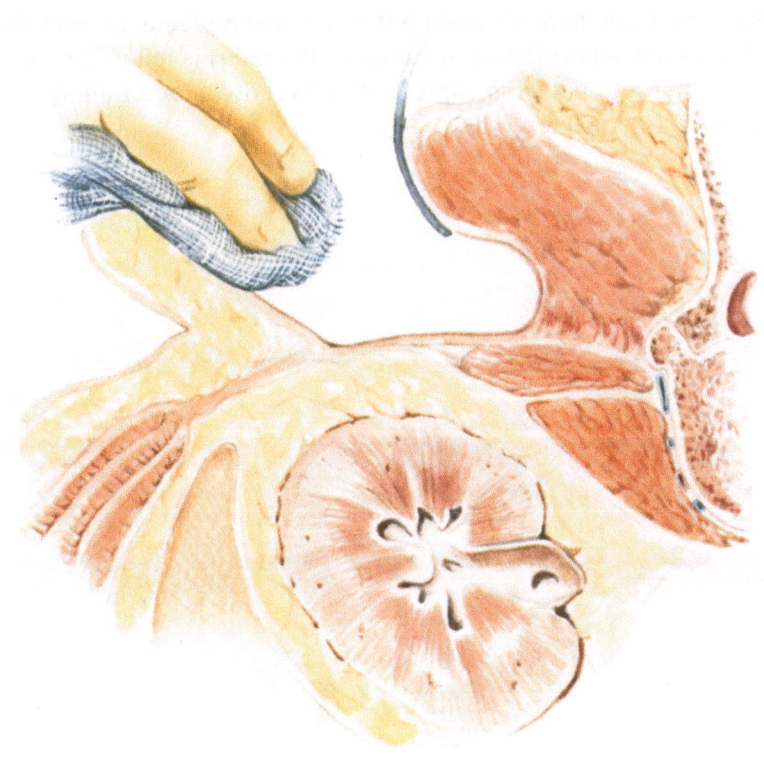

B

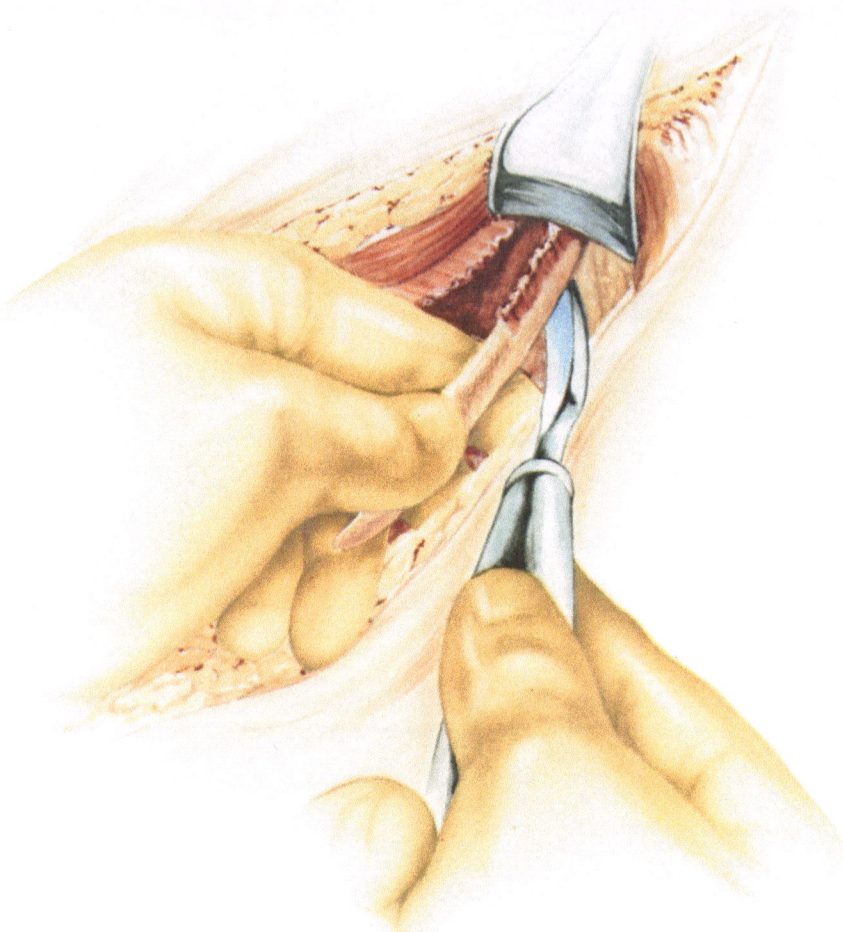

Fig. 3-43. **Removal of the 12th rib.** Several slips of sacrospinalis muscle that insert into the dorsal aspect of the 12th rib are detached. The rib is removed subperiosteally, care being taken to avoid tearing the underlying pleura. Should the pleural space be opened inadvertently, a catheter (16–18 Fr) is left in during closure and removed after residual air is expressed by hyperinflation of the lungs before the skin closure is completed.

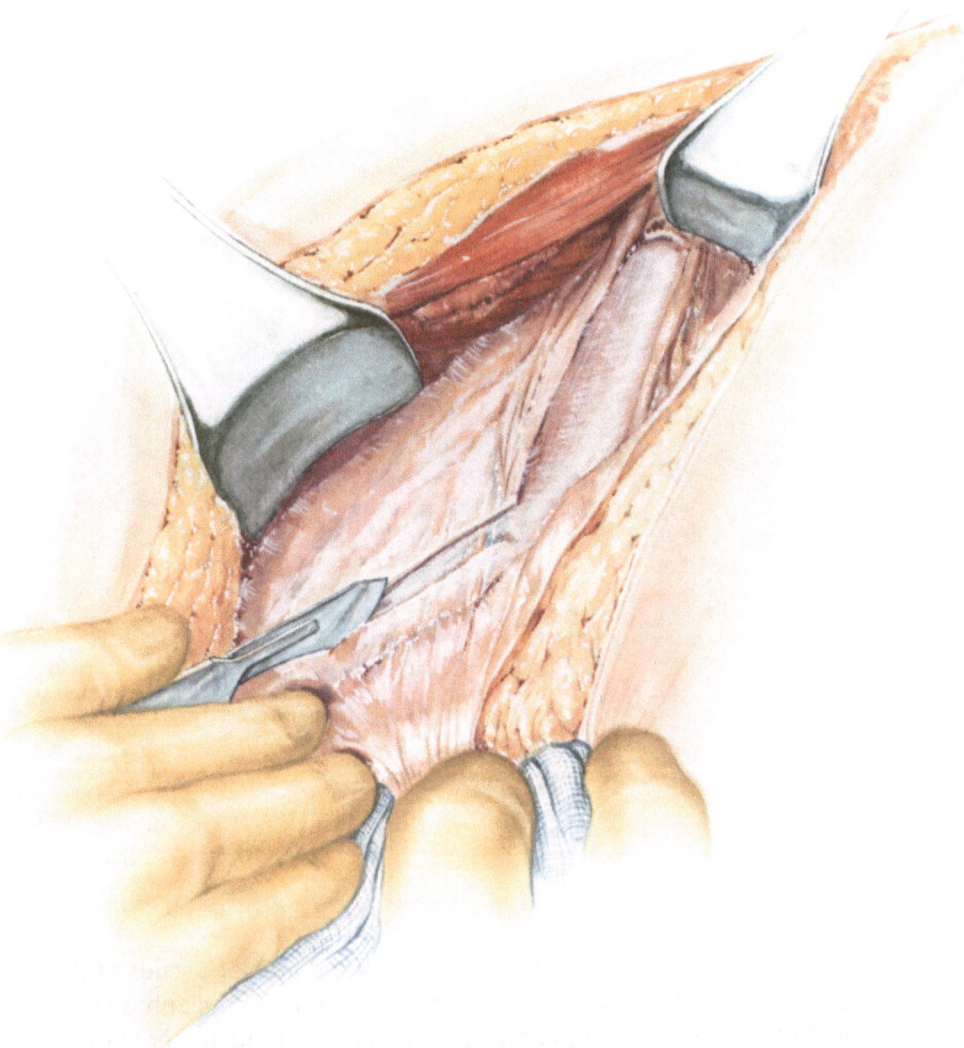

The middle lamella of the lumbodorsal fascia is incised along the lateral border of the quadratus lumborum. The incision usually is carried through the anterior lamella (the transversalis fascia) with the same sweep of the blade. The subcostal vessels run across the field at this point and are dissected free; they are then clamped, divided, and tied. The subcostal nerve parallels the vessels but is separate from them; it is preserved and retracted downward. Although not shown in this figure, the kidney can now be seen invested by Gerota's fascia and surrounded by fat.

Fig. 3-44.

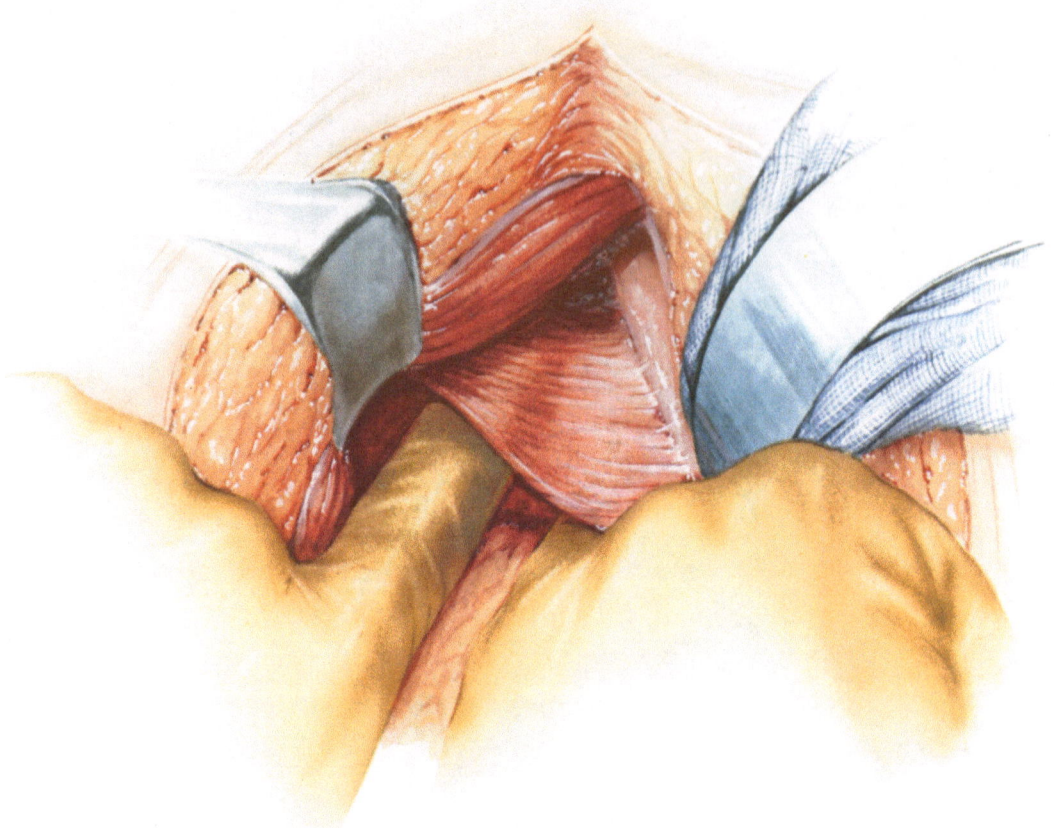

Fig. 3-45. Finger dissection is used as shown to free the fatty and areolar tissues of the suprarenal space from the undersurface of the diaphragm. The diaphragm now forms a shelf of muscle with the parietal pleura adherent to its upper surface.

Fig. 3-46. **Reflection of the pleura.** An important step in obtaining adequate exposure of the adrenal gland is to free the pleura from the diaphragm. This is best accomplished by using a gauze-covered finger to push the pleura upward out of the way.

Fig. 3-47. The diaphragm now can be divided between large metal clips all the way from the free edge to the spine without fear of injuring the pleura.

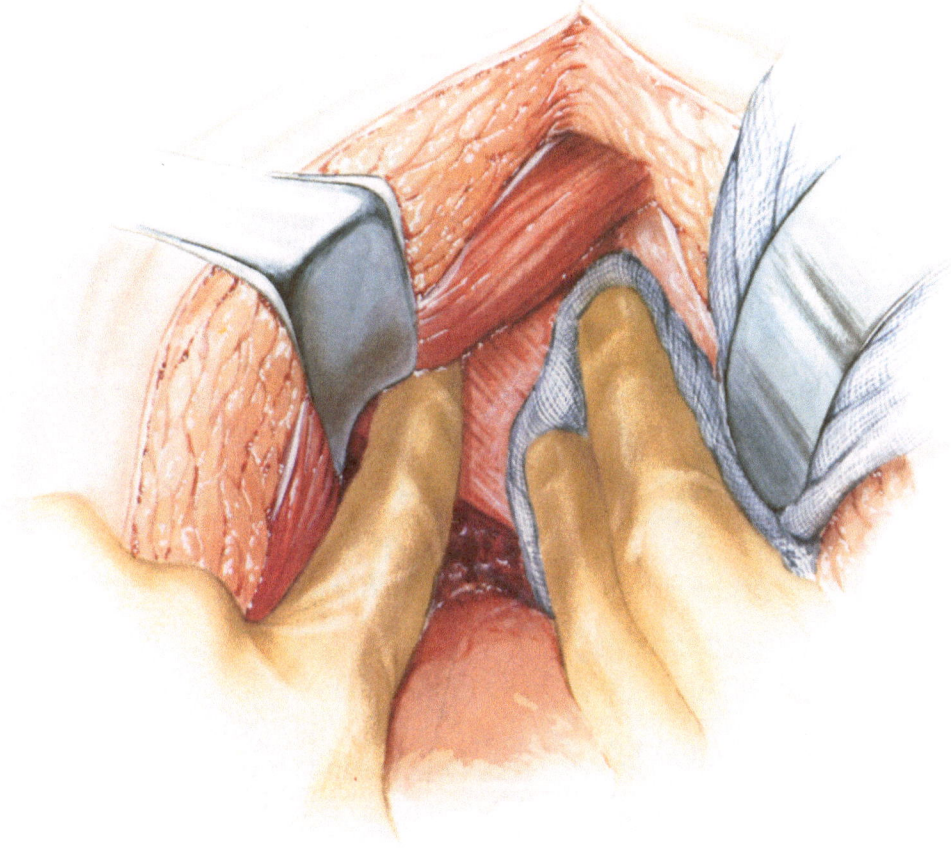

Fig. 3-46.

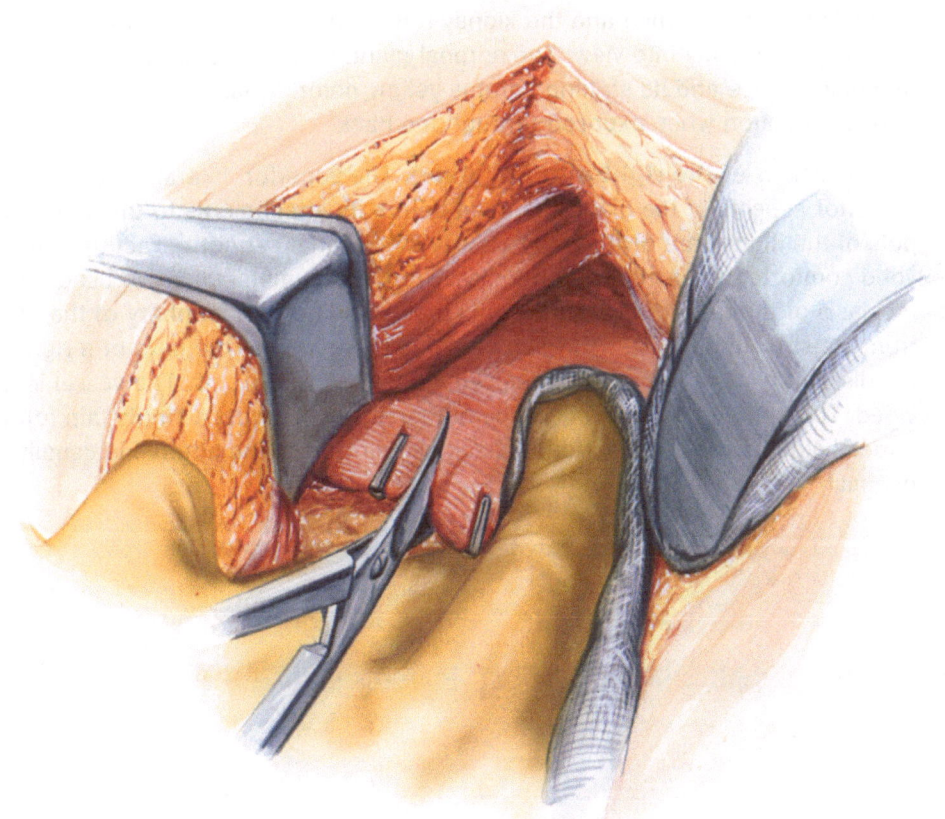

Fig. 3-47.

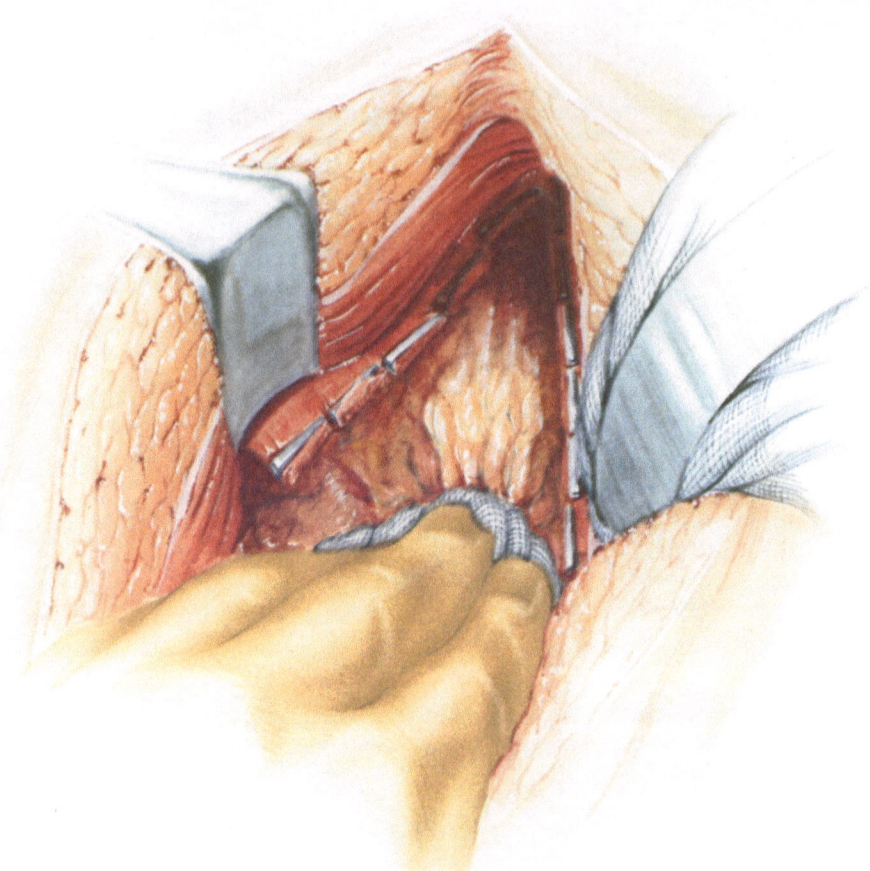

Fig. 3-48. Gerota's fascia is opened and the kidney retracted downward to bring the right adrenal prominently into view. The adrenal gland is recognized by its finely granular surface and its striking chrome-yellow color. It has a surprisingly superficial location when exposed through the back.

Fig. 3-49. **Mobilization of the right adrenal gland.** The superior, lateral, medial, and posterior aspects of the gland are freed before its attachments to the superior pole of the kidney are divided. In this way the adrenal cannot retract upward beyond comfortable reach during the disseciton. Small metal clips are used for hemostasis of the many fine arterial twigs that pass into the periphery of the gland from the surrounding fat. **A.** Each vessel is isolated over the jaws of a right-angle dissector. **B.** Clips are then placed across the vessel. **C.** The vessel is divided. To expedite the dissection, the authors often use just a single clip (on the parietal side) across small arteries; back bleeding from the adrenal is usually minimal.

Fig. 3-49.

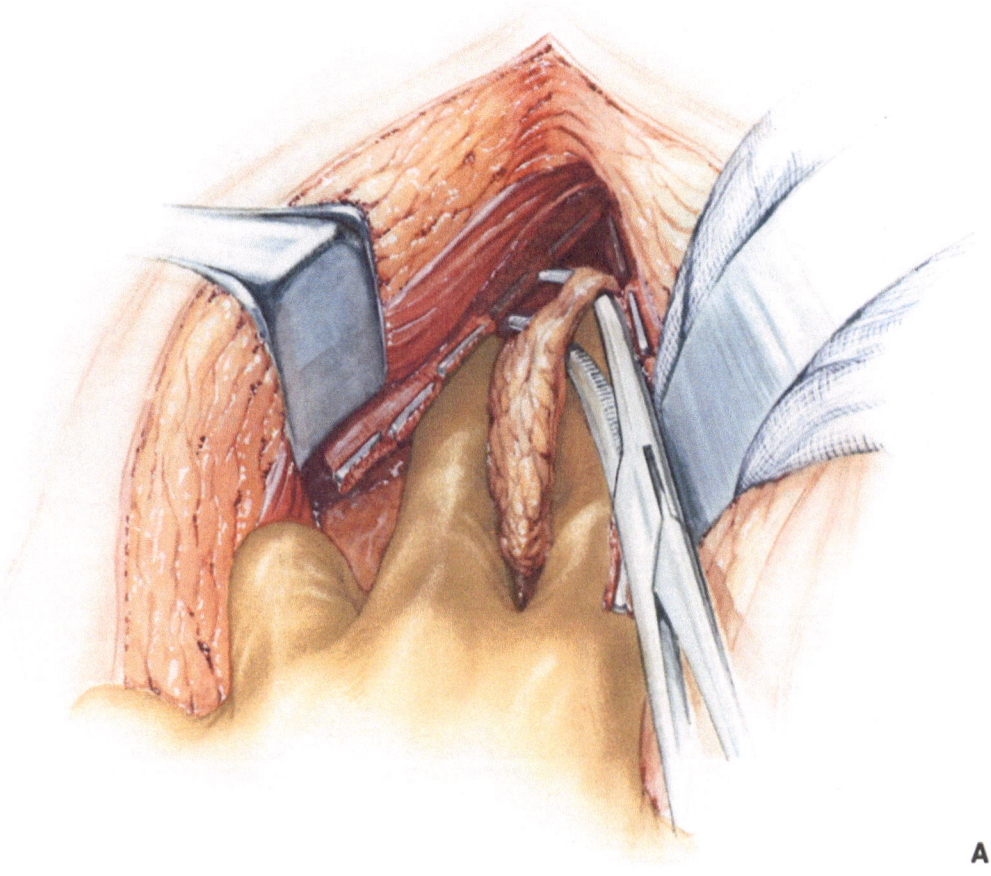

A

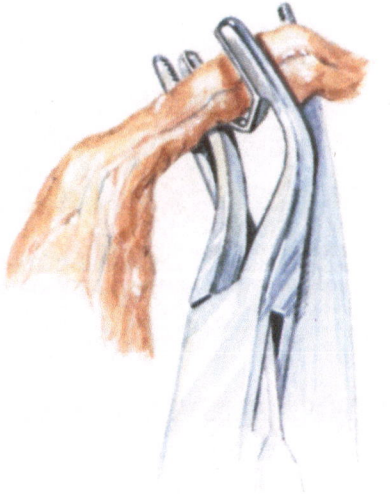

B

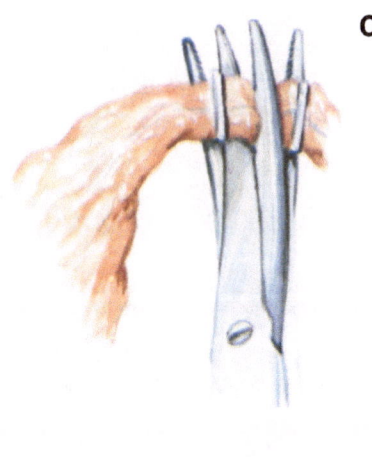

C

Fig. 3-50.

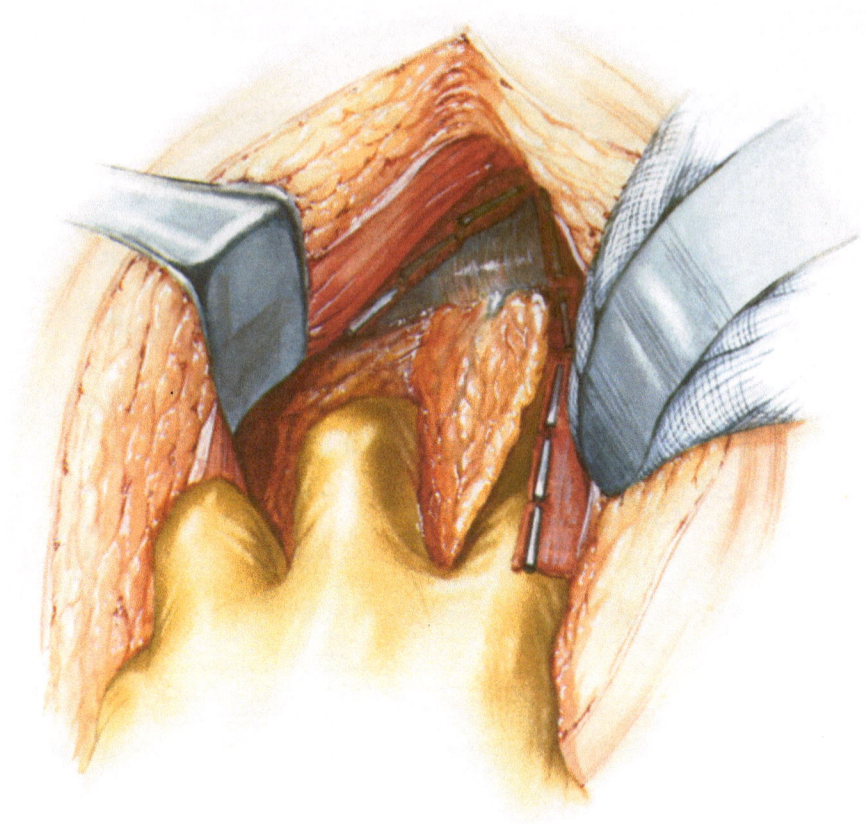

Fig. 3-51.

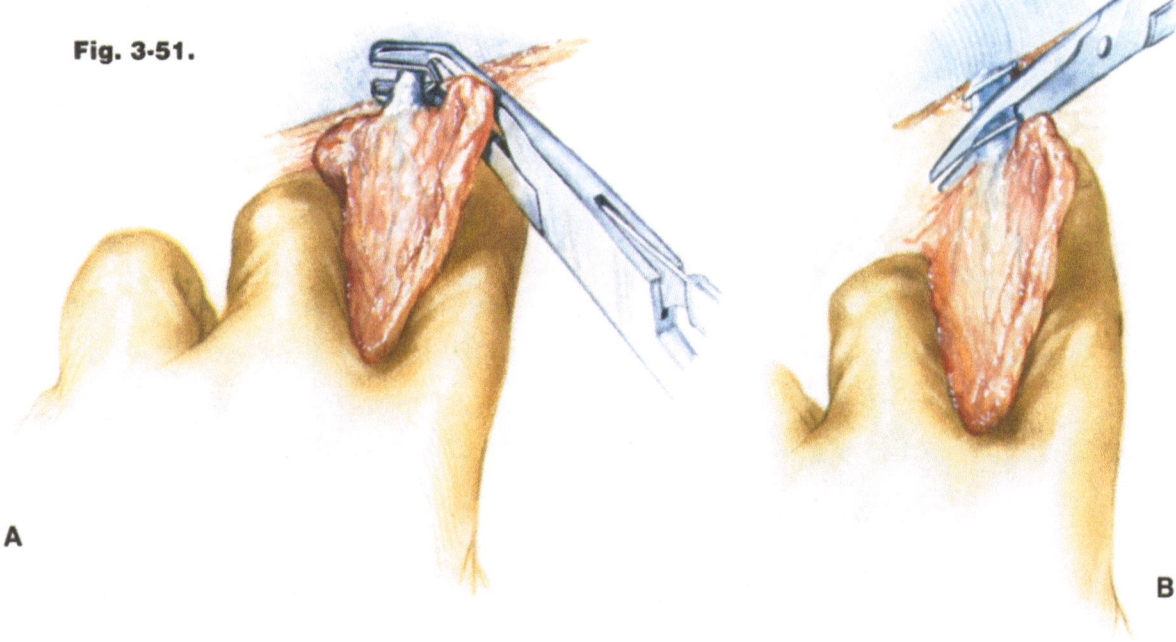

A

B

LEFT ADRENALECTOMY

The left adrenal gland is exposed and mobilized in a similar manner to that depicted for the gland on the right (Fig. 3-52).

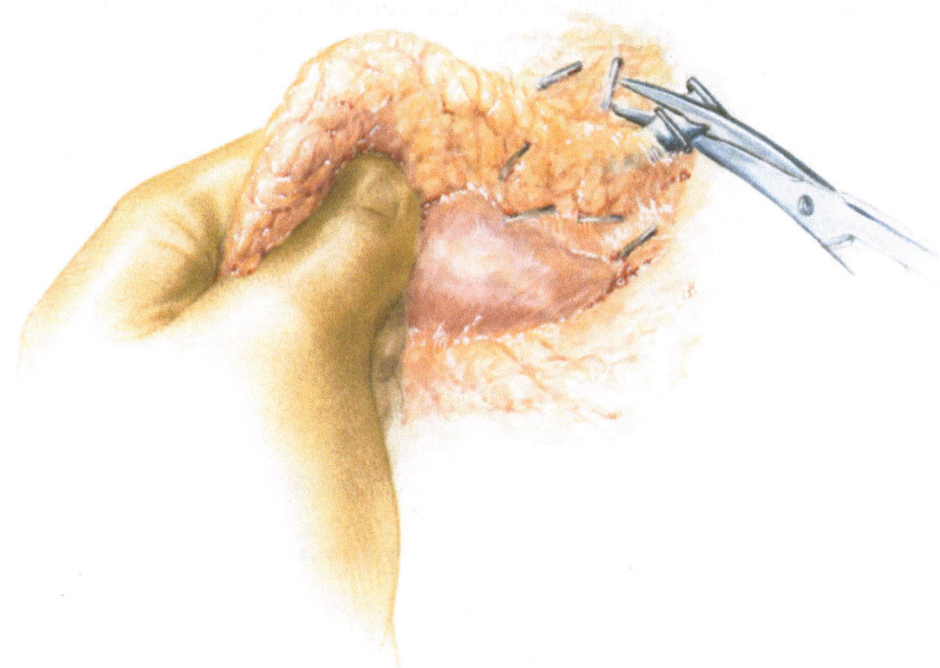

Exposure of the left adrenal gland. The left adrenal gland is a flattened elongated structure. Usually a tongue of adrenal tissue dips down medially toward the hilum of the kidney. It is from this portion of the gland that the main vein emerges, taking an oblique course downward to empty into the left renal vein. With the adrenal gland fully freed, the main venous pedicle is clipped and divided.

Fig. 3-52.

◄ The dissection proceeds methodically until the entire central vein can be safely exposed. The adrenal gland, which is quite friable, should be handled with great care. The authors prefer to manipulate the gland with the fingers of the left hand as shown, rather than to run the risk of fracturing it with forceps or a clamp held by an assistant.

Fig. 3-50.

Ligation of the right adrenal vein. The right adrenal vein is uniformly short and wide; it empties directly into the inferior vena cava. **A.** A large metal clip is placed across the right adrenal vein flush with the inferior vena cava. **B.** Another clip is placed close to the adrenal gland. The vein is severed, the remainder of the peripheral arterial dissection is completed, and the gland is removed.

Fig. 3-51.

CLOSURE

The wounds are irrigated and residual bleeders clamped and tied. Drains are not necessary since the operative field is dry and the abundant perirenal fat obliterates potential dead space. The incision is closed in two layers, using running absorbable sutures (Figs. 3-53 to 3-55).

A postoperative chest x-ray film is taken in the recovery room to check for possible pneumothorax.

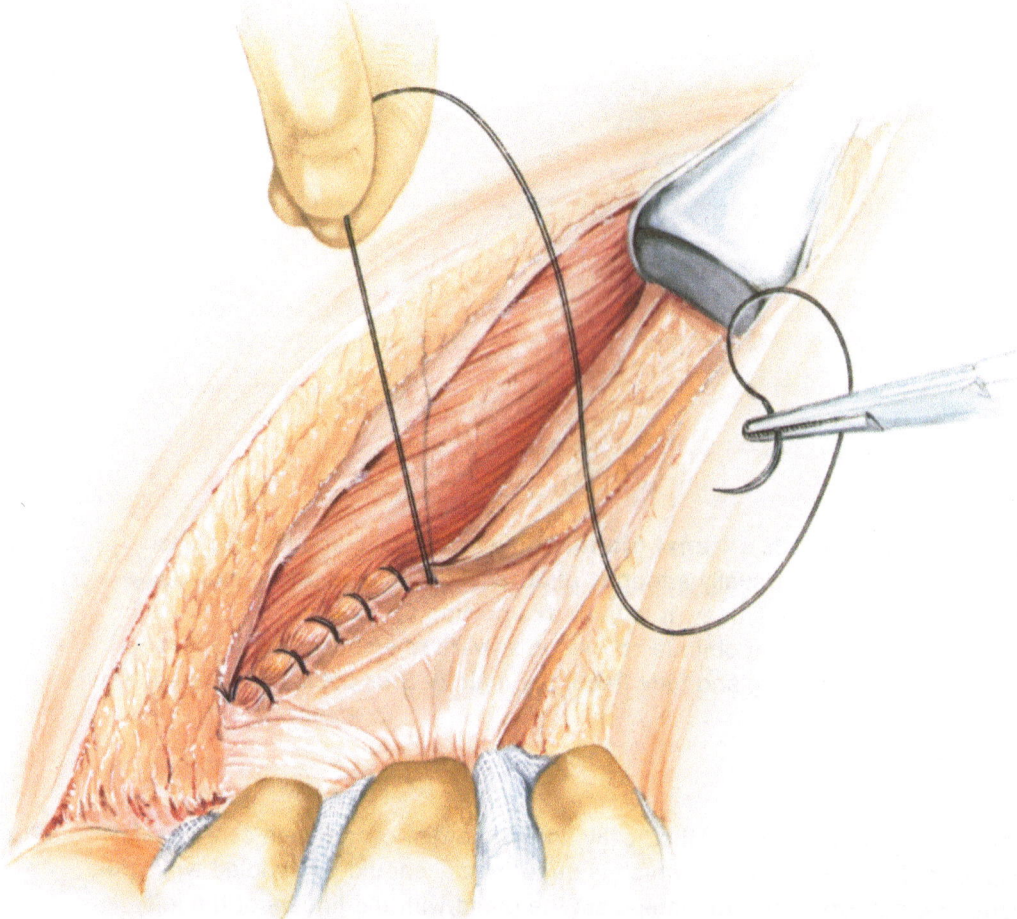

Fig. 3-53. **Closure.** The first layer approximates the external edge of the conjoined anterior and middle lamellae of the lumbodorsal fascia to the belly of the sacrospinalis muscle. A fascia-to-fascia reapproximation at this level usually is not attempted because retraction of the musculofascial planes imposes undue tension on the suture line, causing the stitches to pull out.

Fig. 3-54. The second layer reunites the edges of the divided posterior lamella. The subcutaneous fatty tissues are reapproximated.

Fig. 3-55. Skin closure utilizing synthetic absorbable suture material provides a strong and cosmetically appealing incision.

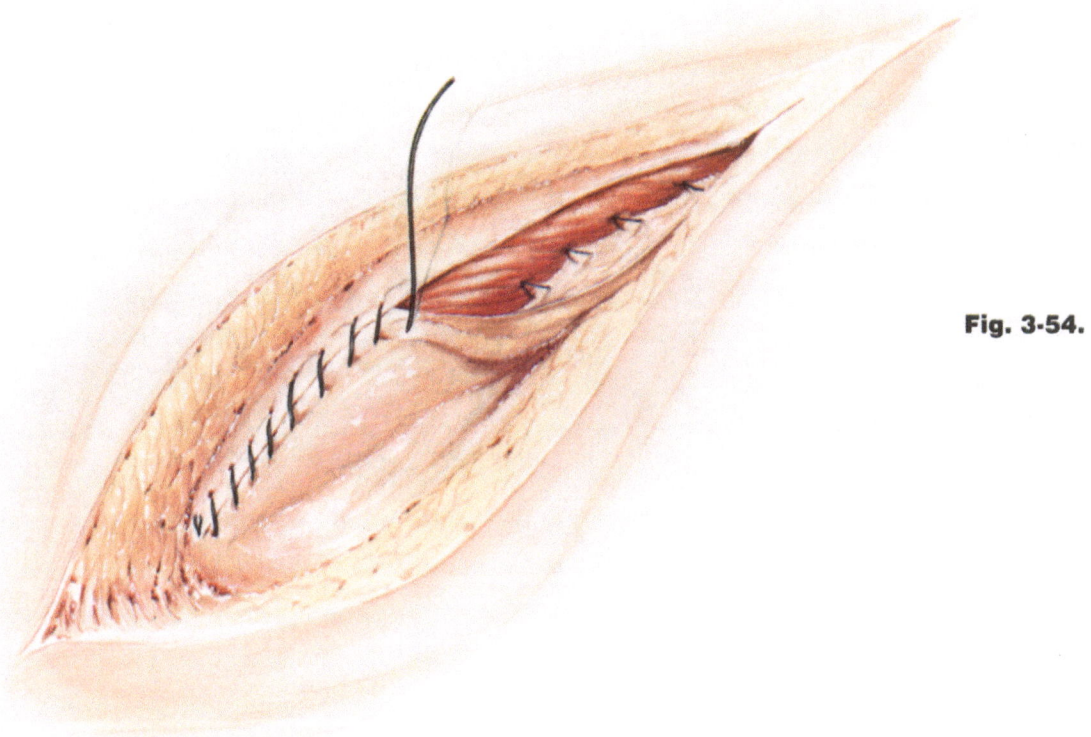

Fig. 3-54.

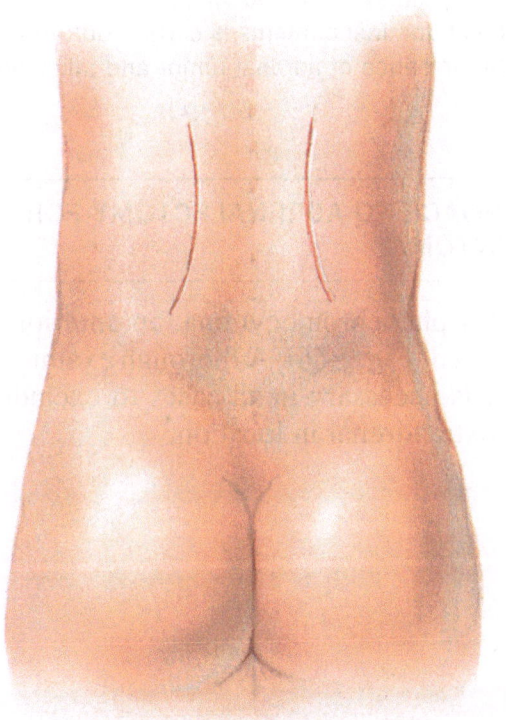

Fig. 3-55.

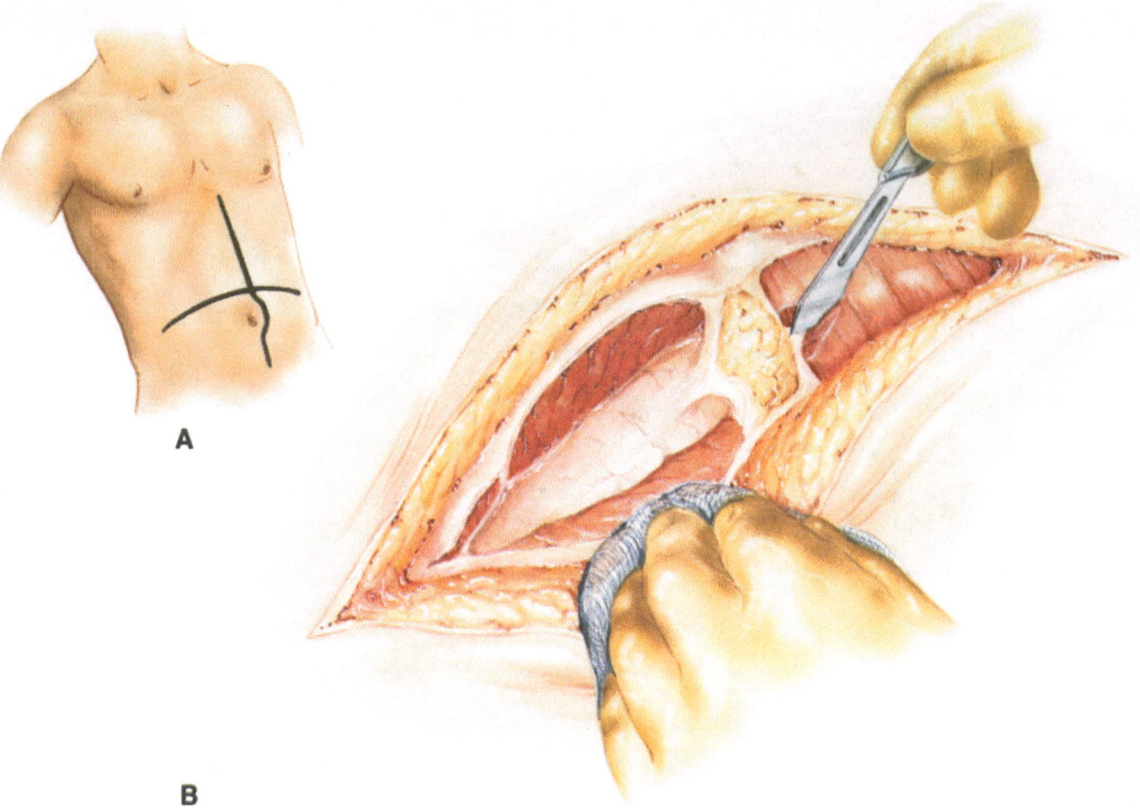

A

B

Fig. 3-56. **Incision.** **A.** A bilateral subcostal incision provides excellent exposure; however, a transverse upper abdominal incision or a long midline incision may be preferred in some patients. **B.** The abdomen is opened and routine inspection and palpation of the abdominal contents is carried out. At this time the surgeon quickly confirms the presence of adrenal tumor and takes note of any other pathology.

ANTERIOR APPROACH TO ADRENALECTOMY FOR PHEOCHROMOCYTOMA

In an operation for pheochromocytoma, an anterior or transabdominal approach is preferred (Fig. 3-56). A thorough examination of the general abdominal cavity is necessary in all cases to exclude the 10% or so of tumors that are extraadrenal in location.

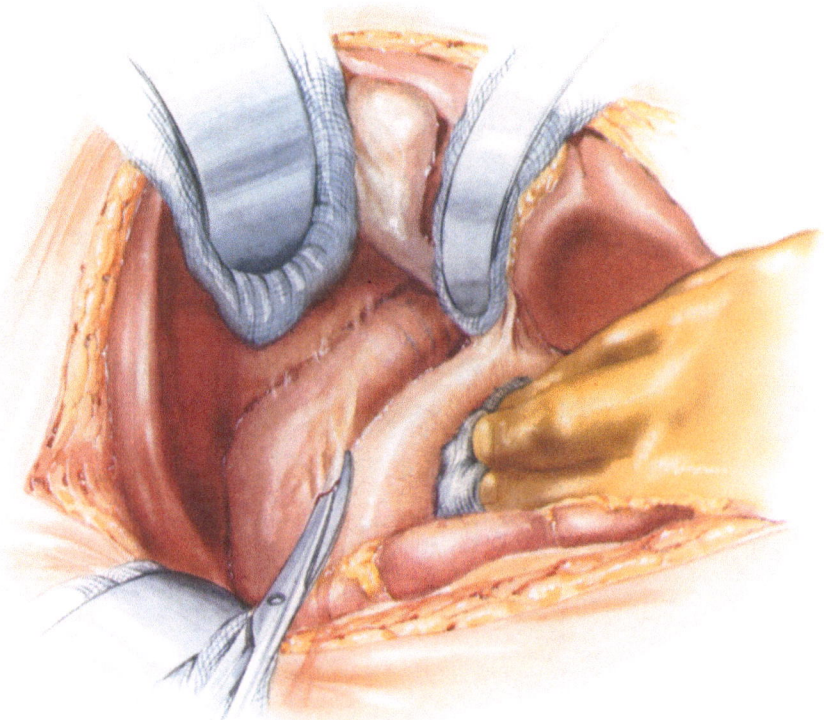

Exposure of a tumor of the right adrenal gland. The hepatic flexure of the colon may be mobilized and retracted downward to expose the duodenal loop. The second portion of the duodenum may be freed by dividing its lateral avascular peritoneal reflection (Kocher maneuver). The right lobe of the liver is retracted upward.

Fig. 3-57.

RIGHT ADRENALECTOMY

The technique for exposure of a tumor of the right adrenal gland is depicted in Figures 3-57 and 3-58.

The principle of early ligation of the adrenal venous drainage is sound, provided adequate exposure allows its safe control. The concept of "dissecting the patient from the tumor" emphasizes the fact that the

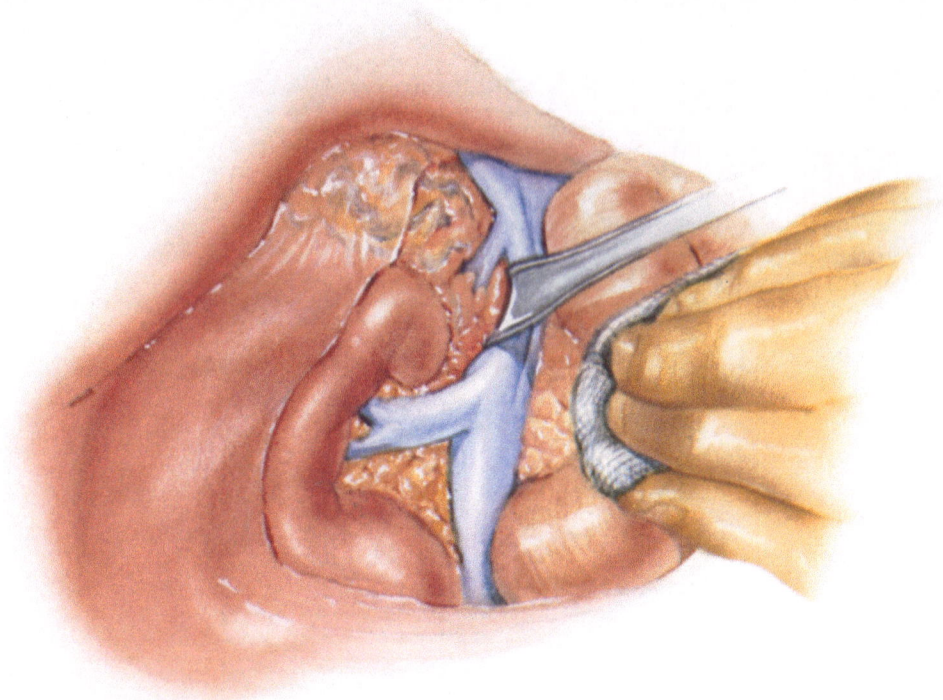

Fig. 3-58. The descending duodenum is separated from the retroperitoneal structures posteriorly by blunt and sharp dissection and is then turned forward and to the left. This maneuver exposes the underlying vena cava and a pheochromocytoma of the right adrenal gland overlying the superior pole of the kidney.

tumor should be manipulated as little as possible. Following dissection upward along the vena cava, and partial freeing of the superior aspect of the adrenal, the right adrenal vein can be safely exposed. A sufficient length of vena cava is exposed to permit side application of a vascular clamp in the event of a caval tear. To facilitate visualizing the adrenal vein, which frequently enters the vena cava somewhat posteriorly, a vein retractor is employed. In this case, the short, wide right adrenal vein is seen clearly as it passes over the front of the medial part of the tumor to reach the vena cava (Fig. 3-59).

With the pheochromoctyoma effectively isolated from the venous side of the circulation, the process of freeing it from its bed can proceed with less concern for the occurrence of paroxysms of hypertension or cardiac irregularities (Figs. 3-60 and 3-61).

LEFT ADRENALECTOMY

The left adrenal gland is exposed as shown in Figures 3-62 to 3-64, and the tumor is removed (Fig. 3-65).

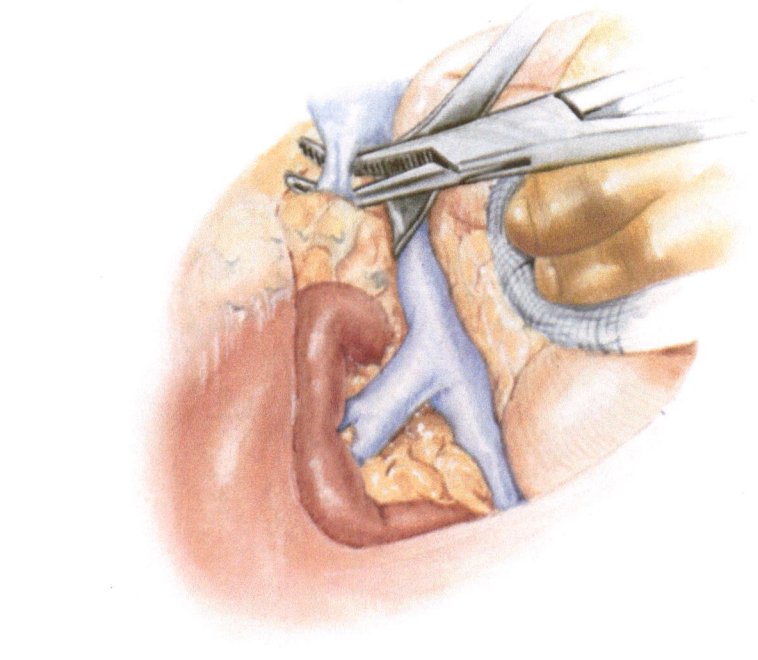

A

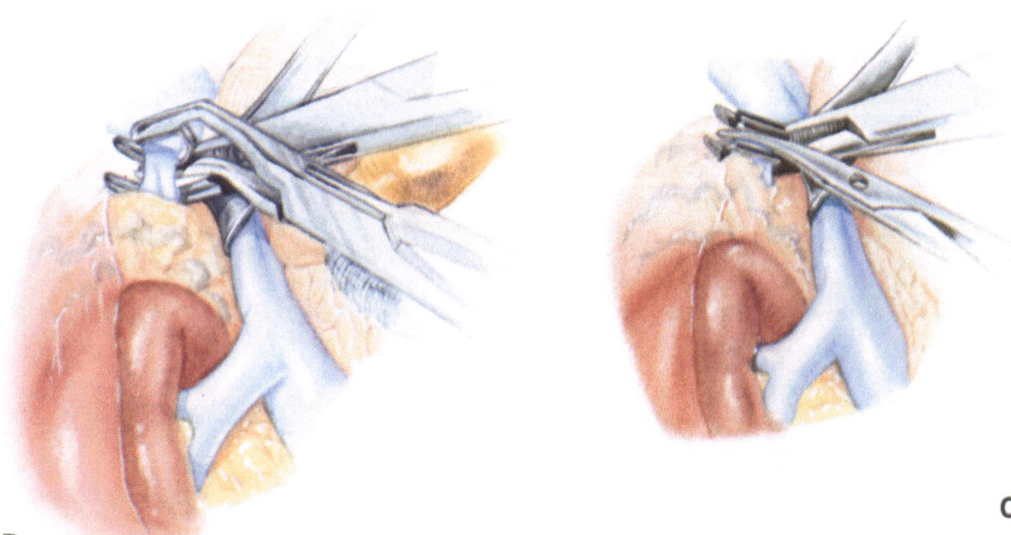

B

C

Ligation of the right adrenal vein. **A.** The adrenal vein is dissected free. **Fig. 3-59.**
B. It is ligated in continuity using large metal clips. **C.** It is severed between
the clips.

Fig. 3-60.

Fig. 3-61.

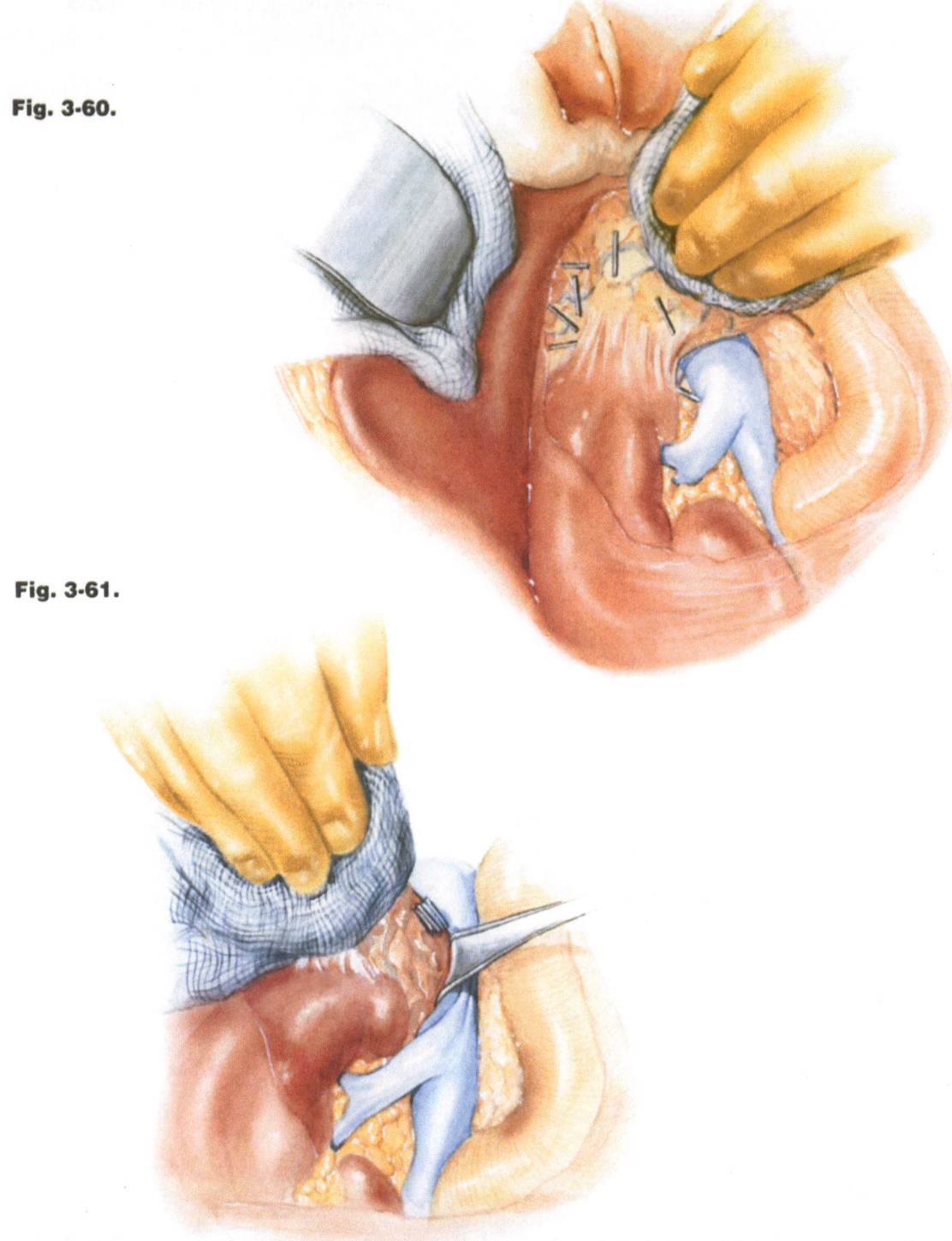

Fig. 3-60. **Excision of tumor.** The entire tumor is dissected free from above downward using metal clips for hemostasis. The authors prefer not to dissect out the lower pole of the tumor until the upper, lateral, and medial borders have been freed.

Fig. 3-61. Quite frequently a tumor of the right adrenal gland extends upward behind the right edge of the vena cava. However, it usually is easily separated from the vena cava by retracting the latter as shown. Finally, the fascial attachments to the kidney are divided and the tumor is removed.

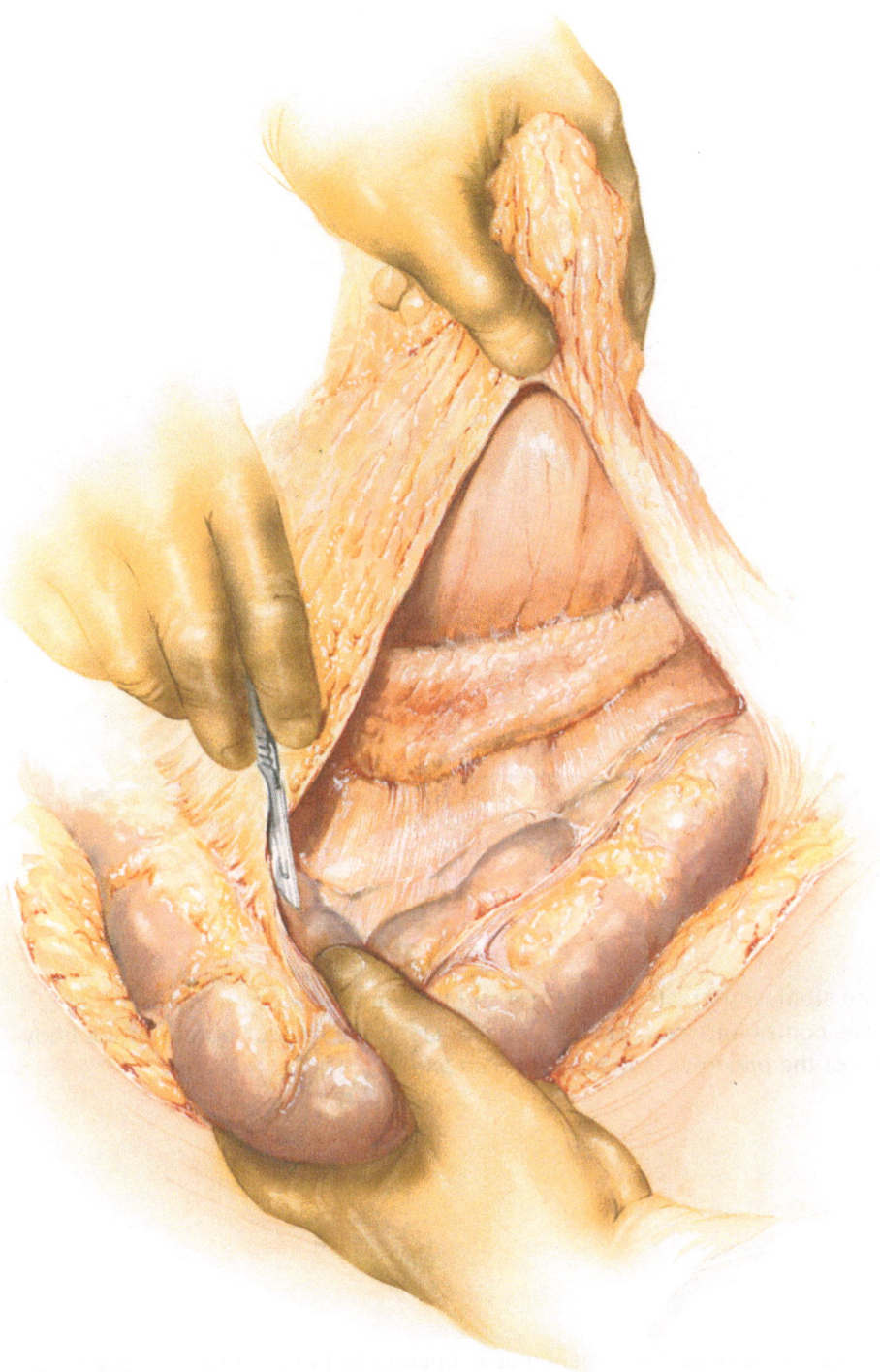

Exposure of a tumor of the left adrenal gland. The left adrenal gland can **Fig. 3-62.**
be exposed safely and conveniently via the lesser sac. By using gentle upward
traction on the greater omentum, its avascular attachment to the distal transverse colon is divided to give direct access into the lesser sac. Care is taken to
avoid excessive traction of the splenocolic ligament for fear of tearing the
splenic capsule. If exposure is not adequate, it is sometimes helpful to mobilize
the splenic flexure of the colon.

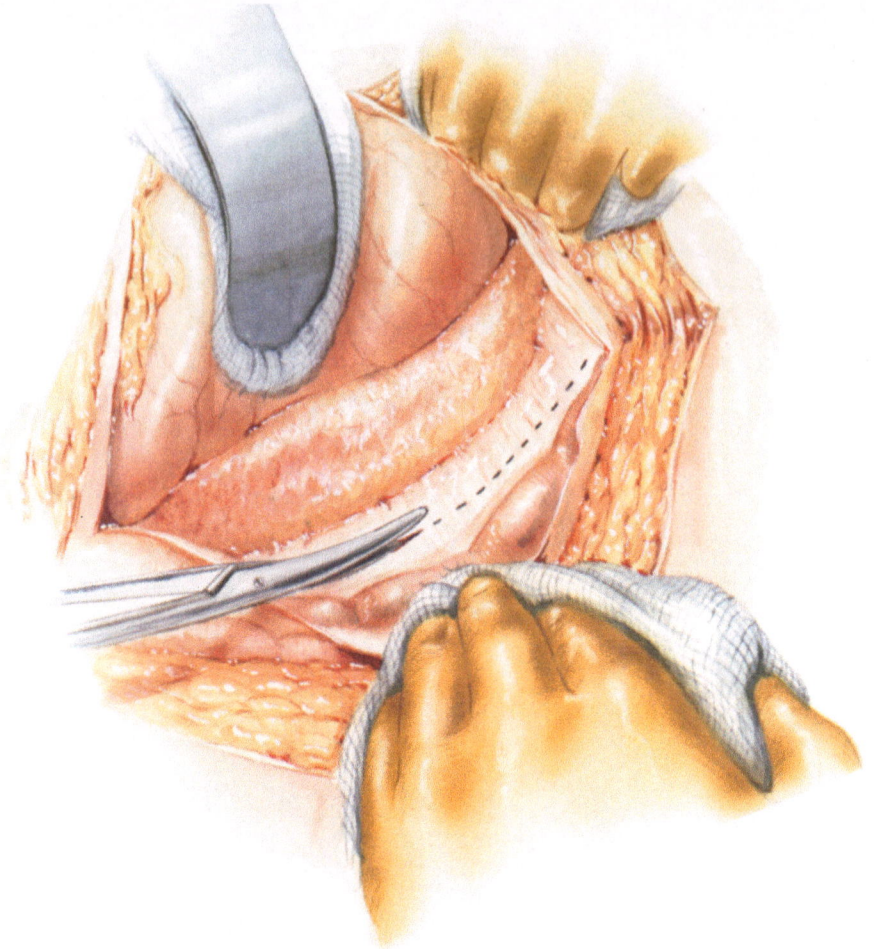

Fig. 3-63. With the stomach retracted superiorly and the transverse colon inferiorly, the pancreas comes into view. The peritoneum along the inferior border of the body and tail of the pancreas is incised (*broken line*).

Fig. 3-64. The areolar plane deep to the pancreas is opened by blunt finger dissection, as depicted. The crooked fingers of the left hand elevate the tail of the pancreas and work in gentle motion, with the fingers of the right hand providing counteraction, to separate the areolar tissues and progressively free the gland.

Fig. 3-65. **Excision of tumor.** With the pancreas freed and retracted upward out of the way, the kidney and a left adrenal tumor lie exposed. The left adrenal vein can be seen entering the left renal vein. It is isolated over a right-angle clamp, clipped in continuity, and divided. As before, the tumor is dissected free from the retroperitoneal fat and, finally, from the kidney, using multiple small metal clips for hemostasis.

Fig. 3-64.

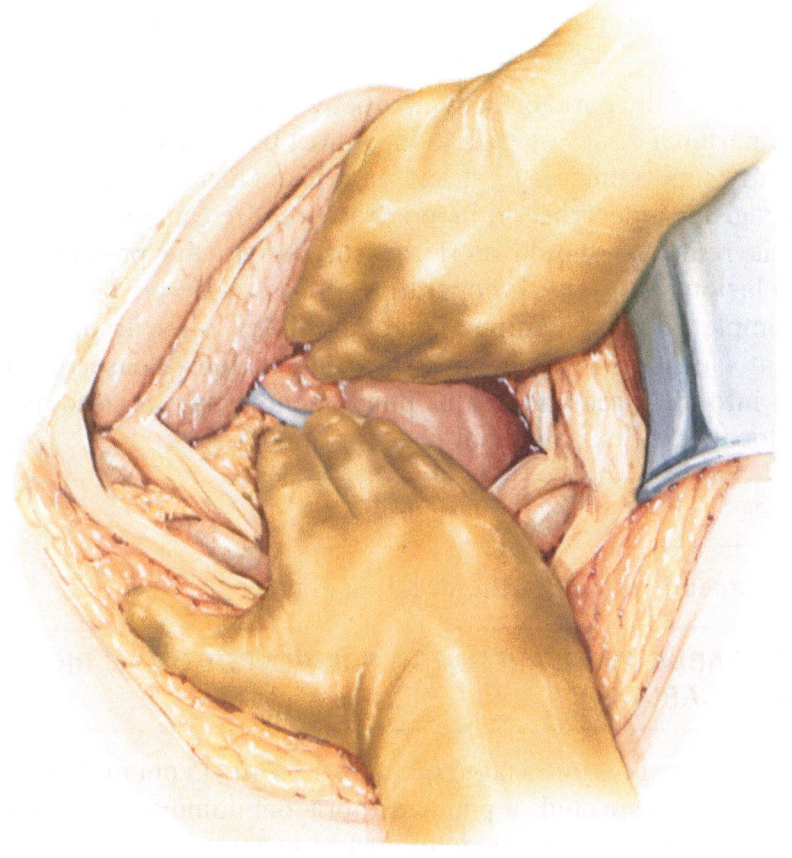

Fig. 3-65.

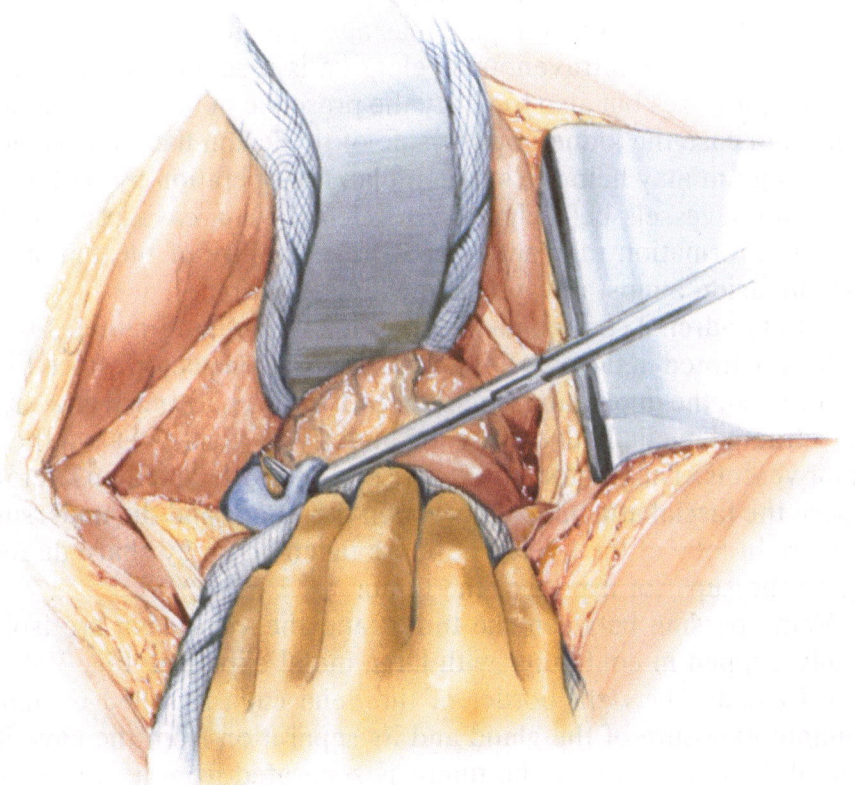

EXPLORATION FOR EXTRAADRENAL PHEOCHROMOCYTOMA

Exploration of the paraaortic sympathetic chains, the opposite adrenal, and the perihilar zones of each kidney must be carried out in every case to exclude supernumerary extraadrenal pheochromocytomas. The failure to register a decrease in blood pressure after an adrenal medullary tumor is removed should alert the surgeon to the possibility that a second lesion is present. Preoperative alpha-adrenergic blockade is seldom complete so that manipulation of a tumor is often associated with a transient elevation in blood pressure due to the release of catecholamines into the circulation. This phenomenon may be used as a guide to the location of extraadrenal pheochromocytomas.

CLOSURE

The abdomen is closed in the usual manner.

THORACOABDOMINAL APPROACH FOR RESECTION OF RIGHT ADRENAL CARCINOMA

When an adrenal tumor is large (greater than 10–15 cm in diameter) and malignancy is suspected, a planned thoracoabdominal approach is employed. This provides the wide exposure necessary for radical en bloc resection of the tumor, which may involve removal of the ipsilateral kidney and/or the tail of the pancreas and spleen.

A preoperative intravenous pyelogram is essential, not only for diagnostic purposes but also to verify the presence of bilateral functioning kidneys in case the kidney on the side of the lesion has to be removed. An aortogram may help the surgeon plan the operation by outlining the large tumor vessels beforehand. An inferior vena cavagram may also provide information relevant to local resectability of the tumor: vena caval invasion almost always dictates unresectability.

A right adrenal carcinoma is exposed as shown in Figures 3-66 to 3-69. As illustrated in the anterior approach to adrenalectomy (see Figs. 3-56 and 3-57), the duodenum is mobilized from its peritoneal attachments and retracted medially to expose the underlying vena cava and the main tumor vessels. The peritoneum is incised superiorly and then laterally to expose the fascial attachments between the tumor and the undersurface of the right lobe of the liver. These are taken down by sharp dissection to free the superior aspect of the tumor.

Veins passing between the tumor and the vena cava are isolated, doubly clipped in continuity with large metal clips (see Fig. 3-59), and then divided. The right border of the vena cava is rolled medially to facilitate exposure of the gland and its separation from the cava itself. Laterally and posteriorly the tumor is separated from its vascular and

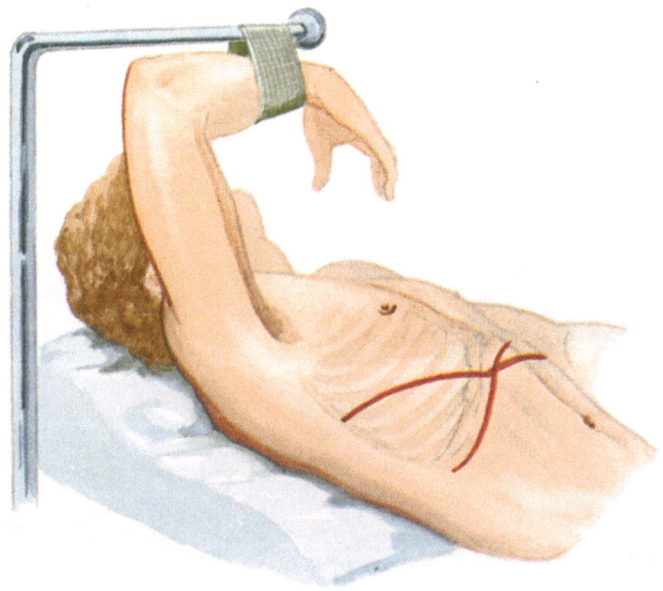

Position. The patient is positioned on the table in the recumbent position with the right side elevated to 45° by a pillow or rolled blanket. The planned incision is indicated by the broken line.

Fig. 3-66.

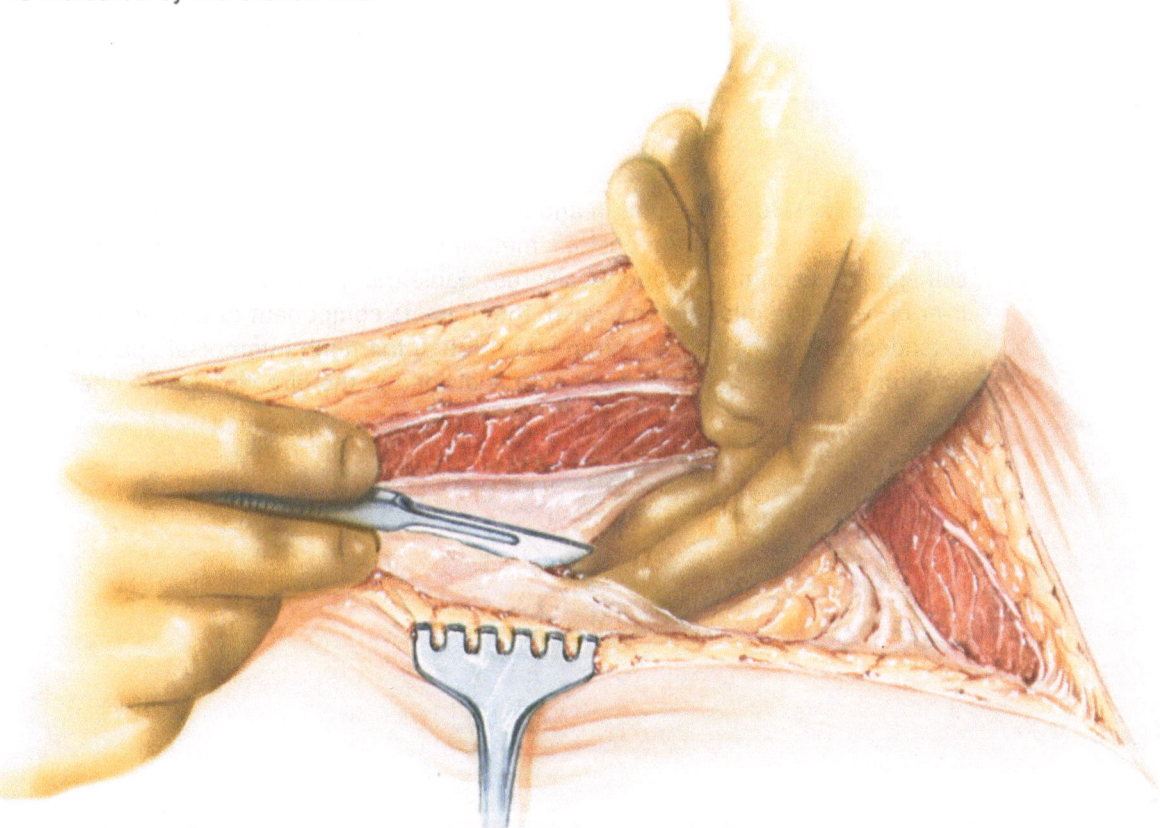

Abdominal incision. The abdominal component of the incision extends transversely across the midline from the lateral edge of the left rectus muscle to the right costal margin opposite the 9th interspace. The rectus muscle on each side has been divided and the incision now is carried down to and through the peritoneum to enter the abdomen.

Fig. 3-67.

229

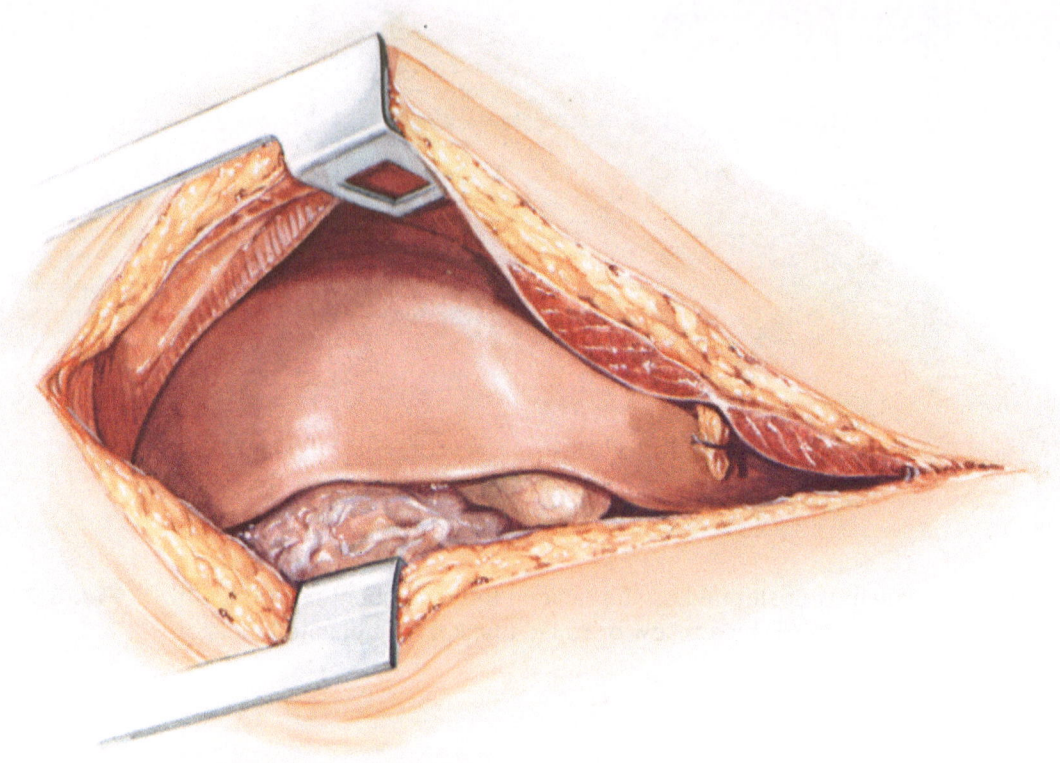

Fig. 3-68.   Thoracic incision. If palpation and inspection of the abdominal organs and lymph node areas reveal no obvious metastatic involvement, and if the tumor itself appears to be mobile and locally resectable (no gross involvement of the liver or adjoining inferior vena cava), the thoracic component of the incision is extended across the costal margin and through the ninth intercostal space into the right pleural cavity. The diaphragm is divided in the direction of the chest incision.

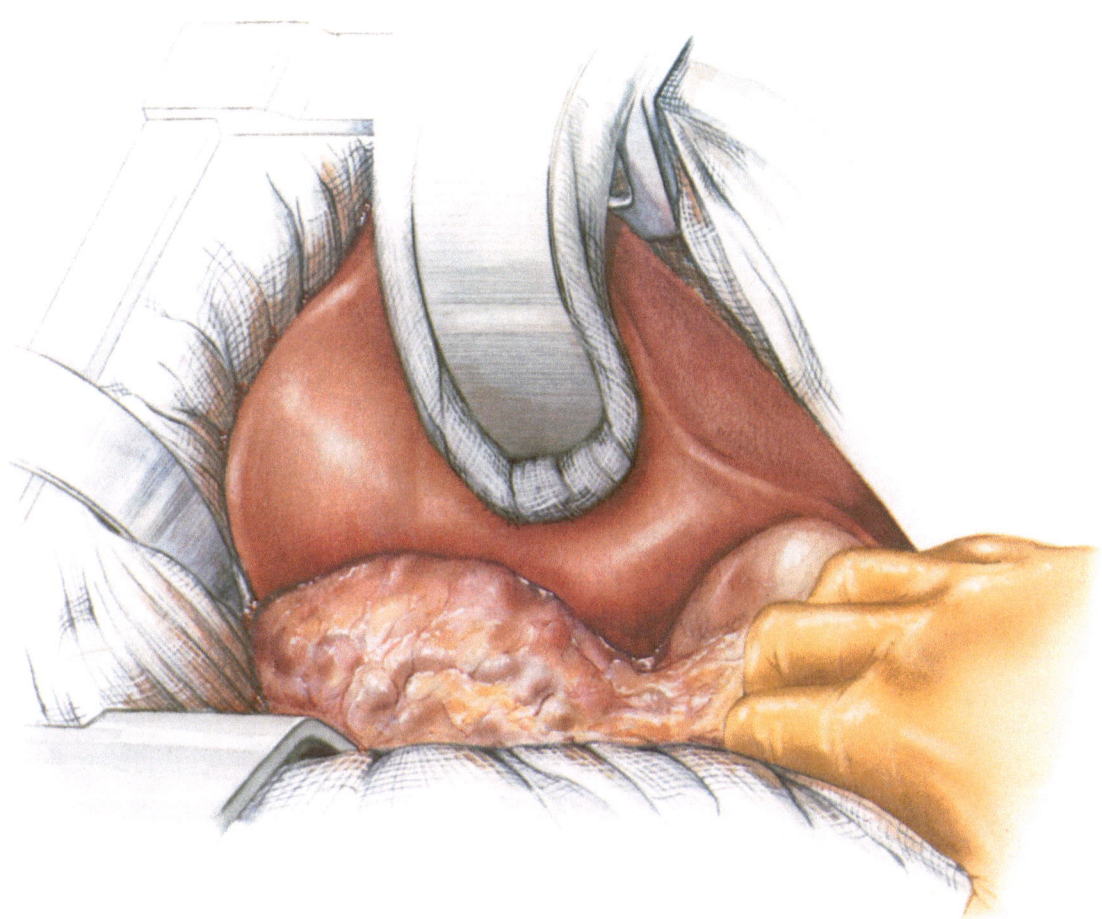

The liver is mobilized by severing the triangular ligament and it is then lifted superiorly using a Deaver retractor. Here, the tumor lies exposed. It is a vascular lesion: large tortuous veins can be seen coursing over its surface directly beneath the posterior parietal peritoneum.

Fig. 3-69.

fascial attachments using sharp and blunt dissection and employing metal clips for hemostasis as shown in Figure 3-60.

Now, the surgeon must ascertain whether there is local involvement of the adjacent kidney. If dissection between the superior pole of the kidney and the tumor reveals malignant invasion, the kidney must be removed in continuity with the adrenal carcinoma (Figs. 3-70 and 3-71).

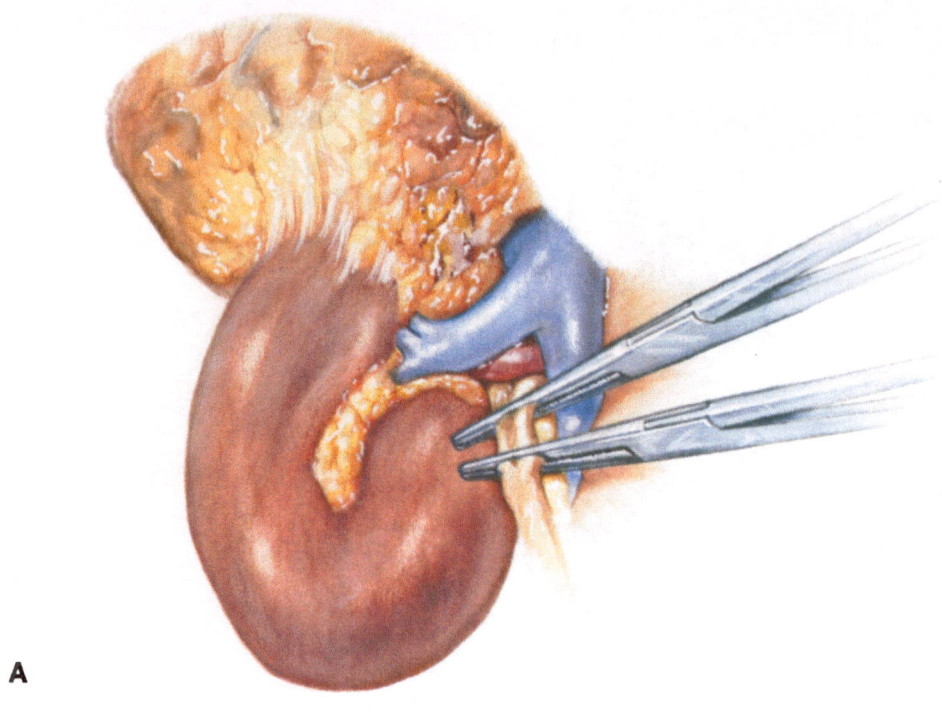

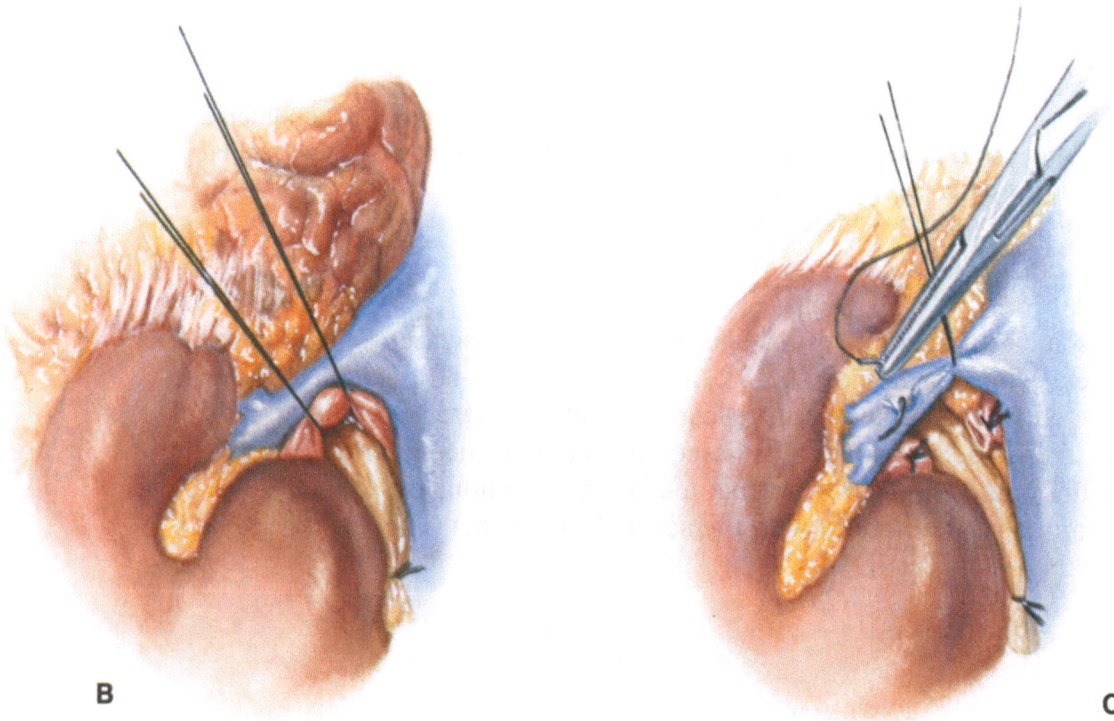

Fig. 3-70. **Removal of the kidney.** **A.** The ureter is first divided. **B.** The right renal artery is then dissected and ligated. **C.** Finally, the right renal vein is isolated, doubly ligated, and transfixed.

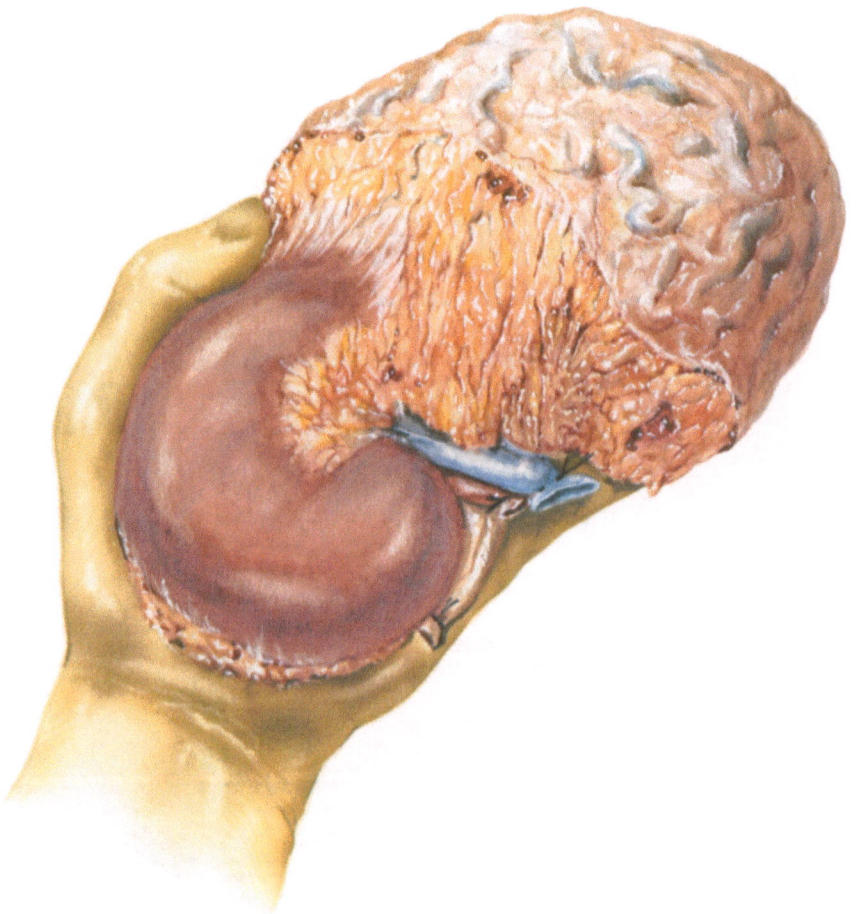

Blunt dissection frees the remainder of the kidney and permits its removal together with the attached tumor.   **Fig. 3-71.**

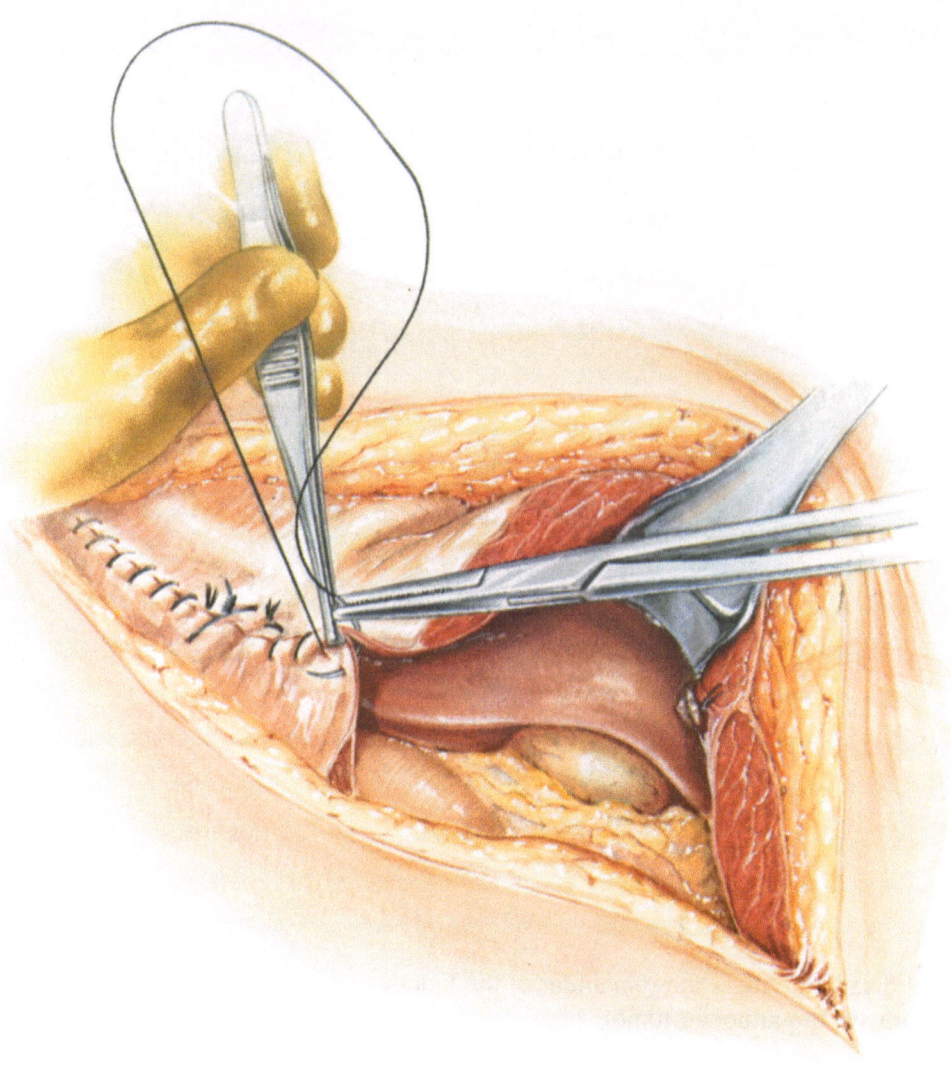

Fig. 3-72.   **Closure.** The wound is closed in layers.

CLOSURE

When hemostasis is judged satisfactory, the field is irrigated, the diaphragm is resutured, and the wound is closed in layers (Fig. 3-72). A chest tube is inserted into the right pleural space during closure. At the completion of the procedure, the lung is hyperinflated to force any residual air from the pleural space, and the tube is removed. A postoperative chest x-ray film is taken to exclude any small residual pneumothorax.

References

1. Weinberger MA: Pheochromocytoma. Arch Intern Med 112:677, 1963.
2. Manger WM, Gifford RW Jr: Current concepts of pheochromocytoma. Cardiovasc Med 3:289–309, 1978.
3. Manger W, Gifford RW Jr: Pheochromocytoma. New York, Springer-Verlag, 1977.
4. Lightman S: Adrenal medulla. *In* James VHT (ed): Comprehensive Endocrinology, The Adrenal Gland. New York, Raven Press, 1979, p 296.
5. Gitlow SE, Mendlowitz M, Bestani LM: The biochemical techniques for detecting and establishing the presence of a pheochromocytoma. Am J Cardiol 26:270–279, 1970.
6. ReMine WH, Chong GC, van Heerden JA, et al: Current management of pheochromocytoma. Ann Surg 179:740–747, 1974.
7. van Heerden JA, Sheps SG, Hamberger B, ReMine WH, et al: Pheochromocytoma: current status and changing trends. Surg 91:367–373, 1982.
8. Scott HW Jr, Oates JA, Nies AS, et al: Pheochromocytoma: present diagnosis and management. Ann Surg 183:587–593, 1976.
9. St John Sutton MG, Sheps SG, Lie JT: Prevalence of clinically unsuspected pheochromocytoma: review of a 50-Year Autopsy Series. Mayo Clin Proc 56:354–360, 1981.
10. Hume DM: Pheochromocytoma in the adult and in the child. Am J Surg 99:458–496, 1960.
11. Mayo CH: Paroxysmal hypertension with tumor of retroperitoneal nerve: report of case. JAMA 89:1047–1050, 1927.
12. Graham JV: Collective review: pheochromocytoma and hypertension: an analysis of 207 cases. Int Abstr Surg 92:105–121, 1951.
13. Stackpole RH, Melicow MM, Uson AC: Pheochromocytoma in childhood. J Pediatr 63:315–330, 1963.
14. Javadpour N, Woltering EA, Brennan MF: Adrenal neoplasms. Curr Probl Surg, 17:5–52, 1980.
15. Van Way CW III, Scott HW Jr, Page DL, et al: Pheochromocytoma. Curr Probl Surg, June, 1974, p 1–59.
16. Scott HW Jr, Reynolds V, Green N, et al: Clinical experience with malignant pheochromocytomas. Surg Gynecol Obstet 154:801–818, 1982.
17. Melicow MM: One hundred cases of pheochromocytoma (107 tumors) at the Columbia–Presbyterian Medical Center, 1926–76: a clinic's pathologic analysis. Cancer 40:1987–2004, 1977.
18. Thompson N: Personal communication, 1983.
19. Crout JR, Sjoerdsma A: Turnover and metabolism of catecholamines in patients with pheochromocytoma. J Clin Invest 43:94–102, 1964.
20. Gifford RW, Kuale WF, Maker FT, et al: Clinical features, diagnosis and treatment of pheochromocytoma: a review of 76 cases. Mayo Clin Proc 39:280–302, 1964.
21. Modlin IM, Famdon JR, Shepherd A, et al: Pheochromocytomas in 72 patients: clinical and diagnostic features, treatment and long-term results. Br J Surg 66:456–465, 1979.
22. Glushien AJ, Mansuy MM, Littman DS: Pheochromocytoma: the relationship to the neurocutaneous syndromes. Am J Med 14:318–327, 1953.
23. Weichert RF: The neural ectodermal origin of the peptide-secreting endocrine glands: a unifying concept for the etiology of multiple endocrine adenomatosis and the inappropriate secretion of peptide hormones by nonendocrine tumors. Am J Med 29:232–241, 1970.
24. Rosati LA, Augua NA: Ischemic enterocolitis in pheochromocytoma. Gastroenterology 60:581–585, 1971.

25. Scharf Y, Nahir M, Plavnic Y, et al: Intermittent claudication with pheochromocytoma. JAMA 205:547, 1968.

26. Gitlow SE, Pertsemlidis D, Bertani LM: Management of patients with pheochromocytoma. Am Heart J 82:557–567, 1971.

27. Harrison TS, Seton JF, Munion GL: High-performance liquid chromatography for urinary catecholamine determination in patients taking alpha-methyldopa. World J Surg 5:462, 1981.

28. Bravo EL, Taragi RC, Gifford RW, et al: Circulating and urinary catecholamine in pheochromocytoma: diagnostic and pathophysiologic implications. N Engl J Med 301:682–686, 1979.

29. Hamberger B, Arver S, Eskilsson P, et al: Plasma catecholamine levels in the diagnosis and management of pheochromocytoma. Surg Gynecol Obstet 152:291–296, 1981.

30. Kopin IJ (moderator): Plasma levels of norepinephrine. Ann Intern Med 88:671–680, 1978.

31. Engelman K, Hammond NG: Adrenalin production by an intrathoracic pheochromocytoma. Lancet 1:609–611, 1968.

32. Mannix H Jr, O'Grady WP, Gitlow SL: Extra-adrenal pheochromocytoma producing epinephrine. Arch Surg 104:216, 1972.

33. Hattery RR, Sheedy PF, Stephens DH, et al: Computed tomography of the adrenal gland. Semin Roentgenol 16:290–300, 1981.

34. Stewart BH, Bravo EL, Haager J, et al: Localization of pheochromocytoma by computed tomography. N Engl J Med 299:460–461, 1978.

35. Thomas JL, Bernardino ME, Samaan NA, et al: CT of Pheochromocytoma. Am J Roentgenol 135:477–482, 1980.

36. Sisson JC, Frager MS, Valk TS, et al: Scintigraphic localization of pheochromocytoma. N Engl J Med 305:12–17, 1981.

37. Valk TW, Frager MS, Gross MD, et al: Spectrum of pheochromocytoma in multiple endocrine neoplasia. Ann Intern Med 94:762–767, 1981.

38. Sutton H, Wyeth P, Allen AO, et al: Disseminated malignant pheochromocytoma: localization with iodine-131-labelled beta-Iodobenzylguanidine. Br Med J 285:1153–1154, 1982.

39. Brogden RN, Heel RC, Speight TM, et al: Alpha-methyl-p-tyrosine: a review of its pharmacology and its clinical use. Drugs 2:81, 1981.

40. Goldfien A: Pheochromocytoma: diagnosis and anesthetic and surgical management. Anesthesiology 24:462–471, 1963.

41. Kreul JF, Dauchot PJ, Anton AH: Hemodynamic and catecholamine studies during pheochromocytoma resection under enflurane anesthesia. Anaesthesiology 44:265–268, 1976.

42. Johns VJ, Brunjes S: Pheochromocytoma. Am J Cardiol 9:120–125, 1962.

43. Scott W, Dean RH, Lea JW, et al: Surgical experience with retrogastric and retropancreatic pheochromocytomas. Surgery 92:853–865, 1982.

44. Sellwood RA, Wapnick S, Breckenridge A, et al: Recurrent pheochromocytoma. Br J Surg 57:309–312, 1970.

45. Beierwaltes WH: New horizons for therapeutic nuclear medicine in 1981. J Nucl Med 22:549–554, 1981.

46. James RE, Baker HL, Scanlon PW: The roentgenologic aspects of metastatic pheochromocytoma. Am J Roentgenol Radium Ther Nucl Med 115:783–93, 1972.

47. Fudge TL, McKinnon WMP, Geary NL: Current surgical management of pheochromocytoma during pregnancy. Arch Surg 115:1224, 1980.

48. Schenker JG, Chowers I: Pheochromocytoma and pregnancy. Obstet Gynecol Surv 26:739–747, 1971.

49. Freier DT, Eckhauser FE, Harrison TS: Pheochromocytoma: a persistently problematic and still potentially lethal disease. Arch Surg 115:388–391, 1980.

50. Harrison TS, Thompson NW: Multiple endocrine adenomatosis. Curr Probl Surg, August, 1975.

51. Sizemore GW, Heath H III, Carney JA: Multiple endocrine neoplasia, type 2. Clin Endocrinol Metab 9:299–315, 1980.

52. Webb TA, Sheps SG, Carney JA: Differences between sporadic pheochromocytoma and pheochromocytoma in multiple endocrine neoplasia, type 2. Am J Surg Pathol 4:121–126, 1980.

53. van Heerden JA, Sizemore GW, Carney YA, et al: Surgical management of the adrenal glands in the multiple endocrine neoplasia type 2 syndrome. In Press.

54. Freier DT, Thompson NW, Sisson JC, et al: Dilemmas in the early diagnosis and treatment of multiple endocrine adenomatosis, type II. Surgery 82:407–413, 1977.

55. Fishman LM, Juchel O, Liddle GW, et al: Incidence of primary aldosteronism in uncomplicated "essential" hypertension. JAMA, 205:497–502, 1968.

56. Laragh JH, Sealey JE, Sommers SC: Patterns of adrenal secretion and urinary excretion of aldosterone and plasma renin activity in normal and hypertensive subjects. Circ Res [Suppl I] 18, 19:I-158–I-174, 1966.

57. Streeten DHP, Touryz N, Anderson GH: Reliability of screening methods for the diagnosis of primary aldosteronism. Am J Med 67:403–413, 1979.

58. Giebink ES, Gotlin RW, Biglieri EG, et al: A kindred with familial glucocorticoid suppressible aldosteronism. J Clin Endocrinol Metab 36:715–723, 1973.

59. Sutherland DJA, Ruse JL, Laidlaw JC: Hypertension, increased aldosterone secretion, and low plasma renin activity relieved by dexamethasone. Can Med Assoc J 95:1109–1119, 1966.

60. Auda SP, Brennan MF, Gill JR: Evolution of the surgical management of primary aldosteronism. Ann Surg 191:1–7, 1980.

61. Grant CS, Carpenter P, Hamberger B, et al: The management of primary aldosteronism. Arch Surg 119:585–590, 1984.

62. Hunt TK, Schambelan M, Biglieri EG: Selection of patients and operative approach in primary aldosteronism. Ann Surg 182:353–361, 1975.

63. Neville AM: The nodular adrenal. Invest Cell Pathol 1:99–111, 1978.

64. Kaplan NM: The steroid content of adrenal adenomas and measurements of aldosterone production in patients with essential hypertension and primary aldosteronism. J Clin Invest 46:728–734, 1967.

65. Ferriss JB, Beevers DG, Brown JJ, et al: Clinical, biochemical, and pathological features of low-renin ("Primary") hyperaldosteronism. Am Heart J 95:375–388, 1978.

66. Mackett MCT, Crane MG, Smith LL: Surgical management of aldosterone-producing adrenal adenomas. Am J Surg 142:89–95, 1981.

67. Beevers DG, Brown JJ, Ferris JR, et al: Renal abnormalities and vascular complications in primary aldosteronism. Evidence on tertiary hyperaldosteronism. Q J Med 45:401–410, 1976.

68. Conn JW: Primary aldosteronism, a new clinical syndrome. J Lab Clin Med 45:3–17, 1955.

69. Delarue NC, Laidlaw JC, Kovacsk K, et al: Hypertension due to "primary" aldosteronism—surgical considerations. Surgery 80:289–296, 1976.

70. Weinberger MH, Grim CE, Hollifield JW, et al: Primary aldosteronism. Ann Intern Med 90:386–395, 1979.

71. Hiramatsu K, Yamada T, Yukimura Y, et al: A screening test to identify aldosterone-producing adenoma by measuring plasma renin activity. Arch Intern Med 141:1589–1593, 1981.

72. Melby JC, Spark R, Cale S, et al: Diagnosis and localization of aldosterone-producing adenomas by adrenal vein catheterization. N Engl J Med 277:1050–1056, 1967.

73. Granberg PO, Adamson U, Cohn KH, et al: The management of patients with

primary aldosteronism. World J Surg 6:757–764, 1982.

74. Melby JC: Assessment of adrenocortical function. N Engl J Med 285:735–739, 1971.

75. Conn JW, Rovner DR, Cohen EC, et al: Preoperative diagnosis of primary aldosteronism. Arch Intern Med 123:113–123, 1969.

76. St. Cyr MJ, Sancho JM, Melby JC: Quantitation of plasma aldosterone by radioimmunoassay. Clin Chem 18:1395, 1972.

77. Ganguly A, Melada GA, Luetsoher JA, et al: Control of plasma aldosterone in primary aldosteronism: distinction between adenoma and hyperplasia. J Clin Endocrinol Metab 37:765–775, 1973.

78. Herf SM, Teates DC, Tegtmeyer CJ, et al: Identification and differentiation of surgically correctable hypertension due to primary aldosteronism. Am J Med 67:397–402, 1979.

79. Vaughan NJA, Jowett TP, Slater JDH, et al: The diagnosis of primary hyperaldosteronism. Lancet, 1:120–125, 1981.

80. Wisgerhof M, Brown RD, Hogan JJ, et al: The plasma aldosterone response to angiotensin II infusion in aldosterone-producing adenoma and idiopathic hyperaldosteronism. J Clin Endocrinol Metab 52:195–198, 1981.

81. Edis AJ: In Discussion of Herwig KR: Primary aldosteronism: experience with thirty–eight patients. Surgery 86:470–74, 1979.

82. Eghrari M, McLoughlin JJ, Rosen IE, et al: The role of computed tomography in assessment of tumor pathology of the adrenal glands. J Comput Assist Tomogr 4:71, 1980.

83. Montagne J, Kressel JY, Korabkin M, et al: Computed tomography of the normal adrenal glands. Am J Roentgenol 130:963–6, 1978.

84. White EA, Schambelan M, Rost CR, et al: Use of computed tomography in diagnosing the cause of primary aldosteronism. N Engl J Med 303:1503–1507, 1980.

85. Gross MD, Greitas JE, Grekin RJ, et al: Letter. N Engl J Med 304:1046, 1981.

86. Miles JM, Wahner HW, Carpenter PC, et al: Adrenal scintiscanning with NP-59: a new radioiodinated cholesterol agent. Mayo Clin Proc 54:321–327, 1979.

87. Herwig KR: Primary aldosteronism: experience with thirty–eight patients. Surgery, 86:470–74, 1979.

88. Adamson U, Efendie S, Granberg PO, et al: Preoperative localization of aldosterone-producing adenomas. An analysis of the efficacy of different diagnostic procedures made from 11 cases and from a review of the literature. Acta Med Scand 208:101–109, 1980.

89. Davis WW, Newsome HH, Wright LD, et al: Bilateral adrenal hyperplasia as a cause of primary aldosteronism with hypertension, hypokalemia, and suppressed renin activity. Am J Med 42:642–647, 1967.

90. Scoggins BA, Coghlan JJ: Primary hyperaldosteronism. Pharmacol Ther 9:367–394, 1980.

91. Kremer D, Boddy K, Brown JJ, et al: Amiloride in the treatment of primary hyperaldosteronism and essential hypertension. Clin Endocrinol 7:151–157, 1977.

92. Russell CF, Hamberger B, van Heerden JA, et al: Adrenalectomy: Anterior or posterior approach. Am J Surg 144:322–324, 1982.

93. Cushing H: The basophil adenomas of the pituitary body and their clinical manifestations (pituitary basophilism). Bull Johns Hopkins Hosp 50:137–195, 1932.

94. Plotz CM, Knowlton AL, Ragan C: Natural history of Cushing's syndrome. Am J Med 13:597–614, 1952.

95. Welbourn RB, Montgomery DAD, Kennedy TL: The natural history of treated Cushing's syndrome. Br J Surg 58:1–16, 1971.

96. Frajria R, Angeli A: Alcohol-induced pseudo-Cushing's syndrome. Lancet 1:1050–1051, 1977.
97. Rees LH, Besser GM, Jeffcoate WJ, et al: Alcohol-induced pseudo-Cushing's syndrome. Lancet 1:726–728, 1977.
98. Thompson NW, Allo MD: Management of acute hypercortisolism. World J Surg 6:748–756, 1982.
99. Orth DN, Liddle GW: Results of treatment in 108 patients with Cushing's syndrome. N Engl J Med 285:243–247, 1971.
100. Thompson JA, Whyte WG, Stirling WB: The treatment of Cushing's syndrome by subtotal adrenalectomy. *In* Binder C, Hall PE (eds): Cushing's Syndrome, Diagnosis and Treatment. London, Heinemann, 1972, pp 126–131.
101. Nelson DH, Meakin JW, Thorn GW: ACTH-producing pituitary tumors following adrenalectomy for Cushing's syndrome. Ann Intern Med 52:560–569, 1960.
102. Hardy J: Transsphenoidal microsurgery of the normal and pathologic pituitary. Clin Neurosurg 16:185–217, 1969.
103. Vale W, Spiess J, Rivier C, et al: Characterization of a 41-residue ovine hypothalamic peptide that stimulates secretion of corticotropin and β-endorphin. Science 213:1394–1397, 1981.
104. Liddle GW, Island D, Meador CR: Normal and abnormal regulation of corticotropin secretion in man. Rec Prog Horm Res 18:125–166, 1962.
105. Samaan NA: Hormone production in non-endocrine tumors. Cancer 273:148, 1977.
106. Rees LH, Bloomfield GA, Gilkes JJH, et al: ACTH as a tumor marker. Ann NY Acad Sci 297:603–620, 1977.
107. Gilby FD, Rees LH, Bondy PK: Ectopic hormones as markers of responses to therapy in cancer. International Congress Series, No. 375. Amsterdam, Excerpta Medica, 1976, pp 132–138.
108. Azzopardi JG, Williams ED: Pathology of "nonendocrine" tumors associated with Cushing's syndrome. Cancer 22:274–286, 1968.
109. Besser GM, Edwards CRW: Cushing's syndrome. Clin Endocrinol Metab 1:451–490, 1972.
110. Reeder HJ, Loriaux DL, Lipsett MB: Severe osteopenia in young adults associated with Cushing's syndrome due to micronodular adrenal disease. J Clin Endocrinol 39:1138, 1974.
111. Scott WH Jr, Foster JH, Rhamy RK, et al: Surgical management of adrenocortical tumors with Cushing's syndrome. Ann Surg 173:892–905, 1971.
112. Liddle GW, Melmon KL: The adrenals. *In* Williams RH (ed): Textbook of Endocrinology (ed 5). Philadelphia, Saunders, 1974.
113. Scott WH Jr, Liddle GW, Harris AP, et al: Diagnosis and treatment of Cushing's syndrome. Ann Surg 155:696–710, 1962.
114. Freeark RJ, Waldstein SS: Present status of the diagnosis and treatment of Cushing's syndrome. Surg Clin North Am 49:179, 1969.
115. Davies CJ, Joplin GF, Welbourn RB: Surgical management of the ectopic ACTH syndrome. Ann Surg 196:246–258, 1982.
116. Crapo L: Cushing's syndrome: a review of diagnostic tests. Metabolism 28:955–977, 1979.
117. Liddle GW: Tests of pituitary–adrenal suppressibility in the diagnosis of Cushing's syndrome. J Clin Endocrinol Metab 20:1539–1560, 1960.
118. White FE, White MC, Drury PL, et al: Value of computed tomography of the abdomen and chest in investigation of Cushing's syndrome. Br Med J 284:770–774, 1982.
119. Dunnick NR, Schaner EG, Doppman JL, et al: Computed tomography in adrenal tumours. Am J Roentgenol 132:43–46, 1979.

120. Muhm JR, Brown LR, Crowe JK, et al: Comparison of whole lung tomography and CT for detecting pulmonary nodules. Am J Roentgenol 131:981–984, 1979.

121. Sheedy PF II, Stephens DH, Hattery RR, et al: Computed tomography of the pancreas. Radiol Clin North Am 15:349–366, 1979.

122. Salassa RM, Laws ER Jr, Carpenter PC, et al: Transsphenoidal removal of pituitary microadenoma in Cushing's disease. Unpublished data, 1983.

123. Salassa RM, Laws ER, Carpenter PC, et al: Transsphenoidal removal of pituitary microadenoma in Cushing's disease. Mayo Clin Proc 53:24–28, 1978.

124. Tyrell JB, Brooks RM, Fitsgerald PA, et al: Cushing's disease: selective transsphenoidal resection of pituitary microadenomas. N Engl J Med 298:753–758, 1978.

125. Bigos ST, Somma M, Rasio E, et al: Cushing's disease: management by transsphenoidal pituitary microsurgery. J Clin Endocrinol Metab 50:348–354, 1980.

126. Scott WH, Liddle GW, Mulherin JL, et al: Surgical experience with Cushing's disease. Ann Surg 185:524–534, 1977.

127. Watson G, van Heerden JA, Grant CS: Adrenal Cushing's disease. Unpublished data.

128. Lawrence JH, Tobia CA, Linfoot JA, et al: Heavy-particle therapy in acromegaly and Cushing's disease. JAMA 235:307–310, 1976.

129. Krieger DT, Amorosa L, Linick F: Cyproheptadine-induced remission of Cushing's disease. N Engl J Med 293:893–896, 1975.

130. Lamberts SWJ, Birkenhager JC: Effect of bromocriptine in pituitary dependent Cushing's syndrome. J Endocrinol 70:315, 1976.

131. Jeffcoate WJ, Rees LH, Tomlin S, et al: Metyrapone in long-term management of Cushing's disease. Br Med J 2:215–217, 1977.

132. Orth DN: Metyrapone is useful only as an adjunctive therapy in Cushing's disease. Ann Intern Med 89:128–130, 1978.

133. Luton JP, Mahoudeau JA, Bonchard PH, et al: Treatment of Cushing's disease by o',p'-DDD: survey of 62 cases. N Engl J Med 300:459–464, 1979.

134. Hamberger B, Russell CF, van Heerden JA, et al: Adrenal surgery: trends during the seventies. Am J Surg 144:523–526, 1982.

135. American Cancer Society. Cancer Facts and Figures. New York, 1981, p 15.

136. McGuire WL: An update on estrogen and progesterone receptors in prognosis for primary and advanced breast cancer. In Iacobelli S, et al (eds): Hormones and Cancer. New York, Raven Press, 1980, pp 337–343.

137. Halsted WS: The results of operation for the cure of cancer of the breast performed at the Johns Hopkins Hospital from June 1889 to January 1894. Johns Hopkins Hosp Rep 4:1–54, 1894.

138. Beatson GT: On treatment of inoperable cases in carcinoma of manima: suggestion for new method of treatment with illustrative cases. Lancet 2:104–107, 162–165, 1896.

139. Huggins C, Bergenstal DM: Inhibition of human mammary and prostatic cancer by adrenalectomy. Cancer Res 12:134–141, 1952.

140. Robin TE, Dalton GA: The role of major endocrine ablation. In Stall BA (ed): Breast Cancer Management—Early and Late. Chicago, Year Book, 1977, p 147–156.

141. Santen RJ, Worgul TJ, Lipton A, et al: Aminoglutethimide as treatment of postmenopausal women with advanced breast carcinoma. Ann Intern Med 96:94–101, 1982.

142. Manni A, Pearson OH: Anti-estrogen induced remissions in premenopausal women with stage IV breast cancer: effects of ovarian function. Cancer Treat Rep 64:779–785, 1980.

143. Pritchard KL, Thompson DB, Myers RE, et al: Tamoxifen therapy in premenopausal patients with metastatic breast cancer. Cancer Treat Rep 64:787–796, 1980.

144. Greenblatt RB, Colle ML, Makesh VB: Ovarian and adrenal steroid production in the postmenopausal woman. Obstet Gynecol 47:383–387, 1976.

145. Judd HL, Barone RM, Laufer LR, et al: In vivo effects of Δ^1-testolactone on peripheral aromatization. Cancer Res [Suppl] 42:3345s–3385s, 1982.

146. Newsome HH, Brown PW, Terz JJ, et al: Medical adrenalectomy and plasma steroids in advanced breast carcinoma. Surgery 83:83–89, 1978.

147. Wells SA, Santer RJ, Lipton A, et al: Medical adrenalectomy with aminoglutethimide. Ann Surg 187:475–484, 1978.

148. Santen RJ, Santner SJ, Tilsen–Mallett N, et al: In vivo and in vitro pharmacological studies of aminoglutethimide as an aromatase inhibitor. Cancer Res [Suppl] 42:3353s–3359s, 1982.

149. Huvos AJ, Hajdu SI, Brosfield RD, et al: Adrenal cortical carcinoma: clinicopathologic study of 34 cases. Cancer 25:354–361, 1970.

150. Lipsett MB, Hertz R, Ross GT: Clinical and pathologic aspects of adrenocortical carcinoma. Am J Med 35:374–383, 1963.

151. McFarlane DA: Cancer of the adrenal cortex: the natural history, prognosis and treatment in a study of 55 cases. Ann R Coll Surg Engl 23:155–186, 1958.

152. van Heerden JA, Henley DJ, Grant CS, et al: Adrenal cortical carcinoma. Surgery 94:926–931, 1983.

153. Richie JR, Gittes RF: Carcinoma of the adrenal cortex. Cancer 45:1957–1964, 1980.

154. Steiner PE: Cancer, Race and Geography. Baltimore, Williams & Wilkins, 1954.

155. Sullivan M, Boileace M, Hodges CV: Adrenal cortical carcinoma. J Urol 120:660–665, 1978.

156. Lewinsky BS, Grigor KM, Symington T, et al: The clinical and pathologic features of "non-hormonal" adrenocortical tumors. Cancer 33:778–790, 1974.

157. Harrison TS, Gann DS, Edis AJ, Egdahl, RH: Surgical Disorders of the Adrenal Gland. New York, Grune & Stratton, 1975.

158. Gabrilove JL, Sharma DC, Wotiz HH, et al: Feminizing adrenocortical tumors in the male, a review of 52 cases including a case report. Medicine (Baltimore) 44:37–79, 1965.

159. Cahill PJ, Sukov RJ: Inferior vena caval involvement by adrenal cortical carcinoma. Urology, 10:604–607; 1977.

160. Geelhoed GW, Dunnick NR, Doppman JL: Management of intravenous extensions of endocrine tumors and prognosis after surgical treatment. Am J Surg 139:844–848, 1980.

161. Didolkar MS, Bescher RA, Elias EG, et al: Natural history of adrenal cortical carcinoma. A clinicopathologic study of 42 patients. Cancer 47:2153–2161, 1981.

162. King DR, Rack EE: Adrenal cortical carcinoma: a clinical pathologic study of 49 cases. Cancer 44:239–244, 1979.

163. Bradley EL: Primary and adjunctive therapy in carcinoma of the adrenal cortex. Surg Gynecol Obstet 141:507–511, 1975.

164. Greenberg PH, Marks C: Adrenal cortical carcinoma: a presentation of 22 cases and a review of the literature. Am Surg 44:81–85, 1978.

165. Hutter AM, Kayhoe DE: Adrenal cortical carcinoma: results of treatment with op'DDD in 138 patients. Am J Med 41:581–592, 1966.

166. Lubitz JA, Freeman L, Okun R: Mitotane use in inoperable adrenal cortical carcinoma. JAMA 2223:1109–1112, 1973.

167. Ostuni JA, Raginsky MS: Metastatic adrenal cortical carcinoma: documented cure with combined chemotherapy. Arch Intern Med 135:1257–1258, 1975.

168. Schteingart DE, Motazidi A, Noonan RA, et al: Treatment of adrenal carcinomas. Arch Surg 117:1142–1146, 1982.

169. Schteingart DE, Tsao HS, Taylor CI, et al: Sustained remissions of Cushing's disease with mitotane and pituitary irradiation. Ann Intern Med 92:613–619, 1980.

170. Cash R, Brough AJ, Cohen MNP, et al: Aminoglutethimide (Elipten-Ciba) as an inhibitor of adrenal steroidogenesis: mechanism of action and therapeutic trial. J Clin Endocrinol Metab 27:1239–1248, 1967.

171. Schteingart DE, Cash R, Coon JW: Aminoglutethimide and metastatic adrenal cancer. JAMA 198:1007–1010, 1966.

172. Russi S, Blumenthal HT, Gray SH: Small adenomas of the adrenal cortex in hypertension and diabetes. Arch Intern Med 76:284–291, 1945.

173. Dobbie JW: Adrenocortical nodular hyperplasia: The aging adrenal. J Pathol 99:1–18, 1969.

174. Prinz RA, Brooks MH, Churchill R, et al: Incidental asymptomatic adrenal masses detected by computed tomographic scanning: is operation required? JAMA 248:701–704, 1982.

175. Bertagna C, Orth DN: Clinical and laboratory findings and results of therapy in 58 patients with adrenocortical tumors admitted to a single medical center (1951–1978). Am J Med 71:855–875, 1981.

176. Smith JM, Keane FB, O'Flynn JD, et al: Primary non-functioning carcinoma of adrenal cortex. Urology 13:253–255, 1979.

177. Young HH: A technique for simultaneous exposure and operation on the adrenals. Surg Gynecol Obstet 54:179, 1936.

Surgery of the Endocrine Pancreas

4

The first association between an endocrine disorder and pancreatic islet cell tumor was made by Wilder and associates (1) in 1927 when they encountered clinical hyperinsulinism in a patient with metastatic islet cell carcinoma; they were able to extract insulin from samples of metastatic tumor. Since this discovery, which has been enhanced by the development and refinement of immunocytochemical techniques and electron microscopy, the gastroenteropancreatic tract has emerged as a major endocrine "organ." It is the source of 15 currently identifiable endocrine cells (2). In addition, it was recognized that similar cells located in other organs possess the capability of producing polypeptide hormones. These cells could take up amine precursors (such as DOPA or 5-hydroxytryptamine), decarboxylate them, and subsequently produce either amines or polypeptides (such as norepinephrine, serotonin, etc). The amine precursor uptake and decarboxylation (APUD) cell system was proposed by Pearse (3), and tumors derived from these cells were referred to as "apudomas" (4) (Fig. 4-1). While controversy exists as to their embryologic origin, the evidence seems strong in support of the neural crest. Neuron-specific enolase, an enzyme present in central and peripheral autonomic nerves, has also been reliably demonstrated in apudomas (2,5). Thus, from the first islet cell tumor in 1927, a widely dispersed but cytochemically similar neuroendocrine APUD cell system has been recognized.

To date, no less than ten different clinical syndromes have been described in association with functioning islet cell tumors of the pancreas (Fig. 4-2). The responsible hormones have been identified: insulin with insulinoma; gastrin with gastrinoma or Zollinger-Ellison syndrome; vasoactive intestinal polypeptide (VIP) with vipoma (WDHA syndrome); glucagon with glucagonoma; somatostatin with somatostatinoma; ACTH with ectopic ACTH syndrome; melanocyte-stimulating hormone with hyperpigmentation; parathyroid hormone with ectopic hyperparathyroidism; 5-hydroxytryptamine with carcinoid syndrome; and cholecystokinin (CCK) with "CCK-oma" (6,7). The same tumor may secrete a number of different hormones owing to the pleuripotential hormone-secreting capability of the cells. No doubt the list of hormones secreted and syndromes recognized will continue to grow.

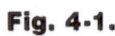

Fig. 4-1.

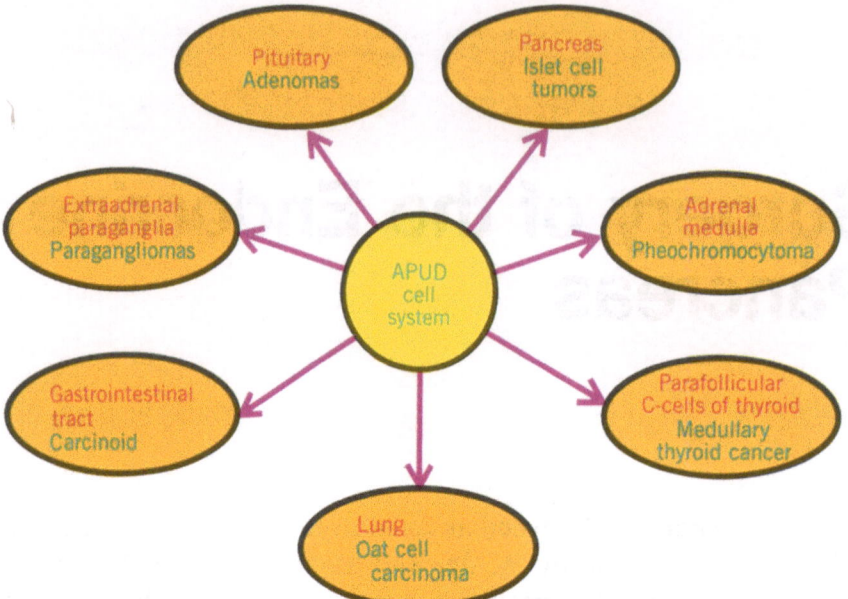

Pituitary
Adenomas

Pancreas
Islet cell
tumors

Extraadrenal
paraganglia
Paragangliomas

APUD
cell
system

Adrenal
medulla
Pheochromocytoma

Gastrointestinal
tract
Carcinoid

Parafollicular
C-cells of thyroid
Medullary
thyroid cancer

Lung
Oat cell
carcinoma

Fig. 4-2.

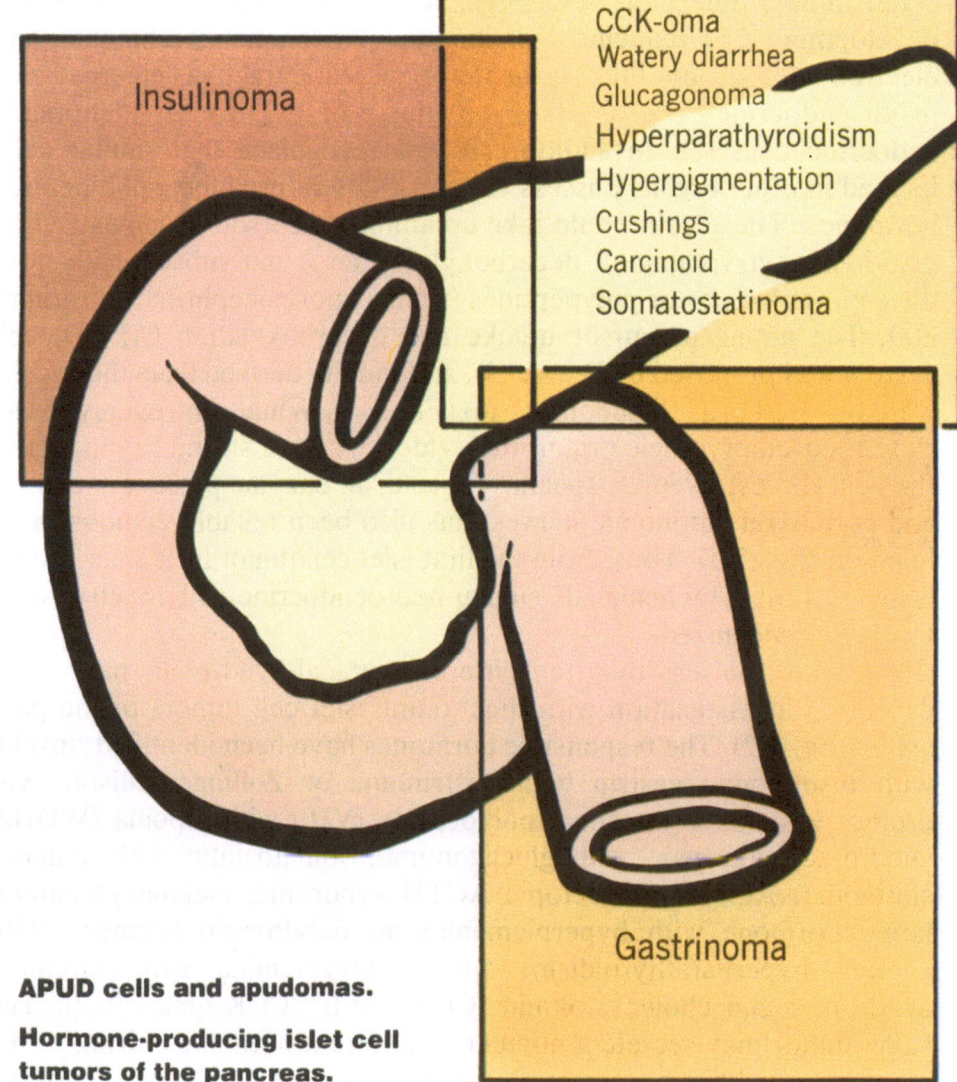

Insulinoma

CCK-oma
Watery diarrhea
Glucagonoma
Hyperparathyroidism
Hyperpigmentation
Cushings
Carcinoid
Somatostatinoma

Gastrinoma

Fig. 4-1. APUD cells and apudomas.

Fig. 4-2. Hormone-producing islet cell tumors of the pancreas.

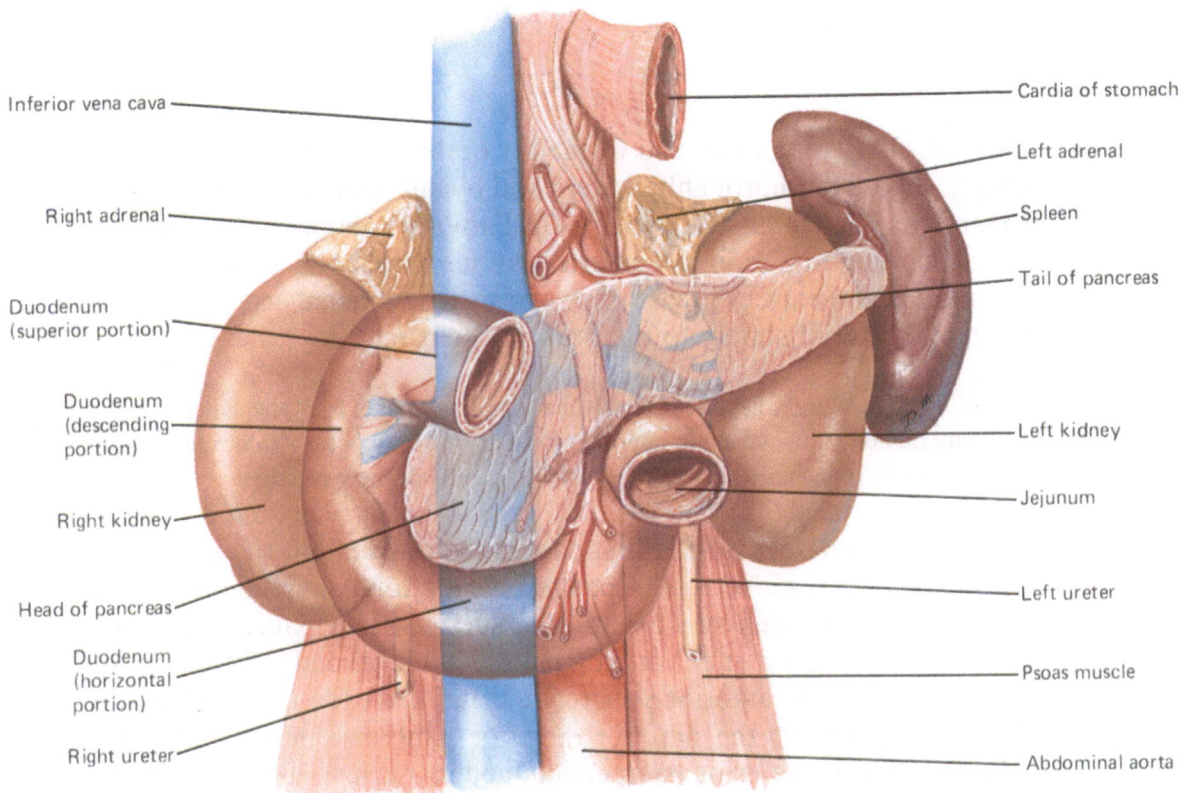

Inferior vena cava

Right adrenal

Duodenum (superior portion)

Duodenum (descending portion)

Right kidney

Head of pancreas

Duodenum (horizontal portion)

Right ureter

Cardia of stomach

Left adrenal

Spleen

Tail of pancreas

Left kidney

Jejunum

Left ureter

Psoas muscle

Abdominal aorta

Posterior relations of the pancreas. For simplicity the common bile duct and the components of the portal venous system are not shown.

Fig. 4-3.

SURGICAL ANATOMY

ORIENTATION

The pancreas occupies a relatively fixed retroperitoneal position in the upper abdomen as it extends obliquely upward at a 45° angle from the duodenal loop to the splenic hilum. It has a thick, wide head and uncinate process and a more slender neck, body, and tail. Posteriorly, the head is related to the inferior vena cava and aorta (Fig. 4-3). The neck overlies and the body and tail extend to the left of the superior mesenteric vessels. Normally, the body and tail may be easily freed from the underlying left adrenal gland, kidney, and renal vessels by blunt dissection. Distal resection of the pancreas extending to the right edge of the portal vein usually incorporates 65%–80% of the gland. The uncinate process refers to that portion of the pancreas that extends around inferiorly beneath the superior mesenteric vein.

BLOOD SUPPLY

Arterial. The complexity and variability of the pancreatic arterial blood supply should be thoroughly understood by surgeons performing major pancreatic resections. The two principal arterial sources are branches of the celiac and superior mesenteric arteries (Fig. 4-4). Typically, the common hepatic artery gives rise to the gastroduodenal artery, which is the major arterial supply to the head of the pancreas.

A "replaced" right hepatic artery—one which originates from the superior mesenteric artery (occurring in approximately 20%)—may occasionally send major pancreatic branches as it ascends behind the head of the pancreas.

After passing behind the first part of the duodenum, the gastroduodenal artery gives rise to the posterior superior pancreaticoduodenal artery, then continues over the anterior surface of the pancreas to bifurcate into the anterior superior pancreaticoduodenal and right gastroepiploic arteries. The anterior pancreatic arterial arcade is completed by the anastomosis of the anterior superior pancreaticoduodenal artery with the anterior inferior pancreaticoduodenal artery, one branch of a common inferior pancreaticoduodenal artery originating from the superior mesenteric artery. Similarly, the posterior arcade is formed by anastomosis of the posterior superior pancreaticoduodenal artery with the posterior inferior pancreaticoduodenal artery (the other branch of the common pancreaticoduodenal artery).

In adults it is nearly impossible to resect either the duodenum or pancreas without seriously compromising the blood supply of the other. It is feasible, however, to resect approximately 95% of the distal pancreas and still preserve the viability of the duodenum, provided a small crescent of the gland is left to protect the pancreaticoduodenal arcades. One must also protect the intrapancreatic common bile duct and its blood supply (the posterior superior pancreaticoduodenal artery) as it courses in or near the posterior pancreaticoduodenal groove.

The blood supply to the neck, body, and tail of the pancreas is derived primarily from branches of the splenic artery. This tortuous vessel courses along the posterior superior border of the gland. The dorsal pancreatic artery typically originates from the first part of the splenic artery and passes vertically downward behind the neck of the pancreas. At the level of the confluence of the splenic and superior mesenteric veins, it branches into minor arteries passing to the right, and the larger transverse (inferior) pancreatic artery, which runs laterally to the left, posterior, and somewhat superior to the lower border of the pancreas. The great pancreatic artery (pancreatica magna) arises

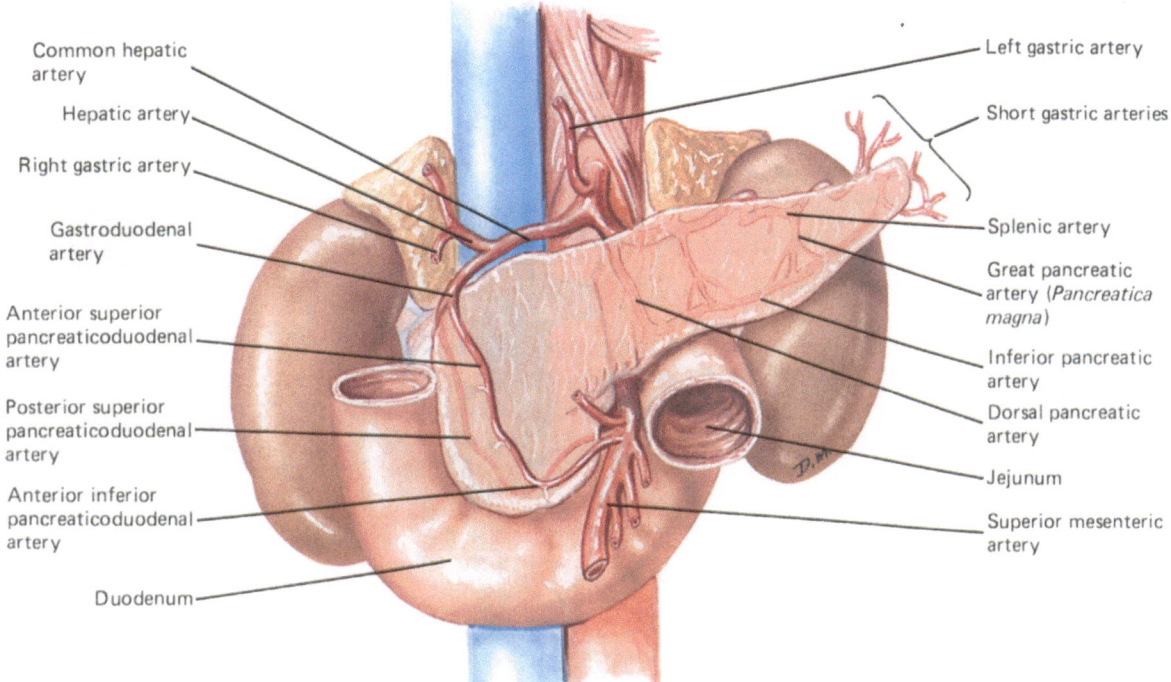

Common hepatic artery

Hepatic artery

Right gastric artery

Gastroduodenal artery

Anterior superior pancreaticoduodenal artery

Posterior superior pancreaticoduodenal artery

Anterior inferior pancreaticoduodenal artery

Duodenum

Left gastric artery

Short gastric arteries

Splenic artery

Great pancreatic artery (*Pancreatica magna*)

Inferior pancreatic artery

Dorsal pancreatic artery

Jejunum

Superior mesenteric artery

Arterial blood supply of the pancreas. **Fig. 4-4.**

from the splenic artery in its distal third and is the major blood supply to the tail of the pancreas.

Venous. While the anatomic pattern of venous drainage generally parallels its arterial counterpart, several features of surgical and radiographic importance should be appreciated (Fig. 4-5).

The portal vein is formed behind the neck of the pancreas by the confluence of the splenic and superior mesenteric veins. The left gastric vein (coronary vein) variably empties either directly into the portal vein or into the splenic vein near its junction with the superior mesenteric vein. The inferior mesenteric vein most commonly joins the splenic vein. Alternatively, it may enter the superior mesenteric vein, or all three may converge together. The anterior surface of the superior mesenteric–portal vein (SMV-PV) behind the neck of the pancreas almost never receives tributaries and may be blindly, gently dissected free unless it is directly involved by a pathologic process.

Veins draining the head and uncinate process of the pancreas include the anterior and posterior pancreaticoduodenal arcades as well as numerous fragile tributaries emptying directly into the lateral aspect of

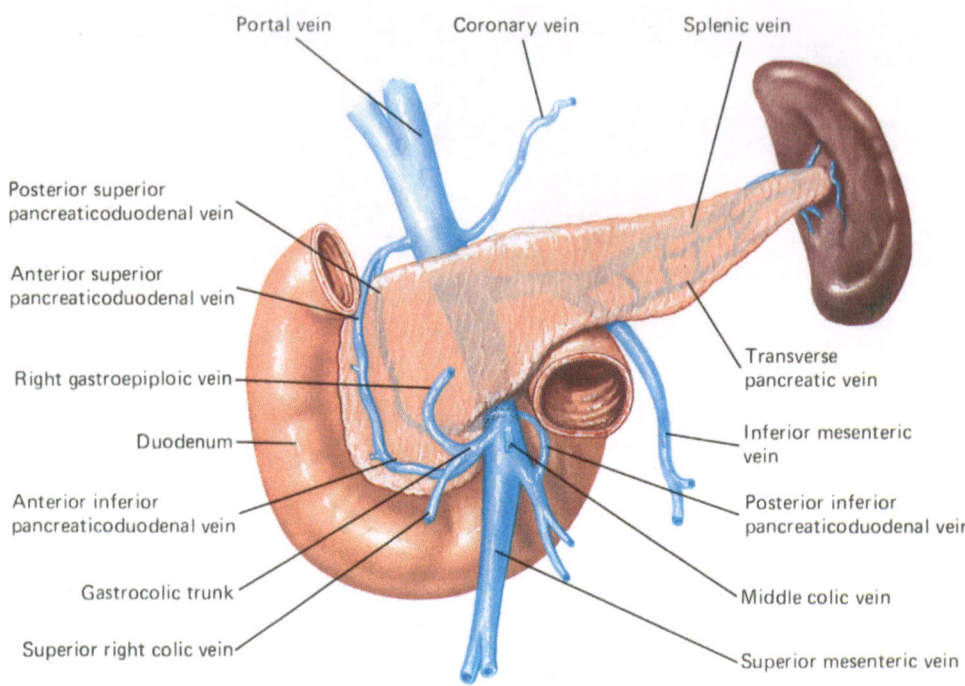

Portal vein   Coronary vein   Splenic vein

Posterior superior
pancreaticoduodenal vein

Anterior superior
pancreaticoduodenal vein

Right gastroepiploic vein

Duodenum

Anterior inferior
pancreaticoduodenal vein

Gastrocolic trunk

Superior right colic vein

Transverse
pancreatic vein

Inferior mesenteric
vein

Posterior inferior
pancreaticoduodenal vein

Middle colic vein

Superior mesenteric vein

Fig. 4-5.   **Pancreatic veins and portal system.**

the SMV-PV. Control of these veins is generally regarded as the most demanding aspect of a pancreaticoduodenal (Whipple) resection.

The junction of the gastrocolic trunk with the superior mesenteric vein is an important surgical landmark. It is a guide to the lower border of the neck of the pancreas, where dissection may proceed safely behind the pancreas, anterior to the SMV-PV. The anterior pancreaticoduodenal, right colic, and right gastroepiploic veins converge to form the gastrocolic trunk, and one must be cautious to avoid tearing these tributaries or the middle colic vein during mobilization of the pancreas.

Venous drainage of the body and tail of the pancreas is collected by a large transverse (inferior) pancreatic vein along the inferior aspect of the gland and through small, short tributaries entering along the course of the splenic vein. Because these tributaries are fragile and easily torn during dissection, resection of the body and tail of the pancreas most commonly includes splenectomy, which shortens and simplifies the procedure.

DUCTS

The main pancreatic duct (Wirsung's) begins approximately 2 cm from the tail of the gland and progressively enlarges until it attains a size of

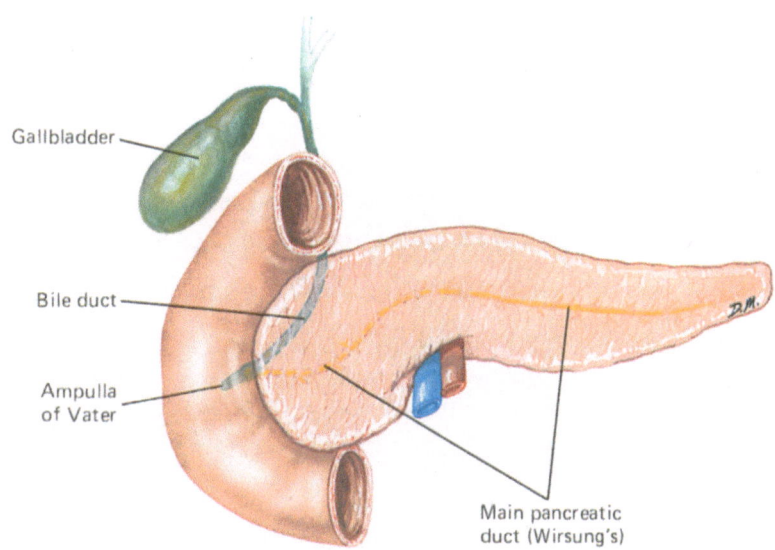

Main pancreatic and common bile ducts.   **Fig. 4-6.**

about 3.5 mm in the head. The accessory duct (of Santorini, not shown) usually connects with the main pancreatic duct in the head of the gland (Fig. 4-6).

The common bile duct descends in a long fissure in the posterior aspect of the head of the pancreas, near the pancreato-duodenal junction. The pancreatic and biliary ducts usually open together at the duodenal papilla.

ISLETS OF LANGERHANS

The pancreas is a composite gland, with exocrine and endocrine components. The exocrine portion comprises the bulk of the gland; the endocrine portion is composed of approximately one million islets of Langerhans (each of which is about 100–200 μm in diameter). These islets are scattered evenly throughout the gland (Fig. 4-7). Five cell types have been identified in human pancreatic islets (Fig. 4-8). These may be differentiated by their ultrastructural, electron microscopic characteristics (Fig. 4-9) or by immunoperoxidase stains for specific hormones (Fig. 4-10). The islets of Langerhans have a rich capillary network to enable rapid transfer of their hormonal secretion into the blood stream. Hypervascularity is a feature of many of the islet cell tumors, which facilitates their localization by angiographic techniques.

Fig. 4-7.

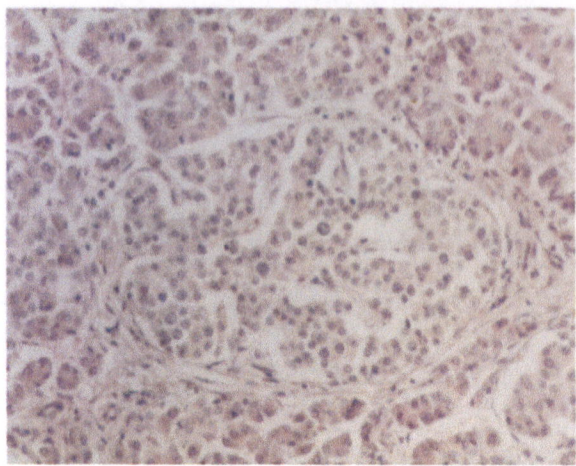

Fig. 4-8.

CELL OF ORIGIN	Alpha	Beta	D₁(PP)	D	Entero-chromaffin (EC)
HORMONE	Glucagon	Insulin	VIP –––––––– Pancreatic polypeptide (PP)	Gastrin Somatostatin	Serotonin ACTH MSH PTH
TUMOR/ SYNDROME	Glucagonoma	Insulinoma	Vipoma WDHA –––––––– No recognized syndrome	Gastrinoma ZES Somatostatinoma	Islet cell tumors

Fig. 4-9.

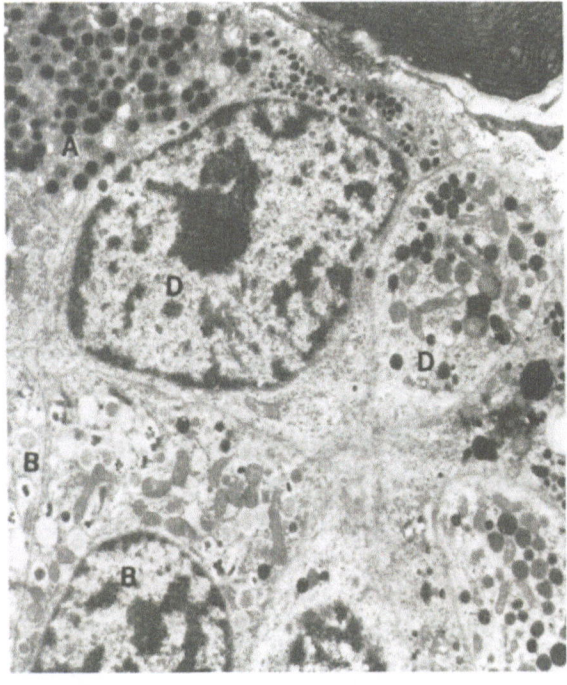

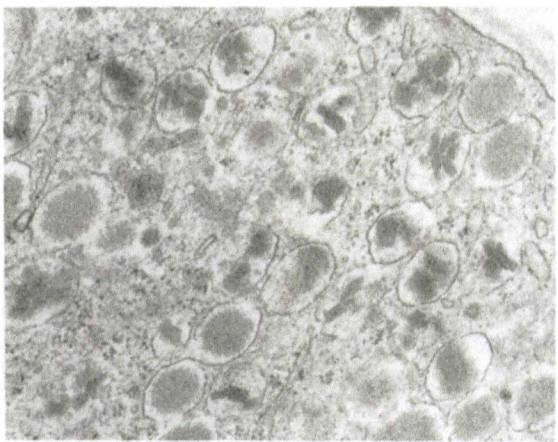

A

B

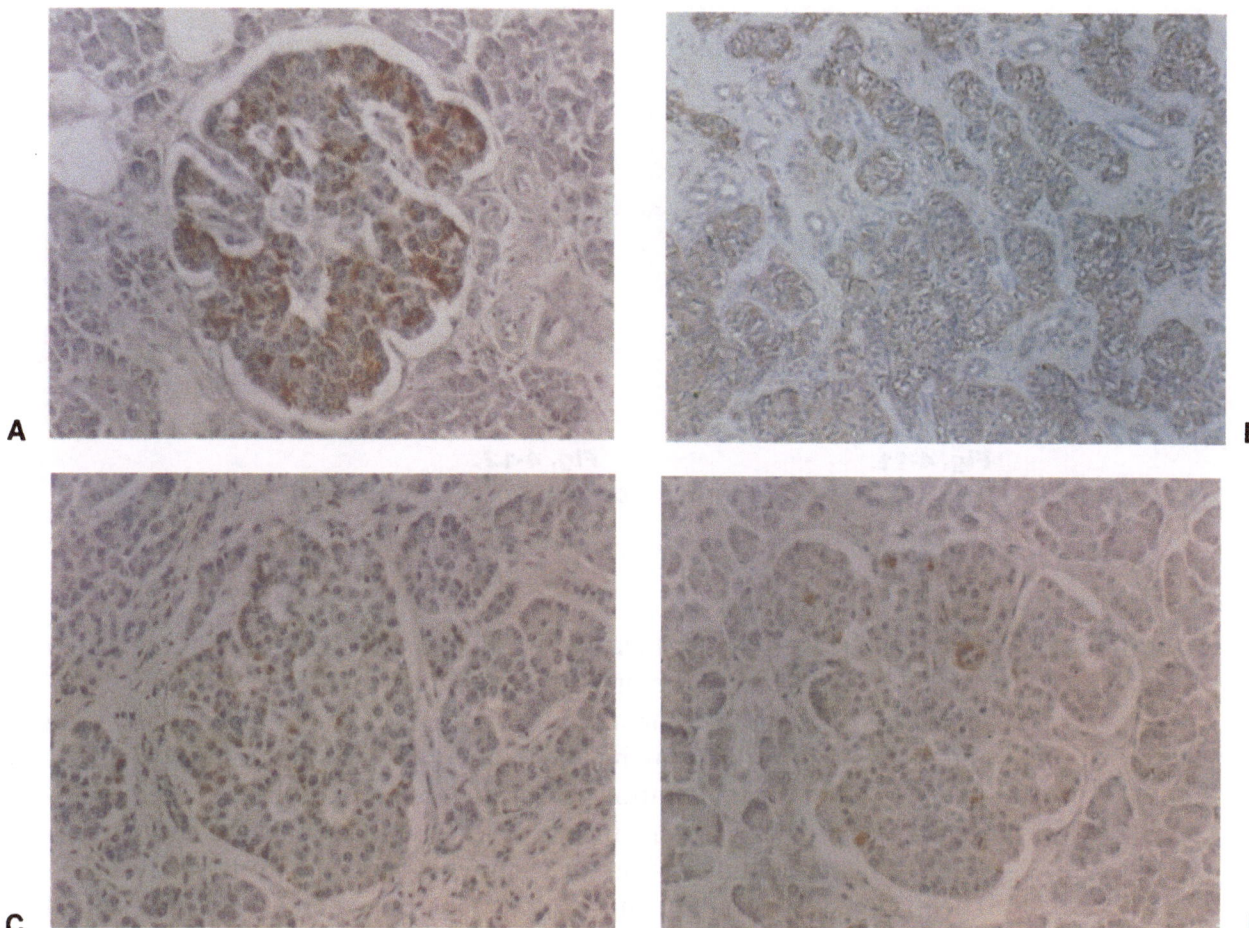

Immunoperoxidase stain for identification of pancreatic cells by **Fig. 4-10.**
specific hormones. **A.** Insulin shows dense staining of the prevalent β islet
cells. **B.** Benign insulinoma shows monomorphic cells with uniform cytoplasmic insulin immunoreactivity. **C.** Glucagon demonstrates the second most
common α islet cell. **D.** Somatostatin identifies the rare D cell. (Gastrin is not
present in the normal adult pancreas.)

Appearance of normal islet. Hematoxylin and eosin stain. **Fig. 4-7.**

Pancreatic islet cells, hormones, and tumors. *ACTH,* adrenocorticotropin; **Fig. 4-8.**
MSH, melanocyte stimulating hormone; *PTH,* parathyroid hormone; *PP,* pancreatic polypeptide; *WDHA,* watery diarrhea, hypokalemia, achlorhydria; and *VIP,*
vasoactive intestinal polypeptide.

Electron micrographic identification of pancreatic cells. **A.** Adult **Fig. 4-9.**
human pancreatic islet. The three cell types—α (A), β (B), and δ (C)—are present,
each of which is identified by the appearance of its secretory granules. ×6040.
(From Handbook of Physiology. Washington, D.C.: American Physiological Society, vol 1, sec 7, 1977, p 97.) **B.** Insulinoma cell. Note the diagnostic crystalline
morphology of many granule cores.

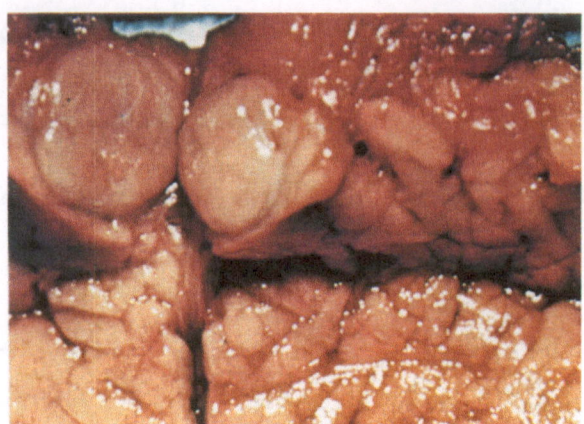 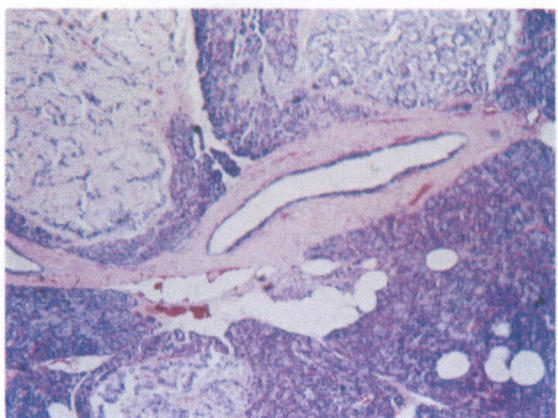

Fig. 4-11. **Fig. 4-12.**

Fig. 4-11. **Gross specimen of an islet cell tumor in resected tail of pancreas.**

Fig. 4-12. **Microscopic specimen showing microadenomatosis of the islet cells.**

Insulinoma   Since 1927, when the first case of insulinoma was recorded at the Mayo Clinic (8), followed by the first successful curative resection of an insulinoma by Graham (9), considerable knowledge and skill in diagnosing and managing insulinomas has been accrued.

The clinical manifestations of these β-islet cell tumors reflect inappropriately elevated plasma insulin levels, typically causing neuroglycopenic and hyperepinephrinemic symptoms induced by hypoglycemia. The diagnosis is strongly suggested by the presence of Whipple's triad (10): (a) symptoms of hypoglycemia provoked by fasting; (b) blood glucose levels at or below 50 mg/dl at the time of symptoms; and (c) the relief of symptoms after the administration of glucose.

PATHOLOGY

Insulinomas in adults may be conveniently thought of as ''10% tumors'': approximately 10% are multiple, malignant, and associated with the multiple endocrine neoplasia type I (MEN-I) syndrome (11,12).

Solitary adenomas are found in about 90% of cases. Grossly, they range from pale yellow (Fig. 4-11) to plum colored or reddish brown; they are somewhat bosselated and usually firmer in consistency than the surrounding pancreas. Most are well encapsulated, which facilitates their enucleation at the time of operation. Most often they are not visible on the surface of the pancreas—they are either covered by a thin layer of pancreas or buried within it.

Nearly 90% of insulinomas are 2 cm or less in diameter; two-thirds are 1.5 cm or less (11,13,14). The size of the tumor is not related significantly to its functional activity nor is there any correlation between size and malignancy (15). Like the islets of Langerhans themselves, the tumors are distributed uniformly throughout the pancreas (13,14). Ec-

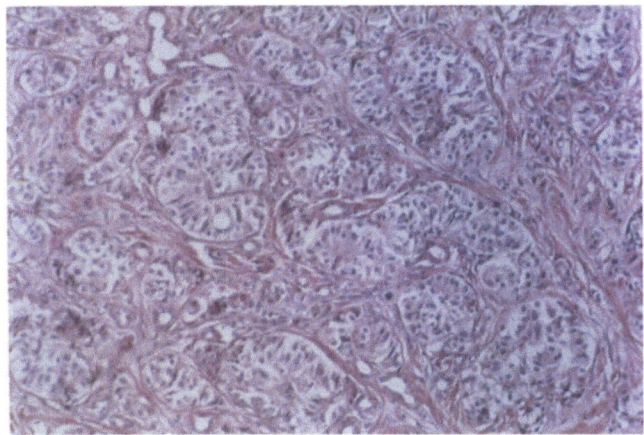

Microscopic specimen of a benign insulinoma. The appearance of malignant lesions may be very similar. Hematoxylin and eosin stain.　　**Fig. 4-13.**

topic insulinomas are rare, constituting less than 2% of cases (14,15) and are located close to the gland.

The incidence of multiple adenomas approximates 10% and should raise strong clinical suspicion of underlying MEN syndrome. Innumerable small macroscopic and microscopic islet cell tumors are sometimes found distributed throughout the entire pancreas (16) (Fig. 4-12). In adults, this entity, known as *adenomatosis* or *nesidioblastosis,* is almost always a part of the more complex syndrome of MEN-I, first described by Wermer in 1954 (17). Nesidioblastosis, thought to be a result of the abnormal persistence of the normal infant pancreatic morphology (when unassociated with MEN-I syndrome) (18), has been recognized extremely rarely (19).

Microscopically benign adenomas (Fig. 4-13) are composed of anastomosing cords of cells lying between vascular channels and supported on a delicate fibrous network. Ultrastructurally, the tumor cells contain secretory granules resembling those of the β cells in adjacent normal islets (20). Specific identification of the insulin in the β-islet cell tumors is possible using immunoperoxidase techniques on fresh or deparaffinized sections (Fig. 4-9).

In common with other endocrine tumors, the usual histologic criteria of malignancy are unreliable when applied to islet cell neoplasms. Approximately 10% of insulinomas are malignant (13,15,22); they tend to be softer, more hemorrhagic, and less well encapsulated than their benign counterparts. Perineural invasion is strong diagnostic evidence for malignancy (23), although the most reliable criterion is the presence of metastases. There is no evidence that benign adenomas ever undergo malignant transformation (24,25).

Islet cell carcinomas spread mainly to regional lymph nodes and via the blood stream to the liver. Metastases may be functioning or non-

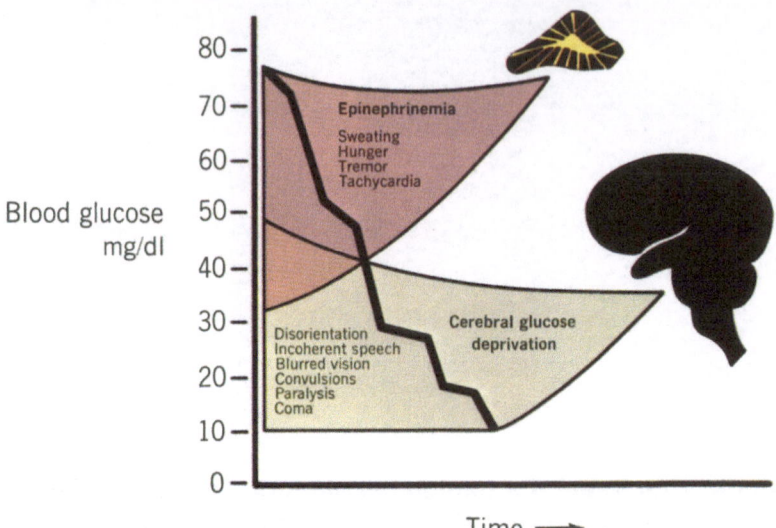

Fig. 4-14. Pathophysiology of a hypoglycemic attack. The initial rapid decline in blood glucose stimulates the reflex release of epinephrine by the adrenal. As the blood glucose level continues to fall, symptoms caused by epinephrinemia merge with those due to cerebral glucose deprivation. (Glucose is the chief energy substrate for the brain.)

functioning; if functioning, they will continue to secrete insulin even after the primary tumor has been removed (15). Even though many cases of metastatic disease may follow an indolent course, with patients surviving many years, median survival may be only 1–2 years (26,27).

DIAGNOSIS

CLINICAL FEATURES

Insulinomas may occur at any age but are most common during the fifth and sixth decades of life, with a mild female sex predominance (11,13). The constellation of clinical signs and symptoms typically becomes apparent in the early morning before breakfast or several hours following a meal, and may be provoked by exercise. Many patients "learn" to avert these symptoms by taking frequent feedings or sweetened drinks, which may cause them to become obese.

The most prominent symptoms are those of neuroglycopenia (11), including diplopia, blurred vision, confusion, abnormal behavior, and amnesia. While these symptoms are usually global and generalized, focal neurologic dysfunction may be seen, frequently leading to an erroneous diagnosis of a primary neurologic disorder. Focal seizures, paralysis, and coma may occur. Activation of the autonomic nervous system with catecholamine release accounts for the accompanying symptoms of weakness, sweating, hunger, tremor, and palpitations (Fig. 4-14).

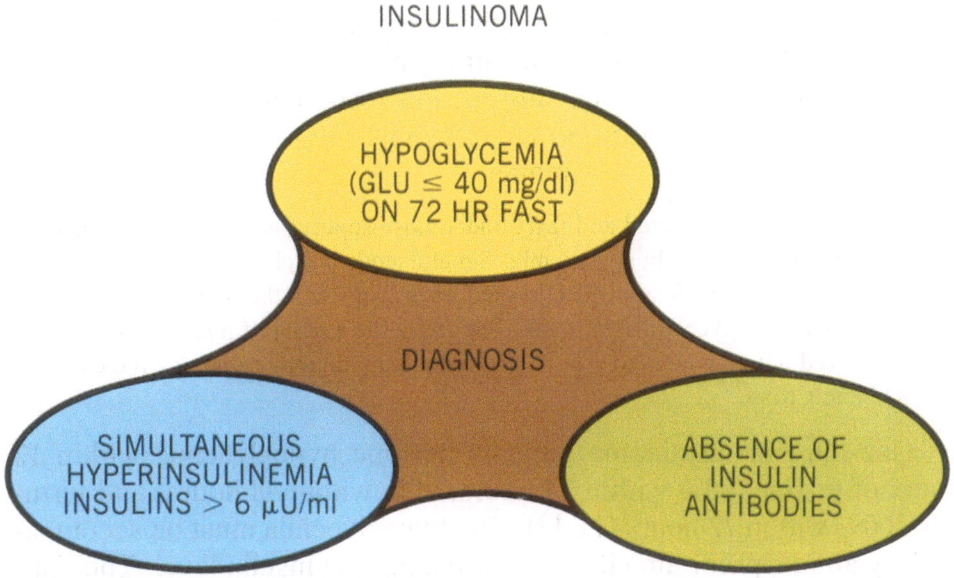

INSULINOMA

Diagnosis of insulinoma. The combination of hypoglycemia, hyperinsuline-mia, and absence of insulin antibodies is diagnostic.

Fig. 4-15.

> The release of epinephrine is a compensatory phenomenon which attempts to re-store blood glucose levels to normal by accentuating the breakdown of hepatic glycogen to glucose. In some patients, this increased glycogenolysis may be suf-ficient to cause spontaneous, temporary recovery.

There is real danger that, with repeated and especially prolonged hypoglycemic attacks, particularly recurring over a long period of time, permanent neurologic damage may be sustained (23,28,29). Delayed diagnosis continues to be a problem, since over one-third of patients may suffer hypoglycemic episodes for 3 years or longer prior to correct diagnosis and treatment (11).

LABORATORY STUDIES

Measurement of plasma insulin by radioimmunoassay has greatly facili-tated and streamlined the diagnosis of insulinoma. Essentially three diagnostic criteria are required to solidify the diagnosis: (a) fasting se-rum hypoglycemia (typically a plasma glucose level at or below 40 mg/dl); (b) concomitant hyperinsulinemia (serum level at or above 6 μU/ml), and (c) absence of insulin antibodies (Fig. 4-15). Some modifi-cations and additions are needed to encompass special circumstances (e.g., insulin-dependent diabetic with an insulinoma; surreptitious self-administration of sulfonylureas).

In general, suppression tests are more reliable than stimulation tests for diagnosing insulinomas. A suppression test provides a means to assess homeostatic control because there is a lack of the normal feed-back inhibition of hormone secretion, which is the sine qua non of an autonomously functioning tumor.

Prolonged Fast. Once an insulinoma is suspected, the diagnosis may be confirmed with a high degree of accuracy by a 72-hour fast (11,13). This is in essence an endogenous suppression test—failure of appropriate insulin suppression in the presence of hypoglycemia—substantiating an autonomously secreting insulinoma.

> The patient is hospitalized and fasts under close supervision. Exercise is encouraged to help stimulate hypoglycemia. Simultaneous samples for plasma glucose and immunoreactive insulin (IRI) should be drawn when the patient develops significant hypoglycemic symptoms. The fast is then stopped and glucose is administered intravenously to relieve the symptoms, thereby satisfying the classic Whipple's triad.

One-third of insulinoma patients become hypoglycemic within 12 hours of fasting; 80% within 24 hours; 90% within 48 hours; and virtually 100% within 72 hours (11,13). The hypoglycemia must be accompanied by an inappropriate elevation of the plasma insulin level. The optimal method of interpreting concomitantly drawn glucose and IRI levels is somewhat debatable.

> Absolute values of glucose at or below 40 mg/dl with simultaneous IRI at or above 6 μU/ml is virtually 100% accurate (11,13). These are the diagnostic criteria favored by the authors. Alternatively, an IRI to glucose ratio of 0.30 or greater has been diagnostically reliable in most patients (30) but may mistakenly exclude some with the disease.

Provided that the surreptitious self-administration of insulin has been excluded by the absence of circulating insulin antibodies, the diagnosis is confirmed. The prolonged fast is so reliable that it forms the "gold standard" to which all other tests must be compared.

Ancillary Tests. A number of ancillary tests may be valuable in the diagnostic evaluation of insulinoma. Proteolytic cleavage of *proinsulin* results in equimolar concentrations and secretion of insulin and connecting peptide (C-peptide). Approximately 85% of patients with insulinomas have elevated plasma levels of proinsulin (31), which is particularly helpful when the fasting IRI is somewhat low or borderline (31,32). Very high proportions of proinsulin are indicative of islet cell carcinoma.

A sensitive and accurate *assay for C-peptide* has become useful in several respects. Since C-peptide is secreted in equimolar amounts as IRI, it also reflects endogenous β-cell secretion. It does not cross-react with insulin antibodies. Thus, *failure* to detect C-peptide during periods of hypoglycemia and hyperinsulinemia indicates that the assayable insulin is *not* endogenous. This would indicate exogenous insulin administration since commercially available insulin does not contain C-peptide. While this situation is rare, it is usually seen in patients with some medical knowledge and has reportedly even led to operation under the mistaken impression that an insulinoma was present (33). Factitial hy-

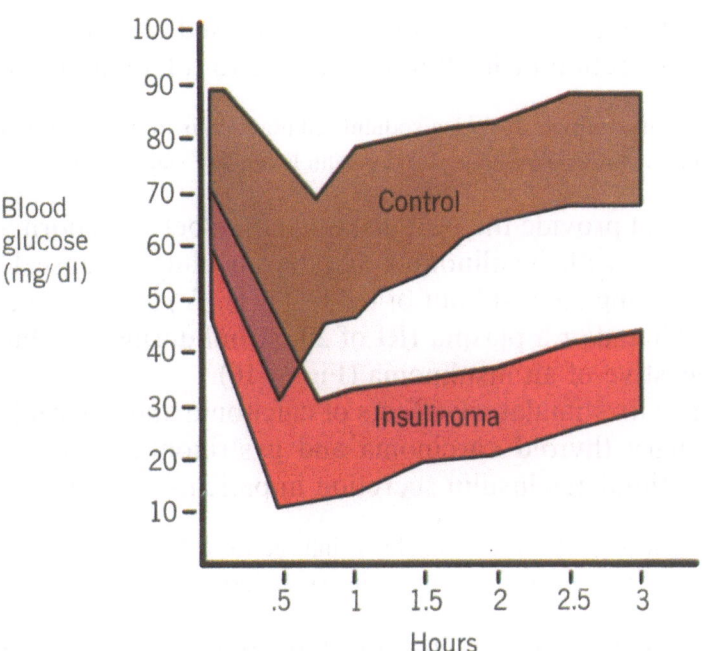

Tolbutamide test. Response in blood glucose level following administration of tolbutamide in normal subjects and in patients with insulinoma (11). Persistent hypoglycemia during the last hour is characteristic of an insulinoma.

Fig. 4-16.

perinsulinism in an insulin-dependent diabetic constitutes a special diagnostic problem because the presence of plasma insulin antibodies in these individuals is to be expected. However, only if there is excess *endogenous* insulin secretion will the C-peptide be elevated (34).

In the *C-peptide suppression test,* infusion of beef or pork insulin with simultaneous assay for C-peptide demonstrates appropriate suppression in normal individuals. Although this test is not 100% reliable, the C-peptide fails to be suppressed in most patients with an insulinoma, consistent with an autonomously secreting tumor.

> **Fish Insulin Suppression Test.** Since there are sufficient immunologic differences between fish and human insulin to allow their separate assay, fish insulin may be used to test for normal suppression (35). Following administration of fish insulin, patients with an insulinoma fail to show normal suppression of assayable human IRI. Fish insulin, however, is not available in the United States, and this test rarely seems necessary due to the development of the C-peptide assay and suppression test.

Provocative Tests. Provocative tests are rarely necessary and are generally less reliable than the 72-hour fast. However, the tolbutamide test and the calcium infusion test offer safe, rapid, and reasonably reliable results. The use of leucine or glucagon for stimulation has virtually been abandoned.

The *tolbutamide test* was the first of the provocative tests to be described (36) and is still used in a supervised, outpatient setting. Patients with insulinomas demonstrate an increased sensitivity and consequent hypersecretion of insulin in response to tolbutamide infusion.

> Following an overnight fast, 1 g sodium tolbutamide is infused intravenously over 2 minutes. Plasma glucose and insulin levels are sampled for 3 hours.

The results that provide the best discrimination between normal individuals and those with insulinomas are the absolute glucose levels and plasma IRI during the last hour of the test (11). A plasma glucose of less than 47 mg/dl and/or a plasma IRI of 20 μU/ml during the third hour is highly suggestive of an insulinoma (Fig. 4-16).

Similar to its stimulatory effects of calcitonin and gastrin in patients with medullary thyroid carcinoma and gastrinoma, *calcium infusion* selectively stimulates insulin secretion in patients with insulinomas.

> Calcium gluconate (5 mg Ca^{++}/kg/hr) is infused for a 2-hour period. Plasma glucose and IRI are drawn at 15-minute intervals during the test.

No significant increases of insulin or decrease of glucose is seen in normal individuals or those with reactive hypoglycemia (37). In contrast, most adult insulinoma patients reliably show a rise in IRI and fall in plasma glucose during calcium infusion (38).

Tests for Malignancy. No blood test presently exists that reliably distinguishes a benign from a malignant islet cell tumor in all cases. As stated previously, a very high level of proinsulin is suggestive of a malignant insulinoma. Kahn et al. (39) reported that human chorionic gonadotropin (HCG) and its subunits have been elevated in malignant insulinoma (immunoreactive HCG elevated in 25%, HCG-β in 21%, HCG-α in 57%) but were normal in all 41 benign insulinomas tested. Thus, an elevated HCG seems very suggestive of malignancy.

Many cases of nonpancreatic tumors associated with hypoglycemia have been reported (40,41). Most have been large retroperitoneal sarcomas, easily identifiable either clinically or by radiographic means. The cause of hypoglycemia associated with these tumors remains obscure. Some tumors have been reported to contain increased biologic insulin-like activity; but plasma IRI levels, when assayed, have been normal or low in these patients (42).

PREOPERATIVE LOCALIZATION STUDIES

With the diagnosis of insulinoma biochemically confirmed, several options are available for localization. While some authors dispute the need or value of preoperative localization (43), most have utilized either visceral arteriography or percutaneous transhepatic sampling. CT and ultrasonography have failed to localize insulinomas in 30%–60% of patients (12) but may improve with technical refinements. Operative, real-time ultrasound has recently been reported to be successful (44,45), but further experience is necessary before its relative value can be assessed (Fig. 4-17). The impetus to proceed with localization seems sound since, in one series, 7 of 34 insulinomas could not be seen or palpated by the surgeon at the time of exploration (46).

PANCREATIC ARTERIOGRAPHY

Selective pancreatic angiography, utilizing stereoscopic filming with magnification and subtraction techniques, identifies between 50% and 90% of tumors with a minimum diameter of 5 mm (43,46). It remains the localizing technique of choice for delineating insulinomas. Their typical angiographic appearance is that of a localized, densely staining tumor blush during the capillary phase (Fig. 4-18). False-positive interpretations are principally caused by lymph nodes, hypervascular lobules of normal pancreas, and accessory spleens.

PERCUTANEOUS TRANSHEPATIC VENOUS SAMPLING

Percutaneous transhepatic portal venous catheterization with subselective sampling of pancreatic venous effluent for hormone assay was first reported in 1975 (47). Many encouraging reports have emerged subsequently, including successful localization of small insulinomas or cases of islet cell hyperplasia that were undetectable by arteriography or intraoperative palpation (48,49). This technique has been successfully utilized in localizing non-β-islet cell tumors of the pancreas. This would seem particularly valuable in those tumors for which angiography is notoriously unsuccessful (i.e., Zollinger-Ellison syndrome).

Transhepatic venous sampling requires considerable angiographic expertise and is tedious, costly, and uncomfortable for the patient. Nevertheless, it appears relatively safe and should be considered when angiographic localization fails or is equivocal.

> The portal vein is catheterized using a percutaneous, transhepatic needle, and the catheter is advanced by fluoroscopic guidance into the multiple small draining veins of the entire pancreas. Blood is sampled at each site, a record of each sample is graphically noted, and simultaneous peripheral samples are taken as controls. Hormonal assays are performed on the blood samples.

Tumors located in the head of the pancreas typically yield elevated hormonal levels in the anterior or posterior pancreaticoduodenal branches; tumors in the neck drain into the confluence of superior mesenteric and splenic veins; tumors in the body or tail drain at the corresponding point along either the splenic or transverse pancreatic veins. It is important to note that the transverse pancreatic vein may join the gastrocolic trunk. Elevated hormone levels at this point of the portal vein must not be mistakenly interpreted as localizing the tumor in the pancreatic head when it actually resides in the body or tail (Fig. 4-19).

Fig. 4-17.

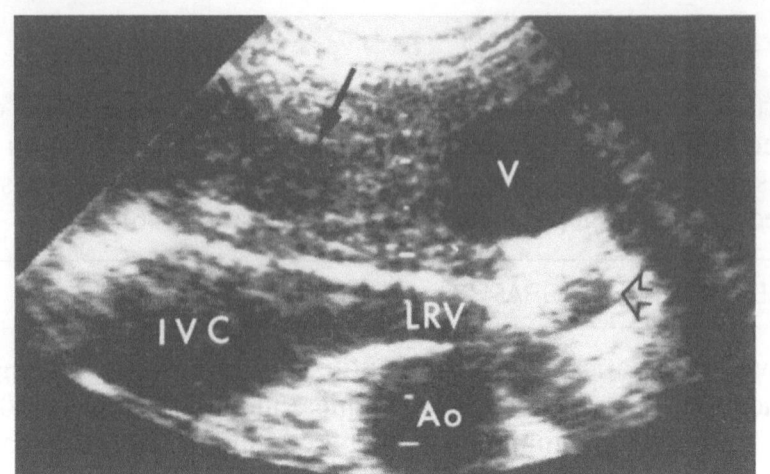

A

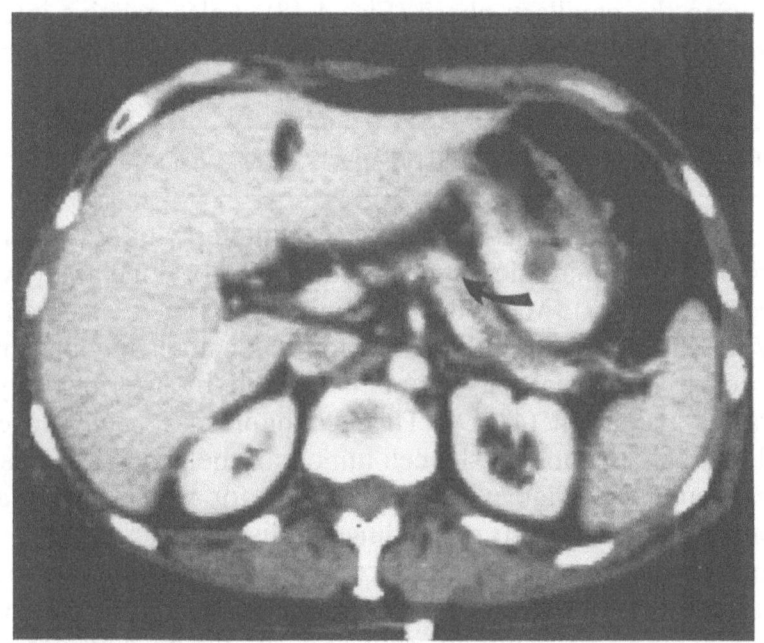

B

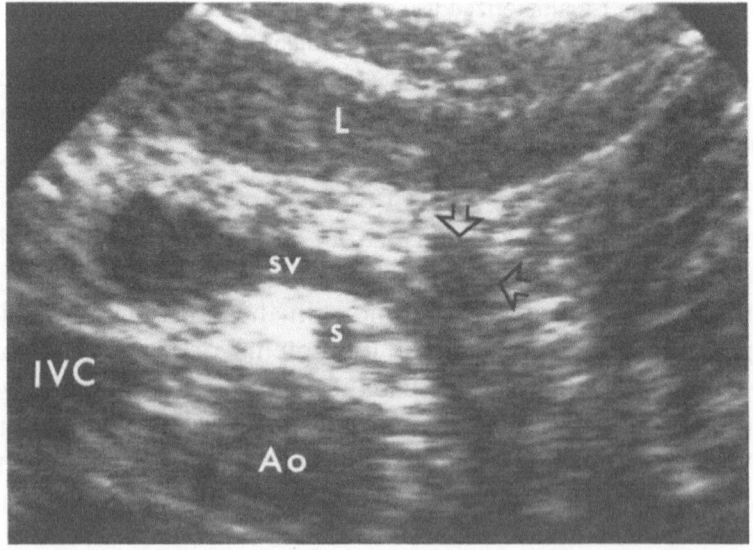

C

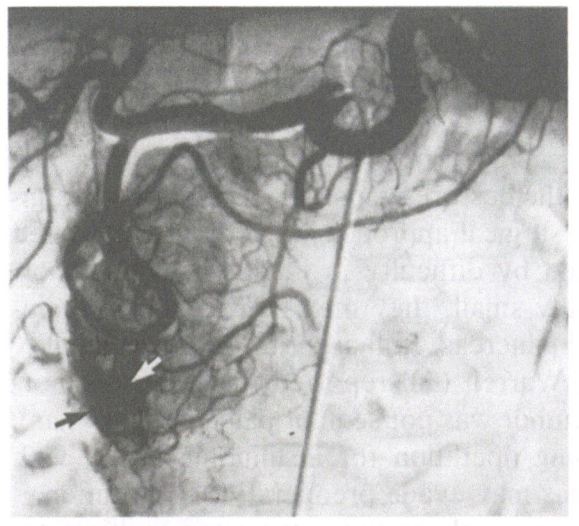
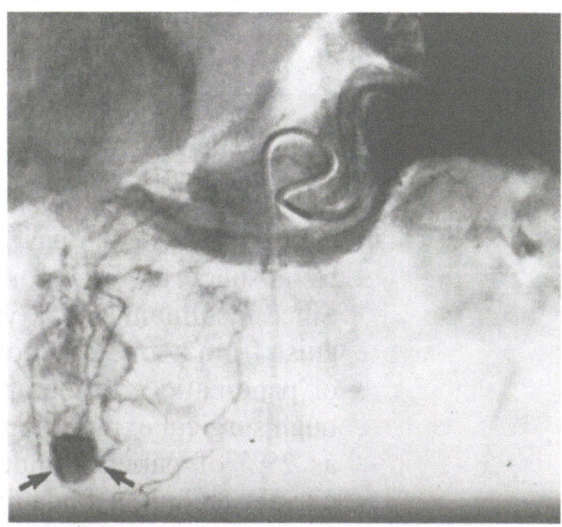

A

B

Celiac axis arteriogram. **A.** Capillary phase shows opacification of an insulinoma in the head of the pancreas (*arrows*). **B.** The valuable addition of
subtraction films clearly demonstrates the insulinoma.

Fig. 4-18.

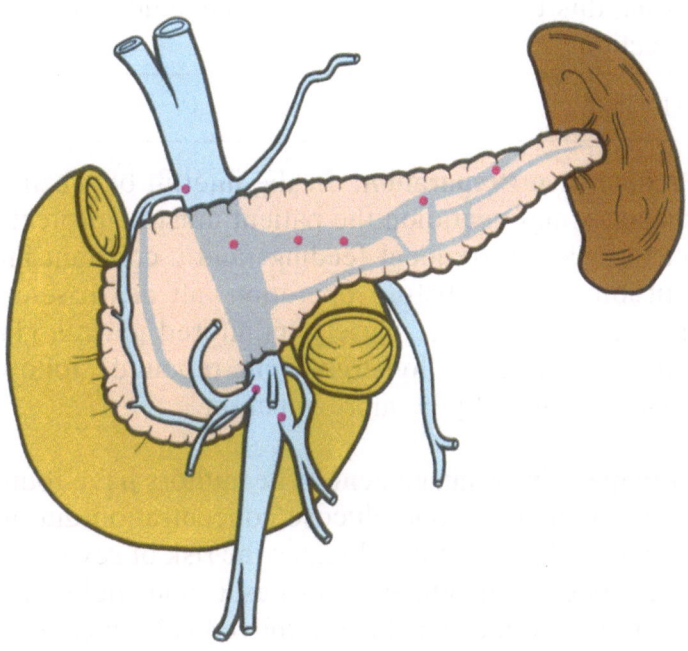

Percutaneous transhepatic venous sampling. Multiple sites of sampling
(•) are necessary for localization.

Fig. 4-19.

◄ **Localization of insulinoma.** **A.** Transverse intraoperative sonogram of the
head of the pancreas and uncinate process demonstrating a subtle, round,
9-mm solid mass—insulinoma (*arrows*). *IVC*, inferior vena cava; *LRV*, left renal
vein; *Ao*, aorta; *V*, superior mesenteric vein; *open arrow*, superior mesenteric
artery. **B.** CT scan with intravenous contrast. A small insulinoma (*arrow*) is
localized in the body of the pancreas. **C.** Preoperative transverse sonogram of
the pancreas (same patient as in B). A 1-cm hypoechoic insulinoma is demonstrated in the body of the pancreas. *L*, left lobe of liver; *SV*, splenic vein; *S*,
superior mesenteric artery; *Ao*, aorta; *IVC*, inferior vena cava.

Fig. 4-17.

261

TREATMENT

The only curative and clearly the best treatment for insulinoma is surgical excision. In the past, the surgical approach was often complicated by an uncertain diagnosis and by difficulty in identifying the tumor. Since insulinomas are typically small, they may be difficult to distinguish from a lobule of normal pancreas. In fact, prior to the availability of pancreatic arteriography, Warren (50) reported that, despite thorough surgical exploration, a tumor was not seen or palpated in as many as 25% of patients undergoing operation for insulinoma. Even with current techniques insulinomas may evade preoperative localization.

In patients with occult tumors, those with suspected multiple tumors or nesidioblastosis, and others in whom serious operative risk is anticipated, a preoperative trial of medical treatment with diazoxide has been advocated (30,43,51). Evaluation of the response and side effects during this trial may provide valuable guidance regarding the extent of resection.

SURGICAL

Preoperative Preparation. In the interim between confirmation of the diagnosis and operation the patient must be protected from hypoglycemic attacks by frequent feedings and a constant intravenous dextrose infusion. Shortly before operation, all dextrose-containing fluids are discontinued and the closely monitored plasma glucose is allowed to fall. The expected "hyperglycemic rebound" following excision of the tumor will thereby be more apparent.

Intraoperative Management. The authors have found it useful to monitor the patient's blood glucose concentration during operations for insulinoma. This practice obviates the risk of severe hypoglycemia occurring undetected under anesthesia and helps to confirm that all functioning tumor has been removed (13,29) (Fig. 4-20).

> During the procedure, blood glucose values are determined every 15 minutes until the tumor is removed; then every 5 minutes thereafter for approximately 1 hour; then as frequently as seems prudent.

The blood glucose level usually rises appreciably within 30–45 minutes if all hyperfunctioning tissue has been removed. An alternative method for monitoring is the use of a computerized, continuous-flow, enzymatic system. This acts as an "artificial β cell," providing either continuous glucose control or continuous glucose monitoring (38).

Intraoperative blood glucose monitoring, however, is not without some problems. There have been reports of hyperglycemic responses despite retained hyperfunctioning islet cell tissue (52,53). Significantly delayed hyperglycemic rebound—a false-negative result—has also

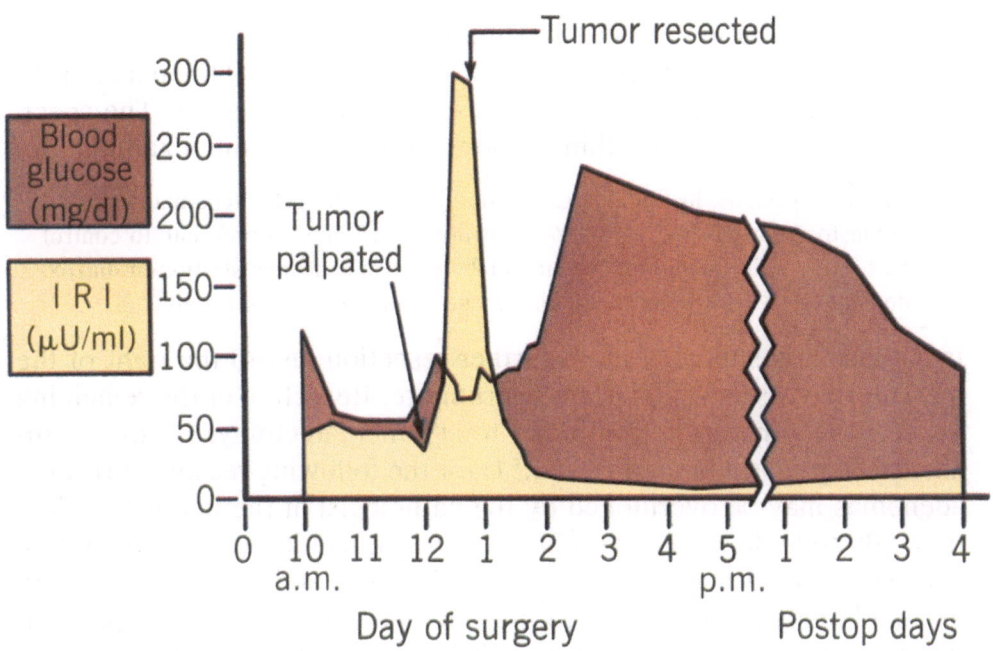

Intraoperative monitoring of blood glucose. Blood glucose and plasma in- **Fig. 4-20.**
sulin (IRI) levels before, during, and after operation for insulinoma. The rebound
in blood glucose concentration after the tumor is removed gives assurance that
no additional tumor is present.

been reported (52,54). Despite these faults, this technique is helpful,
and the authors continue to use it. However, extending a pancreatic
resection based solely on depressed intraoperative blood glucose levels
seems unwise.

Operative Strategy. Even when a solitary insulinoma has been identified by preoperative arteriography, it is essential to explore the entire
pancreas to exclude the possibility of multiple tumors. Kocherization of
the duodenum allows careful examination of the pancreatic head, and
exposure of the body and tail of the pancreas is performed via the lesser
sac by reflecting or dividing the gastrocolic omentum.

When a single tumor is present and palpable near the surface of the
pancreas, it may be safely enucleated. By careful elevation of the
superficial operculum of normal pancreas, the tumor is exposed. Meticulous dissection in the plane between the tumor and normal pancreas
usually prevents damage to the main pancreatic duct. For tumors that
are deeply embedded in the body and tail of the pancreas, distal pancreatectomy is recommended (55). Pathologic confirmation of islet cell
tumor by frozen section is mandatory. Multiple, locally invasive, or
large tumors require resective procedures, rarely necessitating a pancreaticoduodenectomy (Whipple procedure) if the mass is located in the
head of the pancreas. If metastatic islet cell carcinoma is present, resection of the primary neoplasm and any accessible metastatic nodules may
offer significant palliation for an extended period of time.

If an insulinoma cannot be found despite a thorough operative search including ectopic sites, the entire body and tail of the pancreas to the left of the superior mesenteric vessels may be resected. The specimen should be sliced into thin sections for frozen-section examination.

> On rare occasions, histologic examination reveals islet cell adenomatosis or nesidioblastosis for which a 75%–80% resection seems most appropriate to control the hyperinsulinism without causing diabetes (19,53). Administration of diazoxide is advised if the operation fails to control the disease adequately.

If the lesion is still not found, further resection just to the right of the mesenteric vessels would seem appropriate. Resection of the remaining head of the pancreas, resulting in total pancreatectomy, is contraindicated as a primary procedure (38,51) for the following reasons: (a) small adenomas may be overlooked by the pathologist at the initial examination only to be found later on further sectioning (56); (b) intraoperative glucose rebound may be significantly delayed; and (c) treatment with diazoxide may be preferable to incurring permanent insulin-dependent diabetes, exocrine pancreatic insufficiency, and the significant operative mortality and morbidity risks. Total pancreatectomy may subsequently be necessary if medical therapy fails.

Postoperative Management and Results. A transient diabeticlike state is expected postoperatively, presumably due to the suppressive influence of the tumor on extraadenomatous islet cell function. Glucose values ranging from 200 to 300 mg/dl are common; insulin is administered only for significant glycosuria, ketonuria, or electrolyte abnormalities.

Surgical cure of benign lesions is expected in at least 90% of cases, with an operative mortality risk of less than 5% (13). Postoperative complications occur in approximately 15% of patients, the most serious including pancreatic pseudocyst or fistula, and sepsis. Long-term results are usually excellent, with persistent insulin-dependent diabetes occurring in fewer than 10% (29) and neuropsychiatric disorders reported sporadically (57).

Malignant insulinomas are frequently resectable for cure, aggressive resection being well justified. Radical, high-risk procedures for widely metastatic lesions, however, are rarely justified. Palliative resections to reduce hormonal effects are recommended when they may be accomplished safely.

NONSURGICAL

Medical therapy may become necessary in a variety of situations: (a) patient who cannot tolerate general anesthesia; (b) persistent symptomatic hyperinsulinism following 80% resection for nesidioblastosis; (c) unsuccessful abdominal exploration; or (d) metastatic disease.

Diazoxide (a thiazide derivative) increases blood glucose by inhibiting insulin release and decreasing peripheral glucose utilization. Adverse side effects are frequent and may preclude its use. These include salt and water retention, hirsuitism, nausea, bone marrow depression, and hyperuricemia (58). The usual dose is 100 mg, three to four times daily, increasing as needed to control hypoglycemia. A diuretic, trichlomethazide, may be added for both control of edema and a synergistic hyperglycemic effect with diazoxide.

Streptozotocin, an antitumor antibiotic isolated from *Streptomyces acromogenes,* has been widely used in islet cell carcinoma either alone or in combination with 5-fluorouracil (59,60). Streptozotocin is highly toxic to the pancreatic β cells. One-half to two-thirds of patients with metastatic disease have achieved partial remission, and complete remission has been reached in 17%–33% (60,61). Unfortunately, these benefits are attained at the cost of considerable drug-related toxicity: 95% of patients experience nausea and vomiting, sometimes severe, early in the course of therapy. Renal tubular damage is the most serious toxic effect, monitored best by serial urine protein quantitation. Hepatic and, rarely, hematopoietic toxicity has also been observed (60). Despite these side effects, clinical amelioration of hypoglycemia allows most patients to pursue their usual occupations during treatment with the drug.

Hypoglycemia in Children. While exceedingly rare in adults, nesidioblastosis is the most common cause of hyperinsulinism in infants and children under the age of 2 years (62). Differentiation of infants with the more common "idiopathic" hypoglycemia from those with nesidioblastosis is difficult, necessitating keen awareness to prevent serious neurologic damage. Drug therapy has generally been disappointing, although most of these children are successfully treated by 80%–90% pancreatectomy. Rarely, total pancreatectomy may be necessary if adjunctive diazoxide provides insufficient control (63).

Zollinger-Ellison Syndrome

As first described in 1955, Zollinger-Ellison syndrome (ZES) consisted of two patients with the triad of fulminating, atypical peptic ulceration, gastric acid hypersecretion, and a non-β-islet cell tumor of the pancreas (64). Considerable evolution in our understanding and management of patients with ZES has occurred since this landmark report (Fig. 4-21). Of major importance was the development of a radioimmunoassay for gastrin (65), which provided the basis for positively establishing the diagnosis nonoperatively. The present requirements for diagnosis include gastric acid hypersecretion and hypergastrinemia; virulent ulcer disease and demonstration of a pancreatic tumor are no longer prerequisites. The diagnosis of ZES usually refers exclusively to patients with gastrinoma, but some have included the rare entity of antral G-cell hyperplasia. ZES probably accounts for less than 1% of peptic ulcer disease, with an age range of 7–90 years, and a peak age of presentation between the third and sixth decades (66).

PATHOLOGY

Gastrinomas are usually small, pale yellow or plum-colored tumors which may be extremely difficult to identify at operation or even at postmortem examination. Gastrin is not normally present in the adult pancreas (67). That the pancreatic D cell is the origin of gastrinomas bears testimony to the pleuripotentiality of the APUD islet cells. On light microscopy, gastrinomas often bear a striking morphologic resemblance to carcinoid tumors, with small uniform cuboidal cells arranged in a trabecular pattern or in sheets or clumps. Malignant tumors cannot be distinguished from their benign counterparts with any certainty using microscopy alone. As with many other endocrine tumors, the single definitive criterion of malignancy is the presence of metastasis.

DIAGNOSIS

CLINICAL FEATURES

Fox et al. (68) have collected over 800 cases of ZES in the Zollinger-Ellison Tumor Registry (maintained at the Medical College of Wisconsin, Milwaukee); these data, together with many other reports, provide a substantial basis for our understanding of this disease. At least 60%–75% of ZES tumors are malignant (68–70), 50% have metastases at the time of diagnosis, 50% of the pancreatic tumors are multifocal (71,72), up to 30% of ZES tumors are undetected by the surgeon, and over 50% of patients undergoing what was judged a curative tumor excision have persistent or recurrent disease (73). Approximately 20%–30% of gastrinomas are part of the MEN-I syndrome (74) with multiplicity in this setting approaching 100%.

Hyperplasia of pancreatic islets occurs in most patients with gastrinoma and is apparently a consequence rather than a cause of the hypergastrinemia: gastrin has not been found in these hyperplastic islets by immunohistology or by extraction (75). Slightly more than 10% of patients have duodenal wall gastrinomas (66,68), only one-half of which are solitary. The other half have hepatic or regional node metastases or are associated with pancreatic tumors. When contemplating operation one reaches the repeatedly confirmed conclusion that, even following preoperative exclusion of patients with obvious liver metastases and those with MEN-I syndrome, the likelihood of finding a solitary, benign gastrinoma amenable to curative excision is only 20%–25% (66,68,72,75,76).

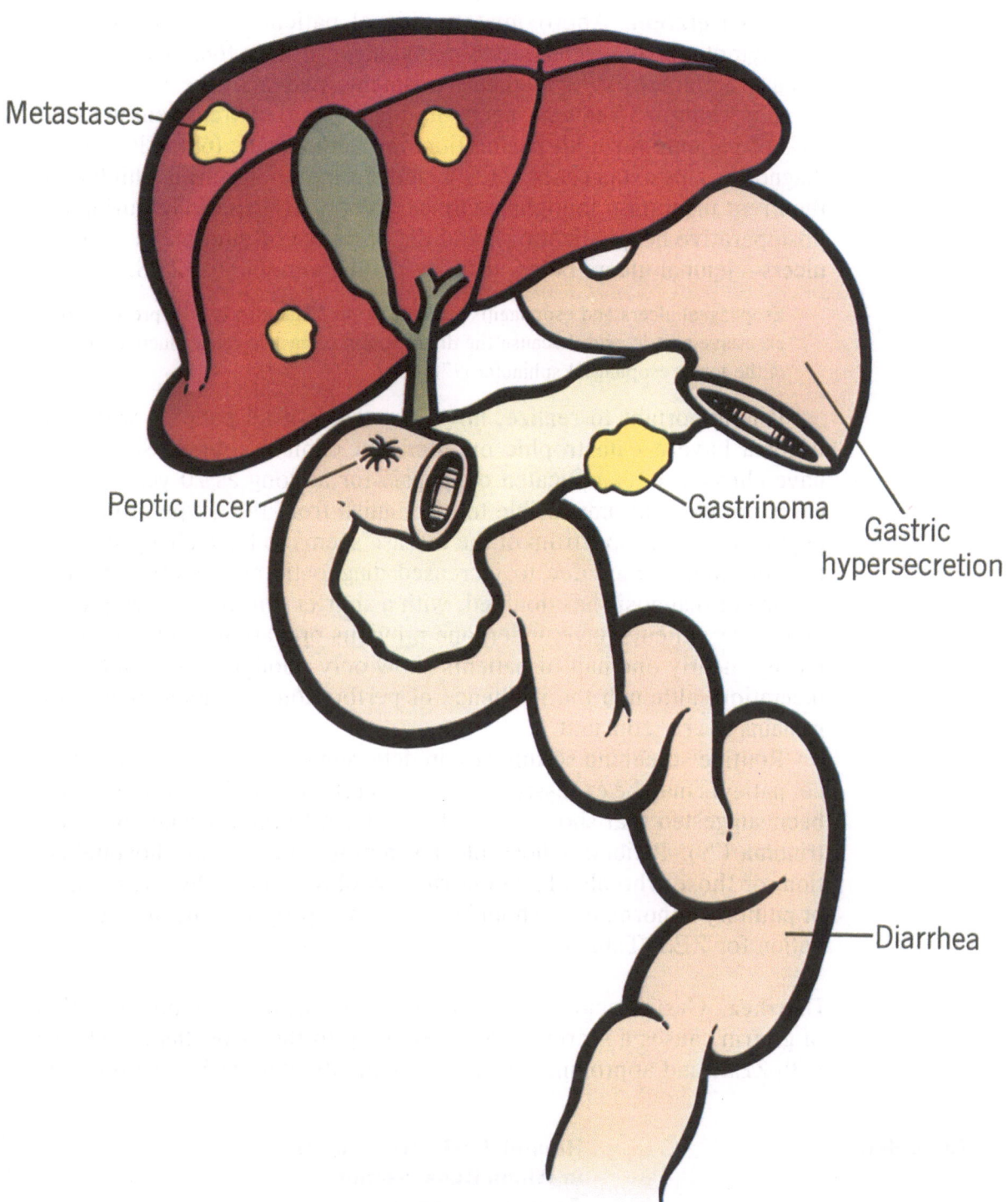

Common features of the Zollinger-Ellison syndrome. **Fig. 4-21.**

Peptic Ulceration. Approximately 90% of patients with ZES present with symptoms and signs due to peptic ulcer disease (68). These ulcers often are refractory to medical treatment; pain may be severe, and complications are frequent, necessitating emergency treatment in about 20% of patients for both perforation and hemorrhage (68). Classically, diagnostic clues suggesting ZES included ulceration during childhood, recurrent ulceration following surgical treatment (especially during the postoperative hospitalization), and the presence of multiple or atypical ulcers—jejunal ulcers being virtually pathognomonic for ZES.

> Esophageal ulcers and esophagitis are unusual findings, despite the presence of excessive gastric acid, because the direct action of gastrin causes increased tone of the lower esophageal sphincter (77).

It is important to realize, however, that not all patients with gastrinoma have a catastrophic or fulminant clinical course. Some may have chronic, uncomplicated dyspepsia for as long as 20 years; these cases are virtually impossible to distinguish from the "type ordinaire" peptic ulcer. The spectrum of the disease seems to have changed in the past decade, in part due to increased diagnostic awareness. The frequency of diagnosis has doubled, with a shorter duration of symptoms, and fewer patients have undergone previous operations (78). Endoscopically, nearly one-half of patients show only duodenitis without frank ulceration, although the incidence of perforation and hemorrhage still remains nearly constant.

Routine screening serum gastrin determinations on all duodenal ulcer patients may be excessive; however, certain associated criteria have been suggested that should alert the clinician to the presence of a gastrinoma (79). Patients whose ulcer symptoms necessitate hospitalization, or those who also have diarrhea, nephrolithiasis, hypercalcemia, or pituitary abnormalities should receive an appropriate diagnostic evaluation for ZES (Table 4-1).

Diarrhea. Gastric acid hypersecretion due to the autonomous secretion of gastrin causes a secretory diarrhea in up to three-fourths of patients with ZES, and approximately 10% of patients with ZES have diarrhea

Table 4-1.

High-Risk (Ulcer) Patients in Whom Basal Serum Gastrin Determination Should Be Obtained

Surgery
Hospitalization
Diarrhea
Hypercalcemia, nephrolithiasis
Pituitary abnormality

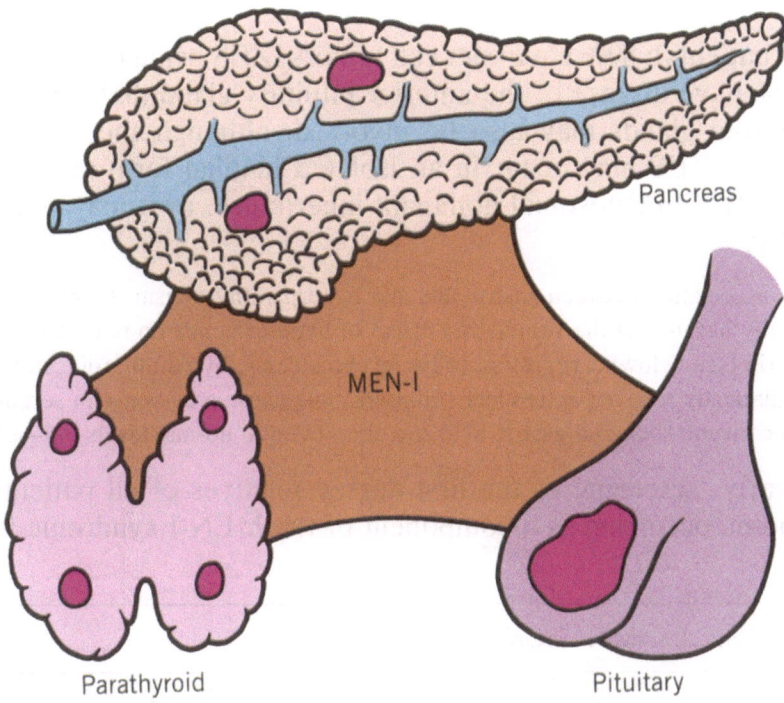

Multiple endocrine neoplasia type I. Tumors, usually multiple, involve   **Fig. 4-22.**
parathyroid, pancreas, and pituitary.

without ulcer disease (72,74). Most patients with diarrhea have about six watery stools daily, with a serum potassium below 2.9 mEq/liter. It may be severe enough to result in severe dehydration and profound hypokalemia.

The diarrhea is temporarily relieved by nasogastric aspiration (80), in contrast to the secretory diarrhea of the Verner-Morrison syndrome (vipoma or WDHA syndrome), which is not. Treatment with cimetidine or total gastrectomy also "cures" the gastrin-induced diarrhea (81).

The excess gastric acid interferes with the digestion and absorption of fat by (a) denaturation of pancreatic lipase (82), (b) interference with bile salt micelle formation by precipitation of glycine-conjugated bile acids (82), and (c) causing intestinal mucosal damage (83). A further contribution to the diarrhea, and possibly the main cause in patients who have diarrhea without steatorrhea, is the direct effect of gastrin on the small intestine, causing impairment of water and sodium absorption (83). Tumor tissue may produce other substances, such as prostaglandins, which affect intestinal motility and secretion, but this possibility is still speculative (84).

ASSOCIATION WITH OTHER ENDOCRINE DISEASE

The association of ZES with other endocrine disease—namely, parathyroid and pituitary—is known as MEN-I syndrome (Fig. 4-22). It is transmitted by an autosomal dominant gene. Hyperparathyroidism is usually manifest earliest and is most common (it is present in nearly

90% of patients); 80% have islet cell tumors (ZES being most common); and 65% have disease of the anterior pituitary gland (85). The adrenal and thyroid glands may also be involved, although this is seen less frequently. ZES may occur in an isolated familial form (about 3% of cases) (72) with autosomal dominant inheritance, or it may occur sporadically.

> The association between gastrinoma and hyperparathyroidism is especially noteworthy because of the stimulatory effect of hypercalcemia on release of tumor gastrin (see below). Correction of the hypercalcemia by parathyroidectomy may dramatically relieve peptic ulcer symptoms and cause a decrease in serum gastrin concentration and gastric acid secretion even to normal levels (86–88).

Clearly, screening of the first-degree relatives of all patients with gastrinoma occurring as a component of the MEN-I syndrome is mandatory.

RADIOLOGIC EXAMINATION

Standard upper gastrointestinal barium contrast studies may not only confirm peptic ulcer disease but sometimes also show features very suggestive of ZES (89). The most frequent abnormalities include a distended, atonic stomach, with a large fasting fluid residue and prominent rugal folds, the radiologic counterpart to increased parietal cell mass.

The duodenum may be greatly dilated—the mucosal folds being thickened due to edema and hyperplasia of Brunner's glands and simulating a cobblestone appearance which may be mistaken for Crohn's disease. There is rapid transit of the contrast material through the small bowel, causing flocculation of the barium. In addition, dilatation of the jejunum and the thickening and edema of the mucosal folds produce a "malabsorption pattern" in some cases (Fig. 4-23). Fewer of these classically described signs are seen with earlier diagnosis (78).

LABORATORY STUDIES

Gastric Secretory Studies. During the era predating reliable gastrin radioimmunoassay, gastric acid secretion studies were valuable. However, there is considerable overlap in test results between patients with idiopathic peptic ulcer disease and those with ZES (90,91). The standard criteria included (a) 12-hour, overnight acid secretion greater than 100 mEq, (b) basal acid output greater than 15 mEq/hr in the intact stomach (or greater than 5 mEq/hr after subtotal gastrectomy or vagotomy), and (c) basal acid output to maximal acid output ratio of greater than 0.6. The value of these uncomfortable and expensive tests has been challenged; they should probably be replaced by the less expensive and more convenient serum gastrin determination, which provides equal diagnostic capability (92).

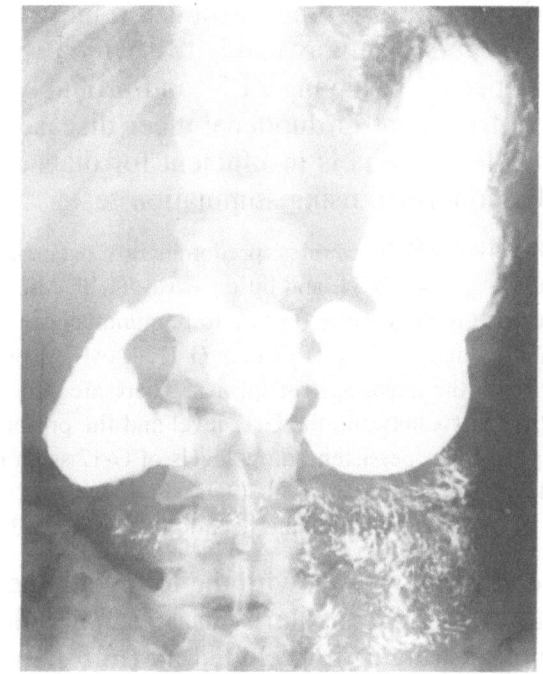

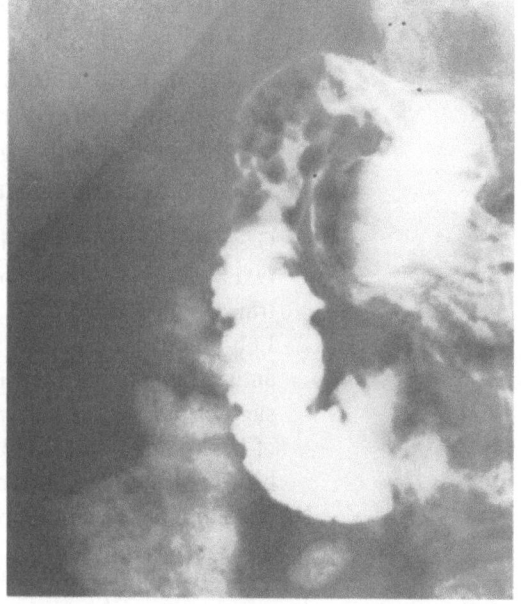

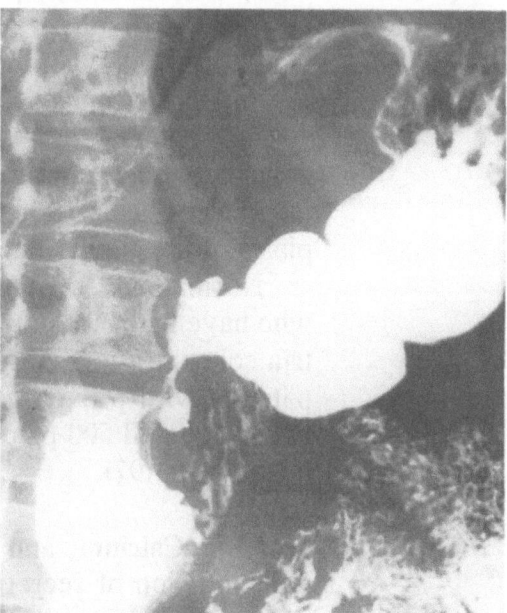

Classic radiographic features of Zollinger-Ellison syndrome. **A.** Ulcera-   **Fig. 4-23.**
tion of the first and second portion of the duodenum. There is dilatation of the
second portion of the duodenum and barium has flocculated in the upper small
intestine to produce a "malabsorption" pattern.   **B.** Cobblestone duodenum
due to mucosal edema and hypertrophy of Brunner's glands.   **C.** Penetrating
ulcer causing marked contraction and deformity of the first portion of the duodenum. There is considerable dilatation of the duodenum beyond the ulcer,
so-called megaduodenum. The mucosal folds in the upper stomach are prominent.

Radioimmunoassay of Gastrin. Fasting serum gastrin is a relatively inexpensive, reasonably reliable, and widely available test which should be obtained in all patients suspected of having ZES, and probably any patient scheduled for surgical treatment of duodenal ulcer disease. An elevated fasting serum gastrin level alone is insufficient for diagnosing ZES; the diagnosis should be confirmed using stimulation tests.

> Gastrin is actually a family of polypeptide hormones, predominantly occurring as two biologically active forms: big gastrin, G-34; and little gastrin, G-17. Minigastrin, G-14, is also active, whereas big-big gastrin appears to be minimally active. In both normal and ZES patients, there is more G-34 than G-17. Most gastrin antisera are equally sensitive to all the major gastrin species. There are data to suggest that a strong correlation exists between the G-17 level and the presence of hepatic metastases (93). Specifically, persistently low levels of G-17 seem to be associated with prolonged, metastasis-free intervals (94), whereas in one series all patients with more than 20% G-17 had definite hepatic metastases (93).

Serum gastrin may be elevated in patients with the following: pernicious anemia (these patients also have achlorhydria); renal failure; chronic gastric outlet obstruction; retained, excluded antrum (patients who have previously undergone a Billroth II partial gastrectomy with residual antral mucosa left attached to the duodenal stump—gastrin is strongly stimulated by the continuous bathing in the alkaline bilious and pancreatic secretions); and antral G-cell hyperplasia (95,96) (immunofluorescent examination of the antral mucosa confirms massive hyperplasia of G cells).

Normal subjects and patients with duodenal ulcer, including those who have had subtotal gastrectomy or vagotomy (64), have fasting gastrin concentrations of 50–200 pg/ml (68). However, as many as 40% of patients with proven gastrinomas may have fasting gastrin levels between 100 and 500 pg/ml. This overlap requires further definitive diagnostic tests (97).

Secretin, Calcium, and Protein Stimulation Tests. The bolus intravenous infusion of secretin (2 U/kg) in patients with gastrinoma reliably produces a prompt, marked, paradoxical increase in the serum gastrin concentration (66,68,75,98,99). Peak response values of gastrin, usually reached within 5–10 minutes after infusion, seem to be the best criteria for confirmation of the diagnosis and may approach 100% sensitivity and specificity (99) (Fig. 4-24). Patients with idiopathic peptic ulcer disease, G-cell hyperplasia, and retained gastric antrum do not show a similar stimulatory response (75,99,100).

In patients with gastrinoma, a continuous infusion of calcium gluceptate (15 mg/kg) over a 4-hour period also produces a gradual, marked increase in gastrin levels (Fig. 4-25). This response is again exclusively limited to gastrinoma patients, showing essentially no overlap with other ulcer patients when peak values are utilized (99). From a practical standpoint, the secretin infusion test is the procedure of choice as it is safer, quicker, more reliable, has fewer false-negative results, and is

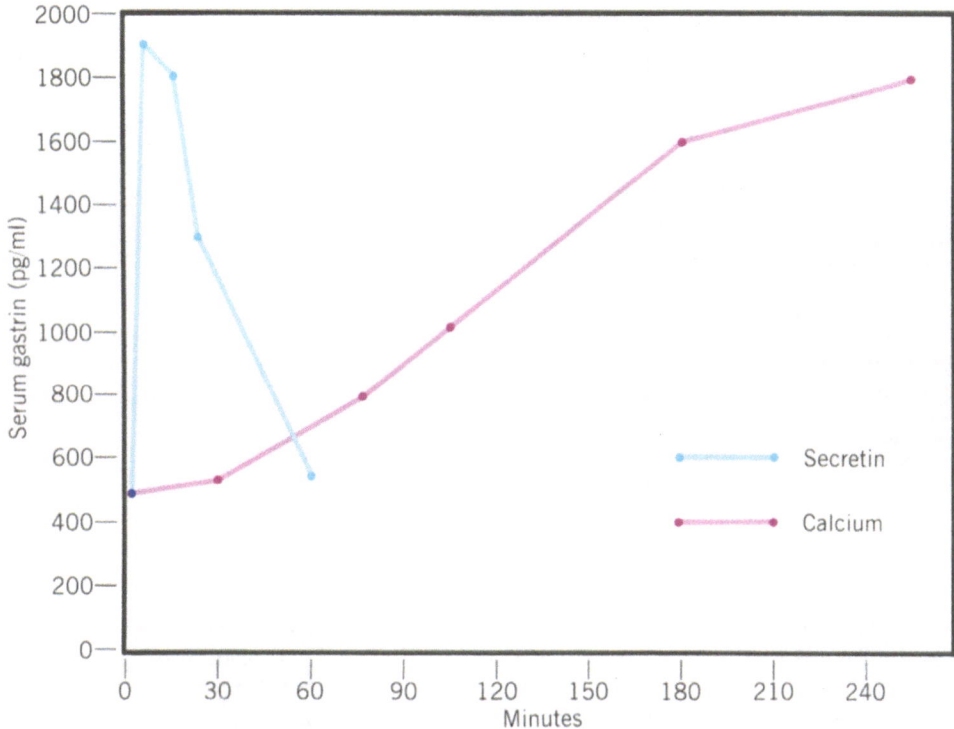

Secretin and calcium stimulation tests. Typical response of serum gastrin to secretin and calcium infusion tests in a patient with gastrinoma. **Fig. 4-24.**

more easily tolerated by the patient (98,99). The calcium infusion test should probably be reserved to help delineate the rare equivocal results obtained using the secretin test.

In normal patients and those with ordinary ulcer disease, serum gastrin increases 50%–100% during the first hour following a protein meal (66,68,75). There is little change, if any, in circulating gastrin in patients with ZES because tumor release of gastrin is unaffected by gastric distention or dietary secretagogues. In contrast, patients with antral G-cell hyperplasia show a markedly accentuated rise in serum gastrin (101) (Table 4-2).

Serum Gastrin Response in the Diagnosis of ZES **Table 4-2.**

Diagnosis	Secretin*	Calcium	Protein
Idiopathic ulcer	↔	↔	↑
G-Cell hyperplasia	↔	↔	↑ ↑
Gastrinoma	↑ ↑ ↑	↑ ↑ ↑	↔

* ↑, increase in gastrin; ↑ ↑, moderate increase in gastrin; ↑ ↑ ↑, marked increase in gastrin; ↔, little or no change in gastrin level.

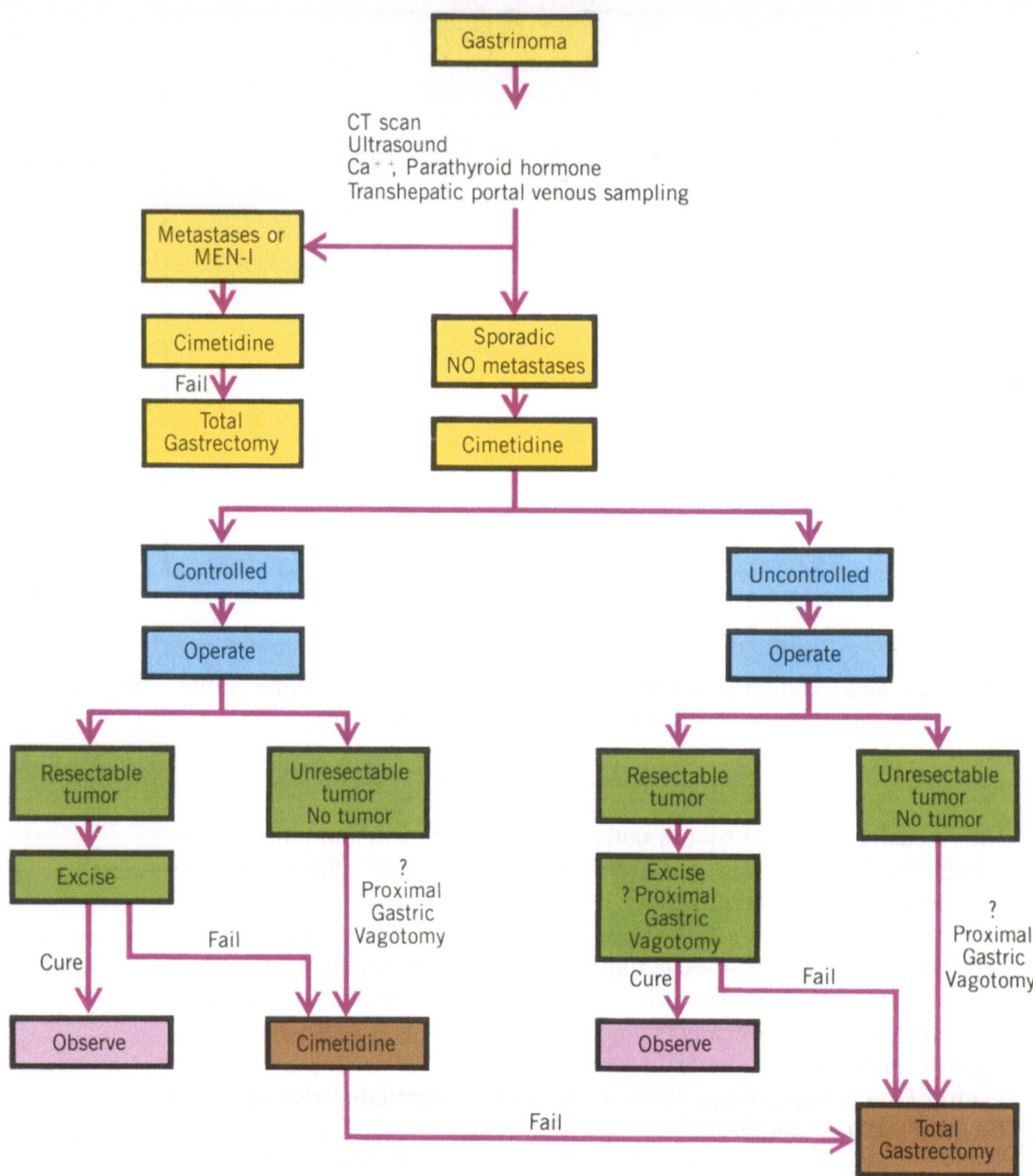

Fig. 4-25. **Gastrinoma: localization and treatment options.** The drugs Ranitidine and Omeprazole may be substituted for Cimetidine.

When the rare diagnosis of G-cell hyperplasia is confirmed by normal secretin and calcium infusion tests, and an exaggerated response to a protein meal, antrectomy is curative.

PREOPERATIVE LOCALIZATION STUDIES

The impetus to pursue preoperative localizing studies for patients with gastrinoma emerged simultaneously with the success of the histamine H_2-receptor antagonist, cimetidine. Treatment could be aimed not only at control of acid secretion but also at possible curative excision of the tumor. Admittedly, the proportion of patients in whom such surgery is feasible is limited—perhaps only 20%–25%—but this is a far higher percentage, with a markedly better prognosis, than those patients with ductal pancreatic carcinoma. Localization need not even be considered if treatment is strictly limited to either extreme of the therapeutic spectrum—either cimetidine therapy or total gastrectomy. However, both of these approaches, if inflexibly applied, deny the patient *any* chance for cure of the tumor and seem highly inappropriate.

Prior to presently available localizing techniques, the most effective modality was intraoperative inspection and palpation by the surgeon. However, up to 50% of these lesions were not found at laparotomy, and support for proceeding with blind distal pancreatectomy seems very tenuous at best (76,102).

Preoperative ultrasound or CT scanning may demonstrate hepatic metastases, thereby excluding curative surgery. However, these modalities have proven unreliable for localization of resectable lesions (103). Whereas arteriography has generally proven efficacious in identifying insulinomas, similar success in attempts to localize gastrinomas has been achieved in only 20%–30% of patients, with false-negative and false-positive error rates of greater than 50% (102, 104,105).

Percutaneous transhepatic selective venous sampling has been used successfully to localize gastrinomas in some cases (106,107,108), including several in which all other modalities had failed (109). When this technique provides strong evidence that the tumor is unifocal, located in the body or tail of the pancreas, with no metastases, a distal pancreatectomy seems justifiable, even if the lesion is nonpalpable.

TREATMENT

The classic therapeutic treatment of total gastrectomy for all patients with gastrinomas was based on the well-established fact that the risks of potentially lethal complications incurred by the ulcer disease outweighed the delayed mortality risk of this rather indolent malignancy. In addition, these tumors are frequently metastatic, multiple, and/or occult, and thus rarely amenable to curative surgery. However, the recognition that nearly all patients could achieve adequate control of the gastric hypersecretion with histamine H_2-receptor antagonists—at least in the short term—has stimulated a total reevaluation of the therapeutic management of these patients (Fig. 4-25).

GASTRINOMA WITH MEN SYNDROME

The patient with ZES and associated primary hyperparathyroidism should first undergo cervical exploration. In a majority of cases correction of the hypercalcemia significantly ameliorates the hypergastrinemia and gastric hypersecretory state (110–112). Attempts at curative surgery seem fruitless as the gastrinomas are virtually always multiple and diffuse (109).

NONSURGICAL

Abundant evidence of successful control of acid hypersecretion by pharmacologic means justifies it as a primary mode of therapy (76,81,113,114). All patients with the confirmed diagnosis of gastrinoma should be initially treated with cimetidine or ranitidine. At least 85% of such patients may be expected to sustain symptomatic relief of dyspepsia and diarrhea, concomitant with a reduction in hyperacidity and ulcer healing. The medication schedule (cimetidine, 300–600 mg every 6 hours) must be assiduously followed, since even short lapses may lead to serious complications. Side effects related to cimetidine have generally been mild and infrequent, predominantly limited to gynecomastia and impotence. Complications that require operation specifically related to failure of adequate cimetidine therapy, at least in the short term, probably occur in less than 10%–15% of patients, and patient acceptance is nearly universal (81,113).

During initiation of medical treatment, one should proceed with evaluation for the presence of multiple tumors, metastatic disease, and MEN-I syndrome. If any one of these is confirmed, curative surgery is virtually impossible; attempts at tumor localization are reserved for the remaining group. After it has been determined whether medical therapy offers sufficient control, those with apparently localized disease and all medical failures should undergo operation.

SURGICAL

Abdominal exploration should be considered for all gastrinoma patients except those with known metastatic disease controlled medically, those with unrelated contraindications to surgery, and probably those with MEN-I syndrome.

Total Gastrectomy. Total gastrectomy is the standard, end-organ ablative treatment for this disease. Postoperative sequelae seem to be better tolerated than when it is performed for gastric adenocarcinoma (68,73), nevertheless, the operative mortality rates range from 2% to 27% in elective cases and may double in the emergency setting (68,76,115,116).

This procedure provides long-term, complete control of gastric hypersecretion. The necessity for patient compliance is limited to monthly vitamin B_{12} injections rather than multiple daily tablets. Total gastrectomy should therefore be considered a primary therapeutic alternative uniquely suited to all patients who have failed medical therapy and any patient who is unable, too unreliable, or unwilling to follow a rigid medication schedule. According to the Zollinger-Ellison Tumor Registry of over 800 case reports (68), the overall 5- and 10-year survival rates after total gastrectomy are 55% and 42%, respectively. Patients with liver metastases have similar survival rates of 42% and 30%, respectively.

Tumor Excision. The use of cimetidine has allowed safe, specific tumor excision and the avoidance of total gastrectomy (114,117,118). With the apparent trend toward earlier diagnosis, improved preoperative localizing techniques, and the safeguard of pharmacologic control of hyperacidity, attempts at complete curative tumor resection—albeit uncommon—seem reasonable. Tumors confined to the duodenal wall, distal pancreas, or even extrapancreatic and extraintestinal locations (119) are amenable to successful removal. Lesions in the head of the pancreas should be treated medically or by total gastrectomy. The chance of curative resection is remote, and the associated morbidity and mortality of pancreaticoduodenectomy is high. In addition, the prospect of subsequent total gastrectomy for recurrent disease would be technically formidable and nutritionally crippling.

Proximal Gastric Vagotomy. Recent, limited experience with proximal gastric vagotomy as a surgical adjunct to cimetidine therapy seems very encouraging (120,121). Consistent reduction in acid hypersecretion has been achieved in a number of patients (121). It may be possible to employ this procedure in gastrinoma patients who require high-dose medical therapy, those undergoing emergency surgery, or those with occult disease.

TREATMENT OF METASTATIC DISEASE

Islet cell carcinomas frequently follow an indolent clinical course, the effects of the malignancy per se being overshadowed by the effects of endocrine hyperfunction. Since gastrinomas are slow growing, this is particularly true of these tumors. Despite the frequency of metastatic spread or the frighteningly high level of serum gastrin, the prognosis generally remains good following the traditional treatment of total gastrectomy (68,72,75). The 5- and 10-year survival rates of 42% and 30%, respectively, in patients *with* liver metastases proven at the time of total gastrectomy support this fact (73). About one-half of the late deaths, however, are due to metastatic spread, although this is often delayed 5–15 years following the initial operation (72,75). Spontaneous regression of metastatic tumor after total gastrectomy has been reported (122) but is rare, occurring in much less than 1% of cases. The high mortality previously associated with gastrinoma has been related more to the sequelae of gastric hypersecretion in the inadequately or untreated case rather than to the presence of metastases.

Once control of gastric hypersecretion has been established either by medical or surgical means, attention may be directed specifically to tumor management. A conservative approach to chemotherapy has been adopted, since the natural history of the untreated tumor is often prolonged. For those whose tumors display more aggressive behavior, treatment with streptozotocin and fluorouracil may offer a 60% chance of tumor regression (123). Side effects include nausea and vomiting, reversible renal toxicity, and bone marrow depression (123).

WDHA Syndrome (Vipoma)

In 1958 Verner and Morrison (124) reported 2 cases of severe refractory watery diarrhea associated with non-β, non-insulin-secreting islet cell adenomas of the pancreas. More than 100 cases of this syndrome have subsequently been described. Various names have been applied to the syndrome, including WDHA (watery diarrhea, hypokalemia, achlorhydria), vipoma, pancreatic cholera, and Verner-Morrison syndrome. The principal characteristics include severe watery diarrhea, marked hypokalemia, and hypo- or achlorhydria.

PATHOLOGY

Approximately 70% of these cases are caused by pancreatic islet cell tumors (D_1 cells) (125), 10%–20% are due to islet cell hyperplasia (126), and 10%–20% are extrapancreatic—originating in ganglioneuroblastomas, adrenal medullary tumors (127), or pulmonary tumors (128). About 50% of the pancreatic tumors are malignant, 75% of which are metastatic at the time of diagnosis. They are infrequently multiple, occur in the body and tail in 80% of cases (126), and have been associated with MEN-I syndrome. Rarely are the extrapancreatic tumors malignant (129). The pancreatic tumors, ranging in size from 1.5 to 7 cm in diameter, are similar to other islet cell tumors in gross and light microscopic appearance. However, the level of vasoactive intestinal polypeptide (VIP) is reliably elevated (129) when chemical extraction is performed on the tumor.

DIAGNOSIS

The age range is from 5 to 72 years, with a mean between 40 and 50 (126). Ganglioneuroblastomas are usually found in children. The sex ratio is about equal.

CLINICAL FEATURES (See Fig. 4-26)

The dominant symptom is a profuse, watery, tea-colored, cholera-like diarrhea (ranging from 1–10 liters/day, typically 4–6 liters/day) that may be episodic or persistent. It is a secretory diarrhea affecting the gut distal to the stomach, and thus is unaffected by nasogastric suction. The resultant massive fecal loss of fluid and electrolytes is potentially life-threatening, leading to significant prerenal azotemia or even refractory renal failure and death (130).

Spontaneous attacks of flushing occur in about 20% of patients; they resemble similar episodes due to carcinoid syndrome (129). This vaso-dilatation may be limited to the face and chest or involve the entire body.

LABORATORY STUDIES

Hypokalemia. Marked fecal potassium loss of 300–350 mEq/day (normal, less than or equal to 15 mEq/day) (126) due to the severe diarrhea leads to muscular weakness, lethargy, and nausea and vomiting. Even with aggressive potassium replacement, serum levels average 2.2 mEq/liter, which may exacerbate renal damage.

Achlorhydria or Hypochlorhydria. Basal achlorhydria occurs in about one-half of the patients. Hypochlorhydria, responsive to histamine stimulation, is more common. Following tumor resection, rebound acid hypersecretion may occur. Acid secretory studies should be obtained during the diagnostic evaluation to help differentiate vipomas from gastrinomas (Zollinger-Ellison syndrome).

Hypercalcemia and Hyperglycemia. Between one-half and two-thirds of WDHA patients are hypercalcemic, with values frequently above 12 mg/dl (126). A parathyroid hormone-like effect on the bone has been postulated to account for this, but these patients have normal parathyroids. Excision of the vipoma cures the hypercalcemia. Similarly, approximately 50% of these patients have fasting hyperglycemia, which also is cured with resection of the primary tumor (126).

Plasma VIP. Little controversy now exists regarding the causative humoral agent. Elevated plasma and tumor levels of VIP have been repeatedly demonstrated in patients with this syndrome (129,131,132).

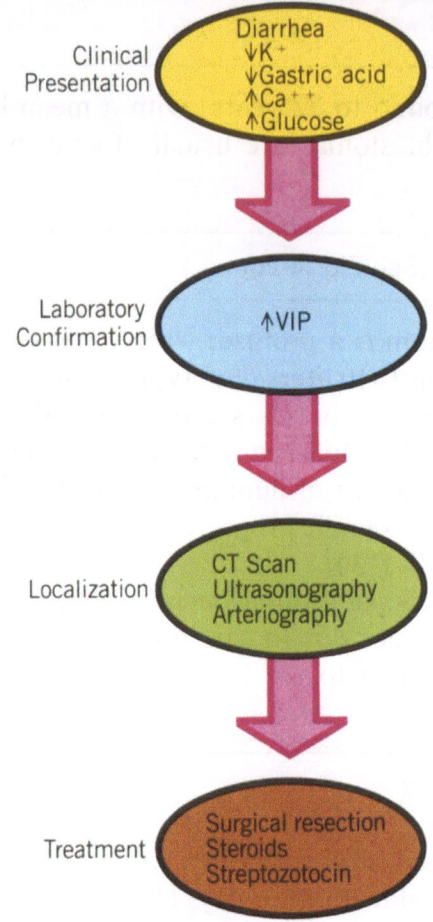

Fig. 4-26.   **Evaluation and management of vipomas (WDHA).**

With rare exceptions, a raised plasma VIP level has been exclusively limited to these patients. Moreover, VIP levels have almost always been normal in patients with a variety of other endocrine and nonendocrine tumors, as well as those with diarrhea of different etiologies (129,133).

Exogenous VIP infusion in humans stimulates intestinal secretion, inhibits intestinal absorption and gastric acid secretion, and stimulates flushing, hypercalcemia, hyperglycemia, bile flow, and pancreatic bicarbonate secretion (125,131,134,135). These effects correlate well with WDHA clinical syndrome. Very similar effects are seen with prostaglandin E_2, which may play some role in the pathogenesis.

Pancreatic polypeptide is also commonly secreted by these pancreatic tumors (extrapancreatic tumors do not secrete this polypeptide). A biologic role for this hormone has not been defined; its value is presently that of a plasma marker.

PREOPERATIVE LOCALIZATION STUDIES

Initially, either CT or ultrasonography should be attempted. Should these fail to localize a tumor, angiography is usually successful (129,132). Transhepatic venous sampling may have a role in difficult cases (136).

TREATMENT

SURGICAL

Following vigorous preoperative resuscitation, surgical excision of both pancreatic and extrapancreatic tumors is the optimal form of treatment (Fig. 4-26). Benign tumors are cured by excision, with correction of all clinical and laboratory abnormalities (provided permanent renal damage has not occurred). If no tumor is found, one should probably regard the pathology as islet cell hyperplasia (nesidioblastosis) and proceed with a subtotal pancreatectomy. Some patients have required a subsequent completion total pancreatectomy for relief of symptoms (130,134,137). If metastatic disease is encountered, cytoreductive surgery for palliation can be effective (138). At operation, the gallbladder is frequently markedly distended (73). Initially this was attributed to a secretin-like effect but it is now attributed to the action of VIP.

NONSURGICAL

Temporary symptomatic control may be achieved using steroid therapy (126,129,130); however, eventual relapse has been the rule. Streptozotocin has been effective in sustaining both objective tumor regression and clinical remission (129,139).

Glucagonoma

Fewer than 100 patients with the glucagonoma syndrome have been reported in the medical literature (140). The first presumed cases of glucagonoma were recorded in 1942 (141), although their association with hyperglucagonemia was not then recognized—the etiology was identified only in retrospect. The composite clinical and laboratory syndrome was first documented in 1966 by McGavran et al. (142) and confirmed by a series of patients with the disease in 1974 (143).

This syndrome is caused by a pancreatic α-islet cell tumor which typically secretes massive amounts of glucagon. It produces a distinctive clinical syndrome, the most prominent features of which are diabetes and a characteristic dermatitis called "necrolytic migratory erythema."

PATHOLOGY

The gross and light microscopic appearance of these α-cell tumors is indistinguishable from other islet cell tumors. Exact identification, however, is possible using electron microscopy, immunofluorescent studies (143–145), and tumor extracts, which invariably demonstrate the presence of glucagon (144). Nearly 80% of these tumors are 3 cm or larger in diameter (140), and 90% are located in the body or tail of the pancreas. From 60% to 75% are malignant (146,147), most frequently metastasizing to regional lymph nodes or the liver. The appearance of metastatic disease may be delayed for years following apparently curative resection (148), and neither tumor size nor plasma glucagon levels are predictive of malignancy.

DIAGNOSIS

CLINICAL FEATURES

The age range spans the second to eighth decades, predominating in the sixth. There is essentially an equal sex ratio. The principal clinical features are listed in Figure 4-27.

Diabetes mellitus is the most frequent component of the glucagonoma syndrome. The diabetes is usually mild; sometimes it is demonstrated only by an abnormal glucose tolerance test. Secondary systemic complications (e.g., nephropathy, neuropathy, opthalmopathy, etc.) and ketoacidosis are rarely present.

Necrolytic migratory erythema is frequently the key to the diagnosis (Table 4-3). Initially it tends to affect the legs, lower abdomen, perineum, and perioral areas. These lesions may heal centrally concurrent with the rash progressing to involve adjacent areas. The lesions usually begin as markedly erythematous macules and papules and progress to blisters that then develop central epidermal erosion (149). They may be very painful, pruritic, and become secondarily infected. As the border of the mascular rash advances, the center heals with a residual brown pigmentation; the entire cycle is complete in 7–14 days. Skin biopsy of the advancing edge is pathognomonic (146). Stomatitis, glossitis, and cheilitis often accompany the rash.

Table 4-3.
Necrolytic Migratory Erythema

Distribution	Appearance	Histology
Lower abdomen, perineum	Raised, reddened edematous patch	Dermis normal
Perioral skin	Epidermis easily rubbed off	Superficial epidermis
Lower limbs	Secondary infection common	necrotic, shows lysis
	Edge of lesion spreads	

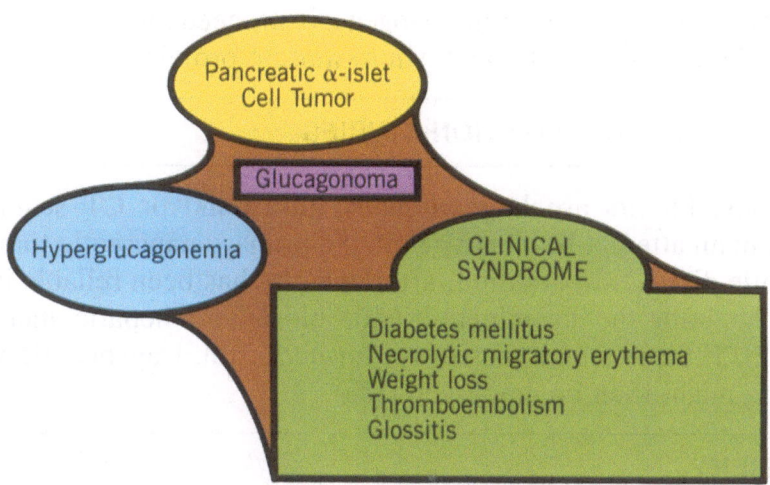

Diagnosis of glucagonoma. **Fig. 4-27.**

Although these patients generally maintain their appetite, significant *weight loss* is a very frequent finding. This is attributed to the marked catabolic effect of glucagon on carbohydrate, protein, and fat metabolism.

Both venous and arterial *thromboembolic complications* have been noted in up to 30% of these patients (143,146). These have been the cause of death in several instances; thus the use of prophylactic anticoagulation is warranted.

LABORATORY STUDIES

Hyperglucagonemia. All patients in whom the syndrome has been prospectively recognized have had elevated basal immunoreactive plasma glucagon levels (140). The vast majority have shown markedly elevated levels averaging in excess of 5000 pg/ml; in normal individuals the level is less than 150 pg/ml (146). Hyperglucagonemia may be found in a number of non-islet cell tumor patients under circumstances of severe stress such as burns, trauma, myocardial infarction, sepsis, diabetic ketoacidosis, cirrhosis, chronic renal failure, and acute pancreatitis (150,151).

Anemia. The commonly encountered normochromic, normocytic anemia may simply reflect the chronically ill state of the patients, or perhaps it is related directly to glucagon excess. Treatment with iron, vitamin B_{12}, and folic acid has usually been ineffective; tumor excision reverses the anemia.

Hypoaminoacidemia. The marked stimulus of gluconeogenesis by glucagon accounts for the severe hypoaminoacidemia and hypoproteinemia regularly found in these patients. It appears that hepatic clearance of plasma aminoacids for gluconeogenesis proceeds more rapidly than the peripheral catabolic breakdown of muscle protein.

PREOPERATIVE LOCALIZATION STUDIES

Since most tumors are large, initially ultrasound or CT scanning is utilized in an attempt to identify both the primary pancreatic tumor and metastatic disease. In addition, arteriography has been reliable in demonstrating both the prominent tumor blush and hepatic metastases (147,152). If these techniques prove unsuccessful, transhepatic venous sampling might then be employed (153).

TREATMENT

SURGICAL

Dramatic and complete reversal of the entire constellation of clinical and laboratory abnormalities follows curative tumor resection. Cytoreductive tumor debulking is generally recommended and seems to ameliorate the clinical syndrome (140,154); however, this palliation frequently lasts less than 1 year.

NONSURGICAL

Used either alone or in combination with 5-fluorouracil, streptozotocin has produced significant tumor regression with concomitant improvement in clinical symptoms (144,146) Plasma glucagon provides an excellent marker for tumor recurrence and should be serially checked. Diamino triazeno imidazole carboxamide (*DTIC*) has proven highly effective with minimal side effects (155). It has been recommended as the drug of choice for this malignancy (146).

PROGNOSIS

Approximately 10% of patients with the glucagonoma syndrome may achieve surgical cure, as judged by prolonged tumor-free survival (140). As in other islet cell malignancies, the tumor may follow a rather indolent course. Even with *no* treatment, one-half of these patients survive more than 5 years (140). This must be borne in mind when one contemplates initiating chemotherapy or evaluates its effects.

Somatostatinoma syndrome is exceedingly rare: only 9 cases have been reported (156) since it was first described in 1977 (157). Most of these patients underwent limited endocrine evaluations since several of the tumors were found incidentally at the time of cholecystectomy.

Somatostatinoma

The clinical presentation is usually subtle and nonspecific, which is at least in part the reason for its rare recognition. Diabetes mellitus, cholelithiasis, steatorrhea, and indigestion associated with a D-islet cell tumor of the pancreas are the main elements of this syndrome.

All tumors have been single and intrapancreatic, and five have been malignant. Uniformly positive immunofluorescent reaction with antisomatostatin antiserum, and tissue extraction for somatostatin have been performed on these tumors to confirm the diagnosis (156).

Many pharmacologic effects of somatostatin have been well characterized (125,158,159). It inhibits release of thyroid-stimulating hormone, growth hormone, insulin, glucagon, pancreatic polypeptide, gastrin, cholecystokinin, secretin, and gastric inhibitory polypeptide. As a result, it suppresses gastric acid secretion, pepsin secretion, gastric emptying, exocrine pancreatic secretion, gallbladder contractility, and intestinal motility. Somatostatinoma has also justifiably been named the "inhibitory syndrome." Plasma somatostatin levels are markedly elevated in these patients. The clinical manifestations of this hormonal excess include mild diabetes, steatorrhea, cholelithiasis, weight loss, indigestion, vomiting, postprandial fullness, and anemia (Table 4-4).

Surgical excision may be curative (160), but most patients have been diagnosed late in the disease course; several have had metastases and died soon postoperatively. Current data are inadequate to assess the effectiveness of chemotherapy or present a meaningful guide to prognosis.

Clinical Features of Somatostatinoma

Table 4-4.

Clinical Manifestation	Etiology: Inhibition of
Steatorrhea	Exocrine pancreas
Mild diabetes	Endocrine pancreas
Cholelithiasis	Gallbladder contractility; cholecystokinin
Indigestion Bloating Vomiting	Gastric emptying, intestinal motility
Anemia, weight loss	(Secondary effects)

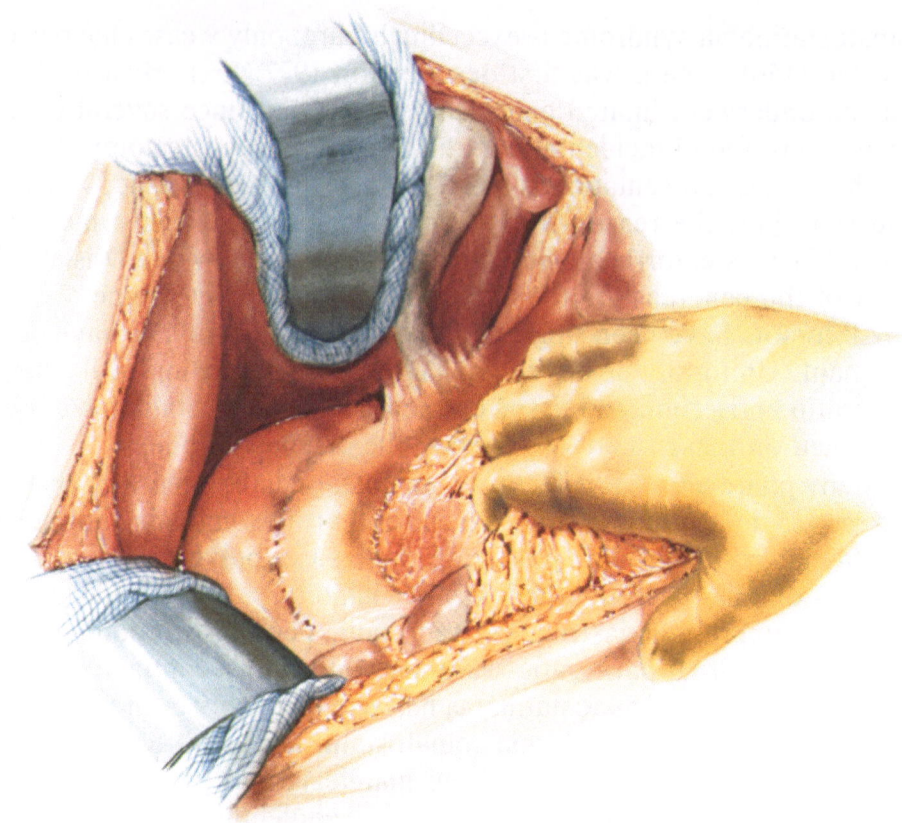

Fig. 4-28. **Inspection and palpation of the pancreas.** Anterior exposure of the head, neck, and ucinate process of the pancreas may be performed by first reflecting the hepatic flexure of the colon away from the underlying duodenum and pancreas. The greater omentum is reflected from its attachments to the colon and mesocolon. Further exposure is achieved by dividing the right gastroepiploic vessels and reflecting the antral and pyloric portions of the stomach superiorly.

Operative Technique

SURGICAL APPROACH FOR INSULINOMA

Surgical excision of insulinomas is the only form of curative treatment. It can usually be performed with a high degree of success and safety, yielding excellent long-term results. Even when the disease is malignant and metastatic, palliative resection may still be indicated and lead to gratifying results.

If the patient is obese (not an uncommon finding with insulinoma), a bilateral subcostal incision provides the best access to the pancreas. A high transverse or a generous upper midline incision may be preferred in the nonobese individual. Once the abdomen is opened, routine inspection and palpation of the abdominal contents are carried out. Multiple

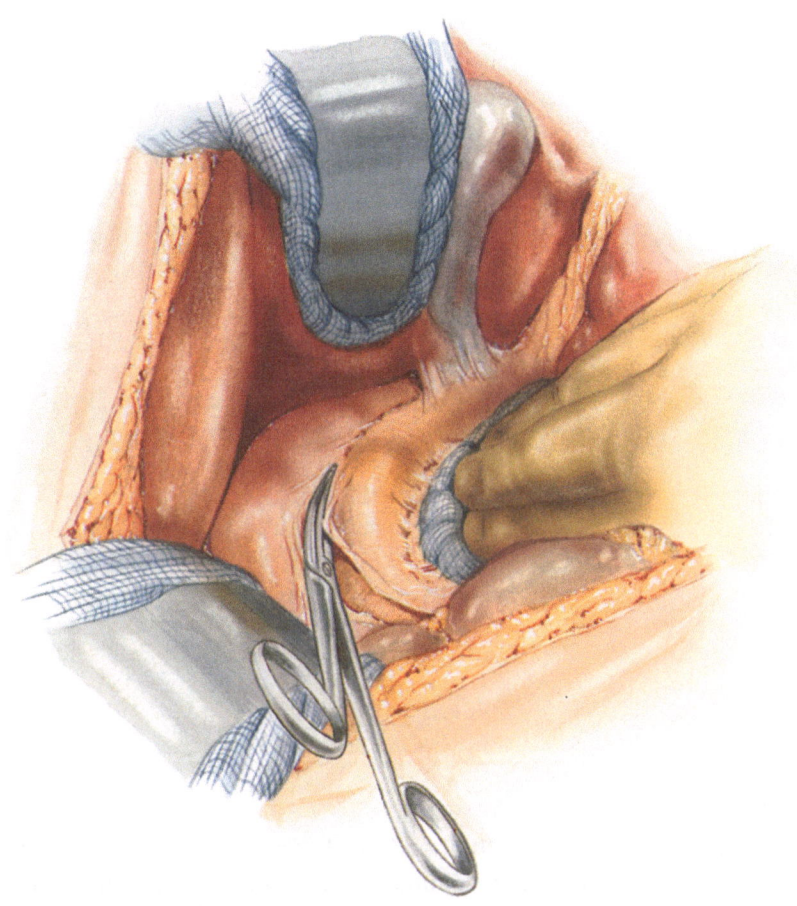

The peritoneum along the lateral aspect of the duodenal loop is incised. The duodenum and pancreas are freed from the underlying vena cava and aorta by a combination of blunt and sharp dissection.

Fig. 4-29.

tumors of varying size are found in about 10% of cases. Thus, even if a tumor has been identified by preoperative arteriography, small supernumerary lesions must be excluded by careful examination of the entire pancreas as shown in Figures 4-28 to 4-32. If the pancreas is more firmly tethered posteriorly, adequate palpation is possible only after thorough mobilization of the gland (Figs. 4-33 to 4-35).

Most commonly, the removal of an insulinoma is accomplished by simple enucleation (Fig. 4-36). After the tumor is excised, the pancreatic wound is inspected carefully for evidence of injury to the main pancreatic duct (see below). If no ductal injury is found, the pancreatic wound is closed with interrupted silk sutures and the area is drained (Fig. 4-37).

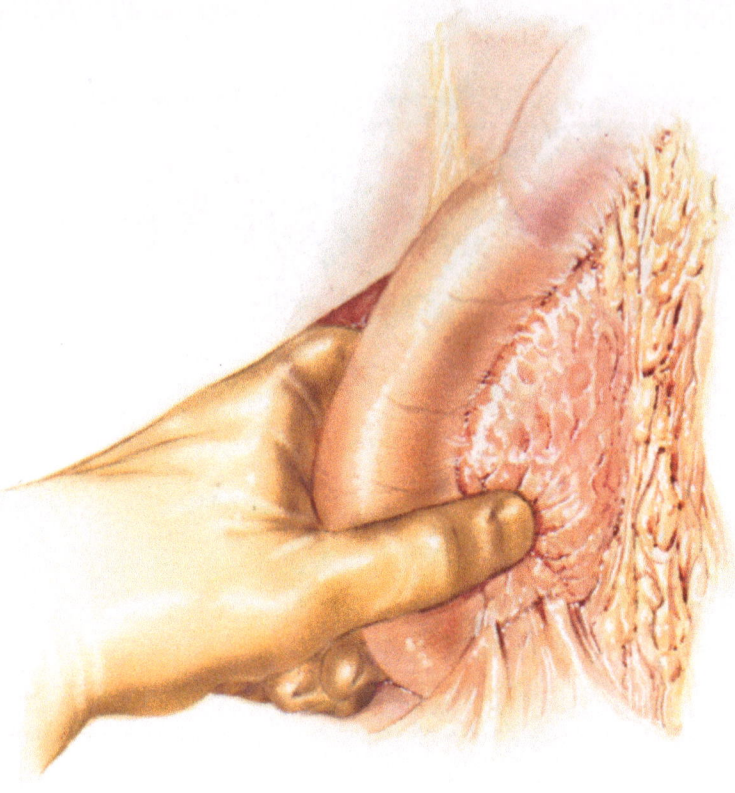

A

Fig. 4-30. **A.** It is now possible to palpate the head, neck, and uncinate process of the pancreas between the fingers and thumb of the left hand. **B.** This cross-sectional view shows palpation of an islet cell tumor in the head of the pancreas. **C.** In cases in which the uncinate process is inaccessible to palpation or feels suspicious, it should be exposed by an upward mobilization of the entire right colon and its attached mesentery.

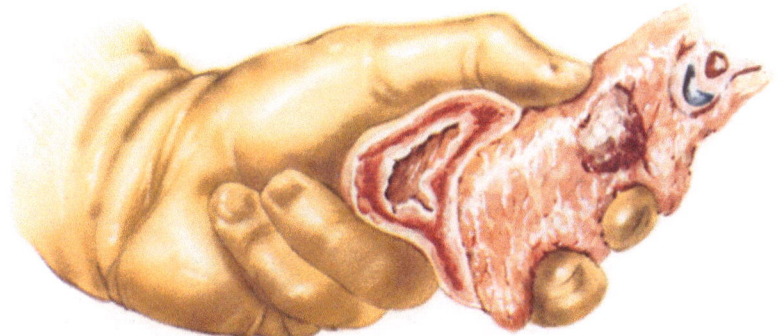

B

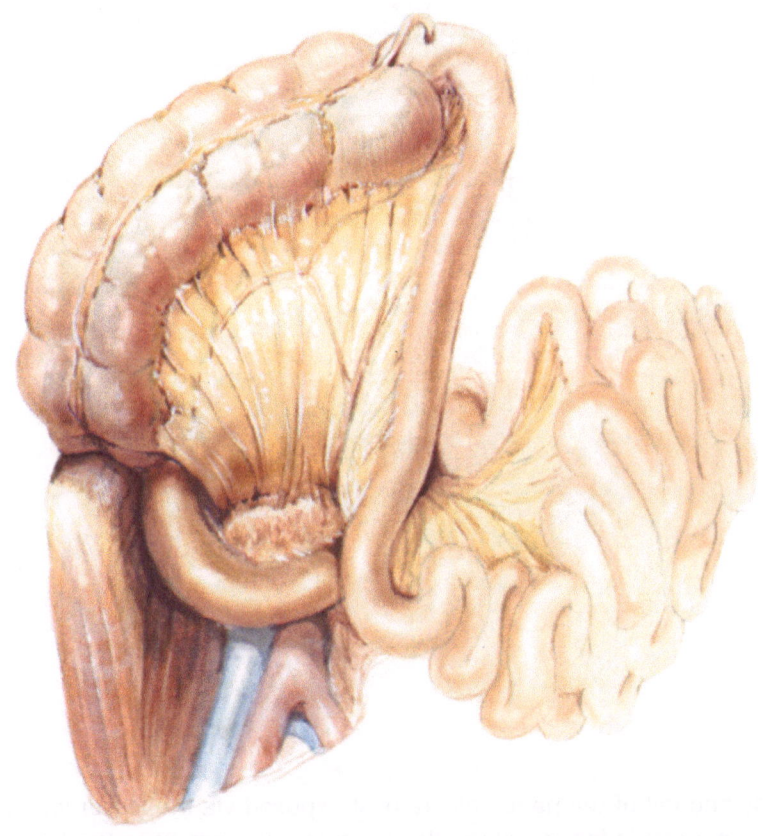

C

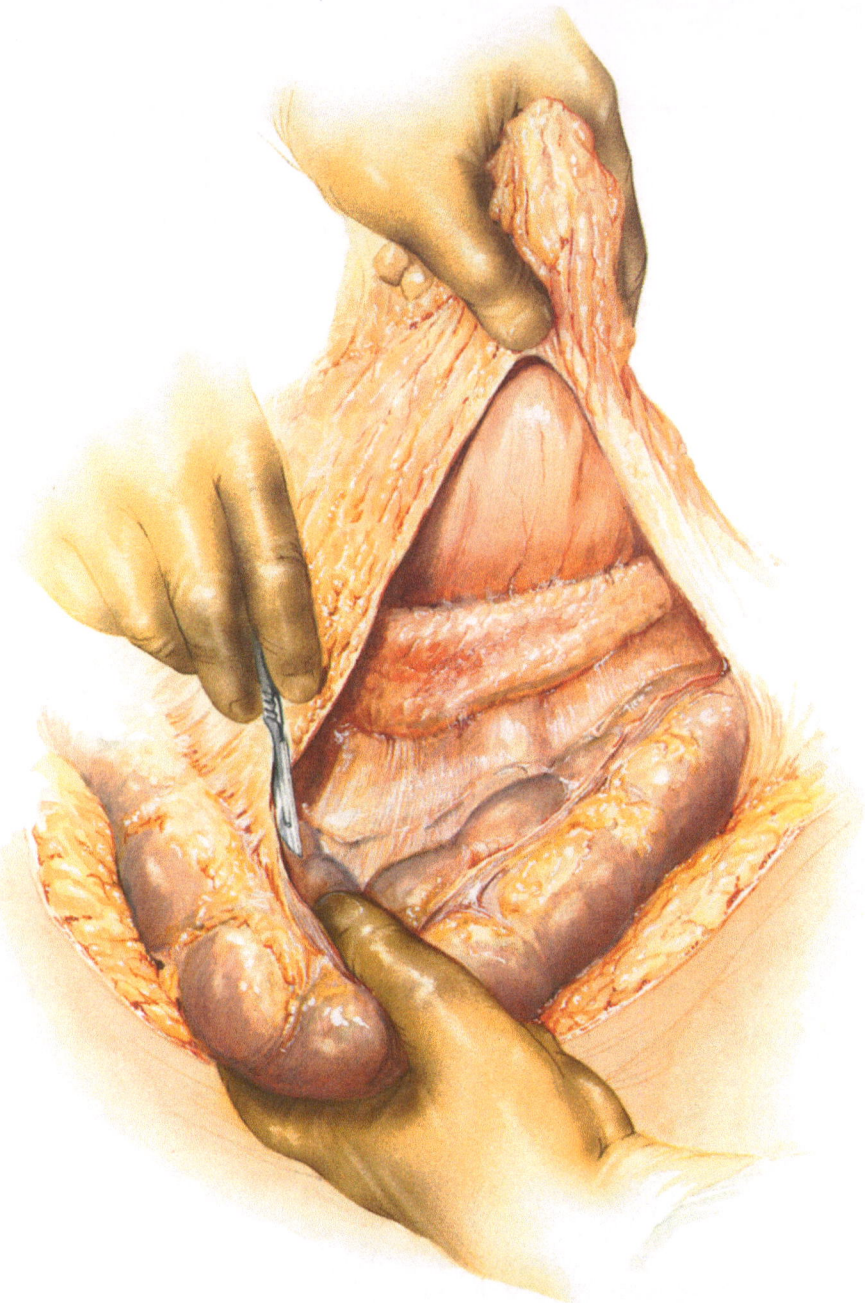

Fig. 4-31. The body and tail of the pancreas are best exposed via the lesser sac. The gastrocolic omentum is incised along its avascular attachment to the transverse colon. To avoid injury to the spleen by excessive traction on the splenocolic ligament, the splenic flexure of the colon is mobilized.

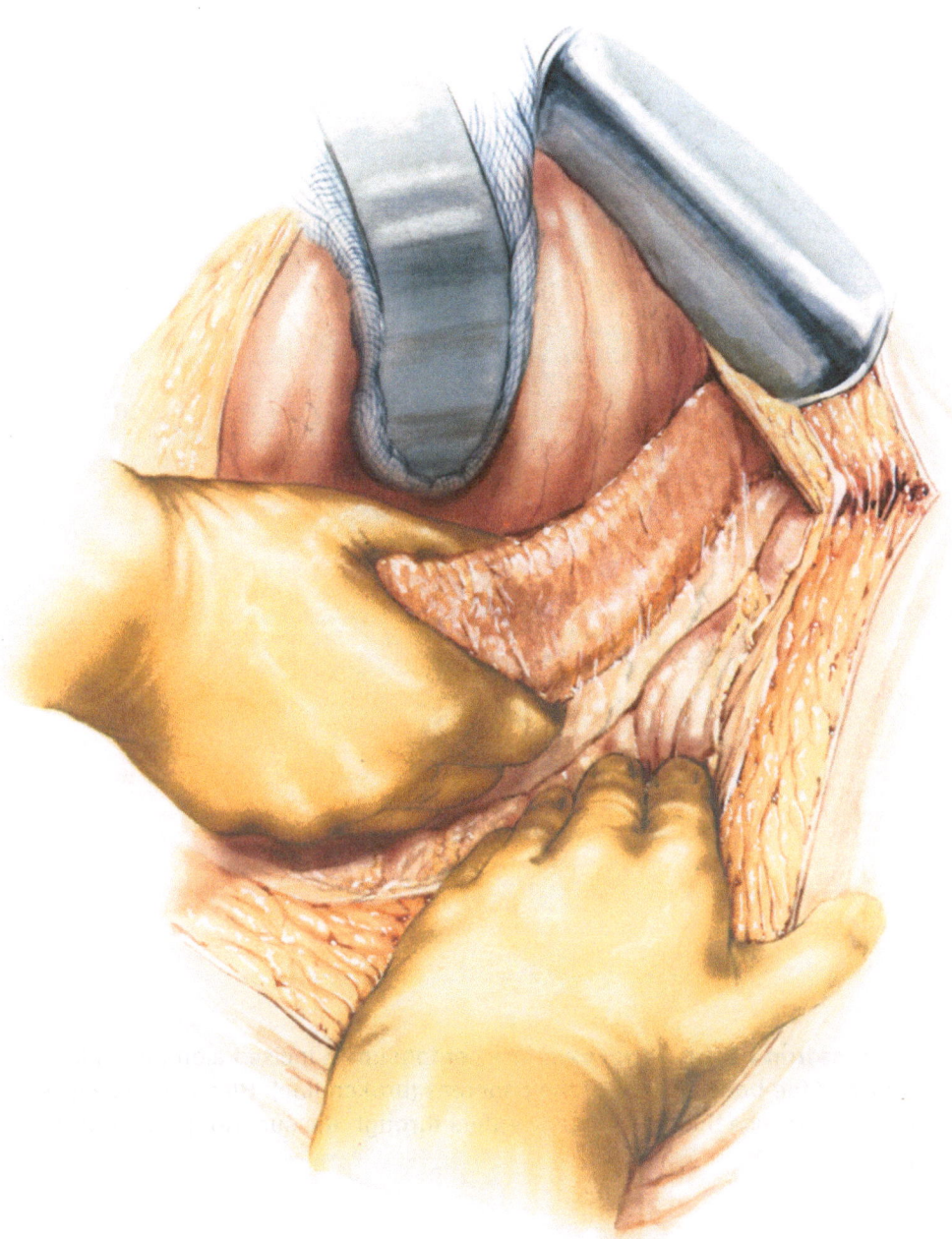

The stomach is retracted superiorly and the transverse colon inferiorly (by the assistant's left hand) to expose the pancreas. The loose areolar attachments between the body and tail of the pancreas and the retroperitoneal parietes usually permit palpation of the gland between the fingers and thumb of the right hand.

Fig. 4-32.

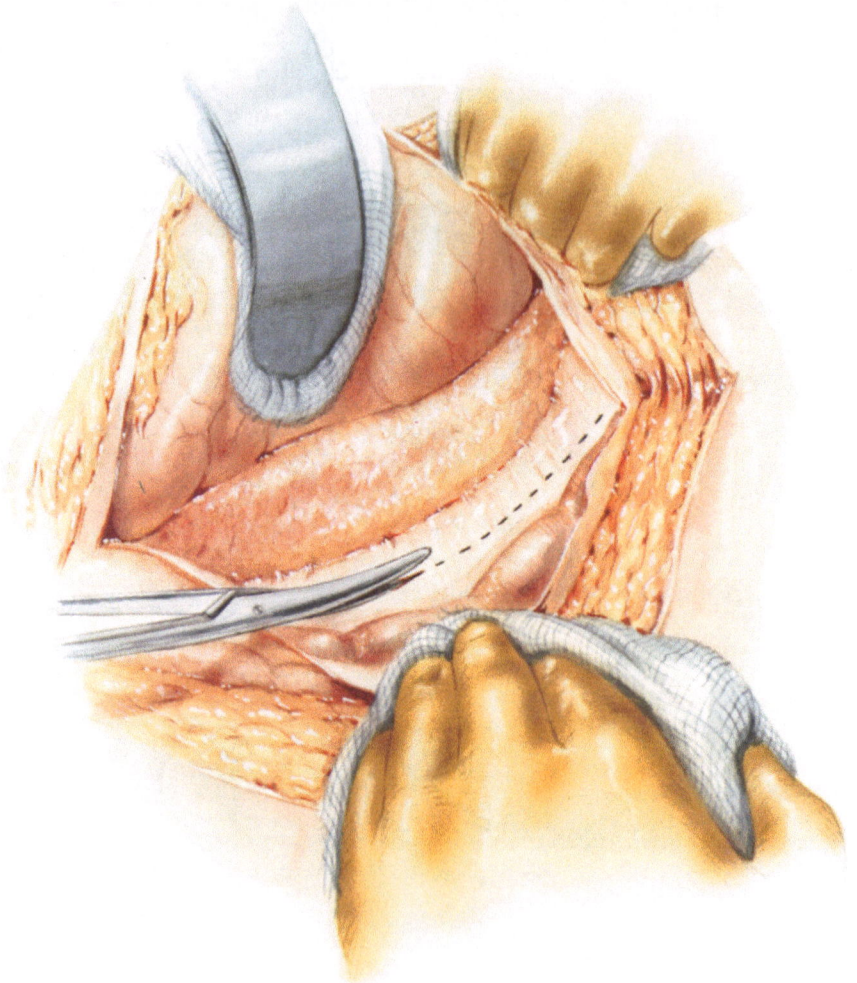

Fig. 4-33. **Mobilization of the pancreas.** The peritoneum is incised along the inferior border of the body and tail of the pancreas (broken line). Bleeding usually is minimal because the blood supply enters through the superior portion of the gland.

Fig. 4-34. **A and B.** The areolar plane deep to the pancreas is now opened by blunt finger dissection, as depicted. The crooked fingers of the left hand elevate the tail of the pancreas and work in gentle motion, with the fingers of the right hand providing countertraction, to separate the areolar tissues and progressively free the gland.

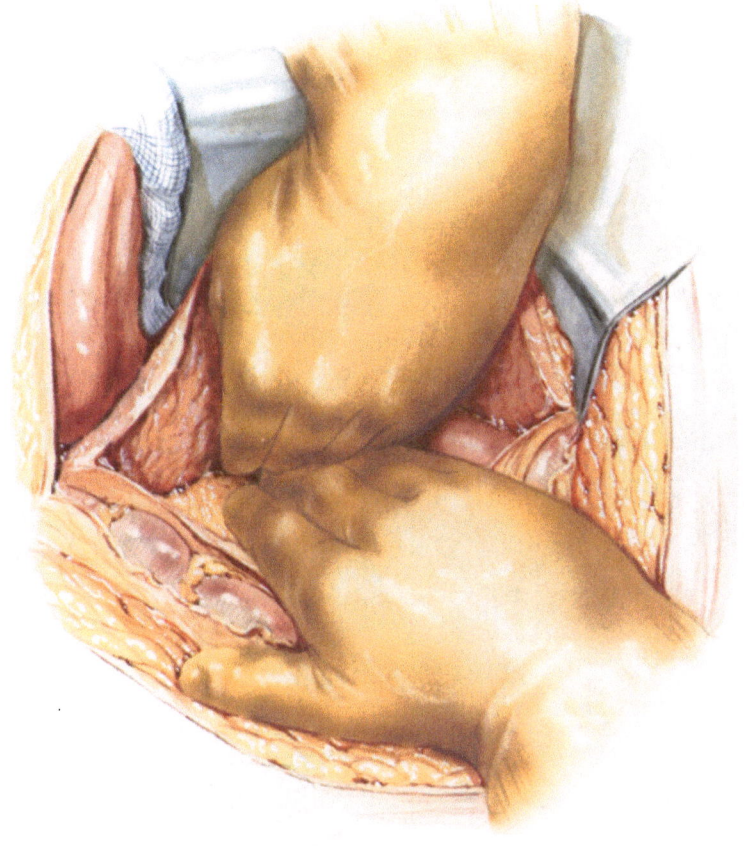

Fig. 4-34.

A

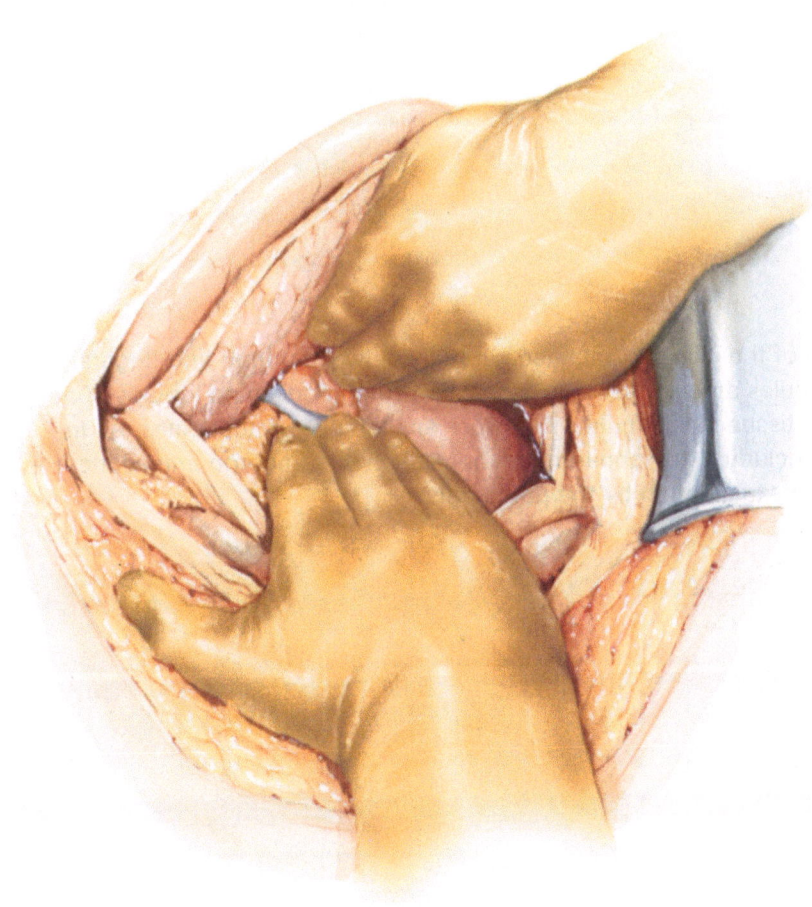

B

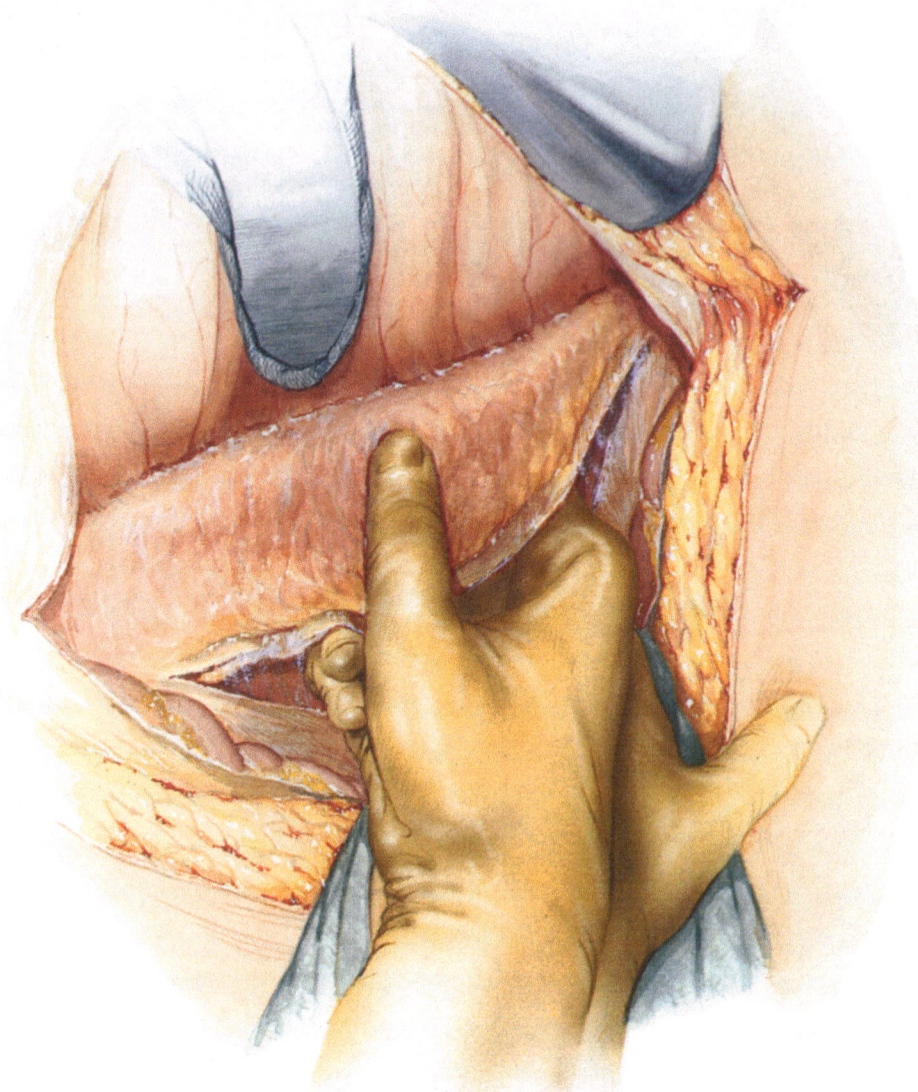

Fig. 4-35. The substance of the gland is palpated carefully between thumb and fingers. Suspicious nodules are exposed and biopsied. Lymph nodes and lobules of normal pancreatic tissue may simulate the gross appearance of adenomas. All tissue removed (including any apparent adenomas) should undergo immediate frozen section and examination by the pathologist.

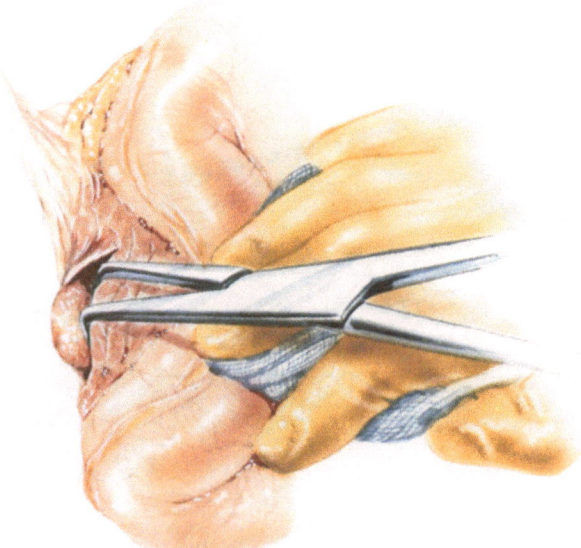

Enucleation of an islet cell adenoma from the posterior aspect of the head of the pancreas. An Adson right-angle clamp is a useful dissecting instrument in this situation. Bleeders are controlled by cautery or ligated with silk; nonabsorbable sutures should be used whenever there is risk of exposure to the digestive effects of pancreatic juice.   Fig. 4-36.

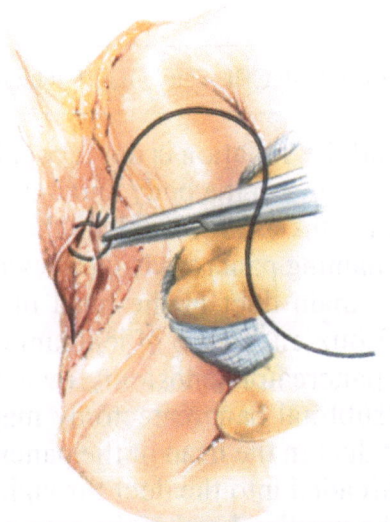

Closure. The pancreatic wound is closed with interrupted silk sutures.   Fig. 4-37.

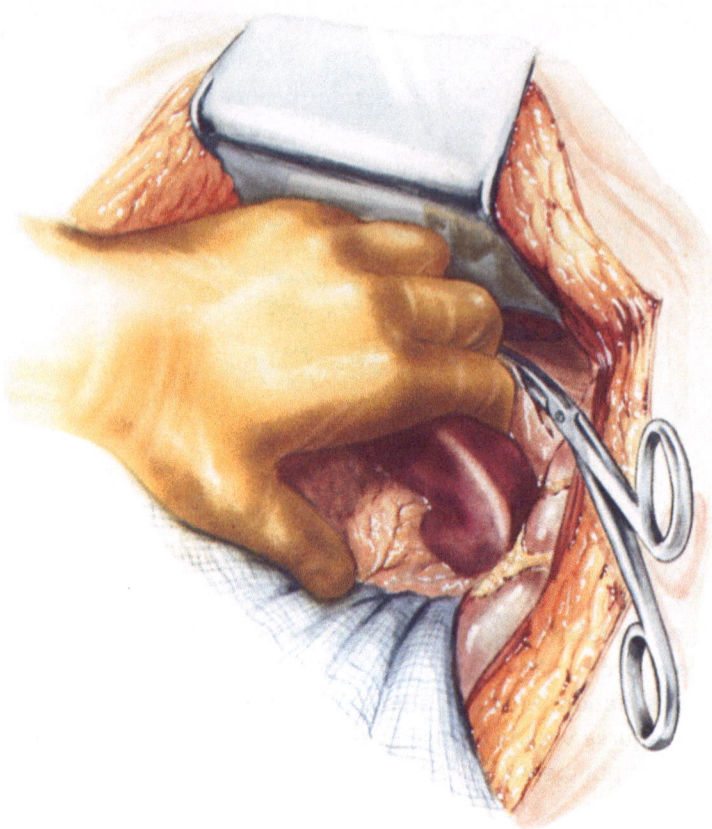

Fig. 4-38. **Distal pancreatic resection.** The lienorenal ligament is divided to mobilize the spleen and tail of the pancreas. The short gastric vessels are divided and ligated, freeing the spleen from the stomach.

REPAIR OF INADVERTANT PANCREATIC DUCT INJURY

If the duct is injured and the situation is not recognized, a fistula inevitably results. Injury to the duct in the body and tail of the pancreas is best managed by amputating the gland distal to the side of damage. The severed end of the remaining pancreas is oversewn (see Fig. 4-41B–C).

Transection of the main duct in the head of the pancreas is best treated by bringing a Roux-en-Y limb of jejunum up to the site of damage and fashioning a pancreatojejunostomy over the wound. If this is not feasible, total or subtotal pancreatectomy may be required. For a minor tear of the main duct in the head of the pancreas, a fine polyethylene catheter can be threaded into the duct through the duodenal papilla to serve as a splint. The proximal end of the catheter is brought through the pylorus into the stomach and out via a gastrostomy tube to the surface. After 10–14 days of gastric decompression and local suction

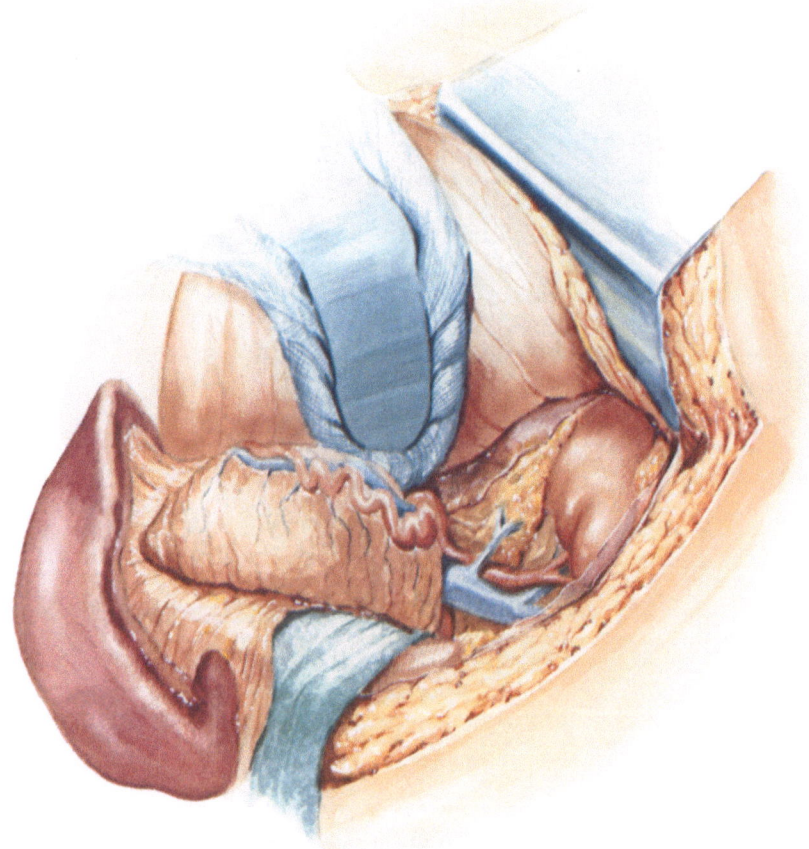

The peritoneum along the upper border of the pancreas is incised and the spleen, pancreas, and associated vessels are reflected from left to right. (The pancreas has already been mobilized from below; see Fig. 4-34.)

Fig. 4-39.

drainage of the operative site the duct injury should be healed. A catheter pancreatogram can be performed to determine whether the leak is indeed healed; the catheter and gastrostomy tube are removed subsequently.

DISTAL (75%) PANCREATIC RESECTION

Although most adenomas located in the body and tail of the pancreas can be enucleated without difficulty, multiple or large tumors are probably better treated by distal pancreatectomy. *Blind distal pancreatectomy,* which removes all of the pancreas to the left of the mesenteric vessels, seems indicated when a tumor is not palpable. Although it is possible to perform a distal pancreatectomy without sacrificing the spleen, the operation is greatly simplified by concomitant splenectomy (Figs. 4-38 to 4-41).

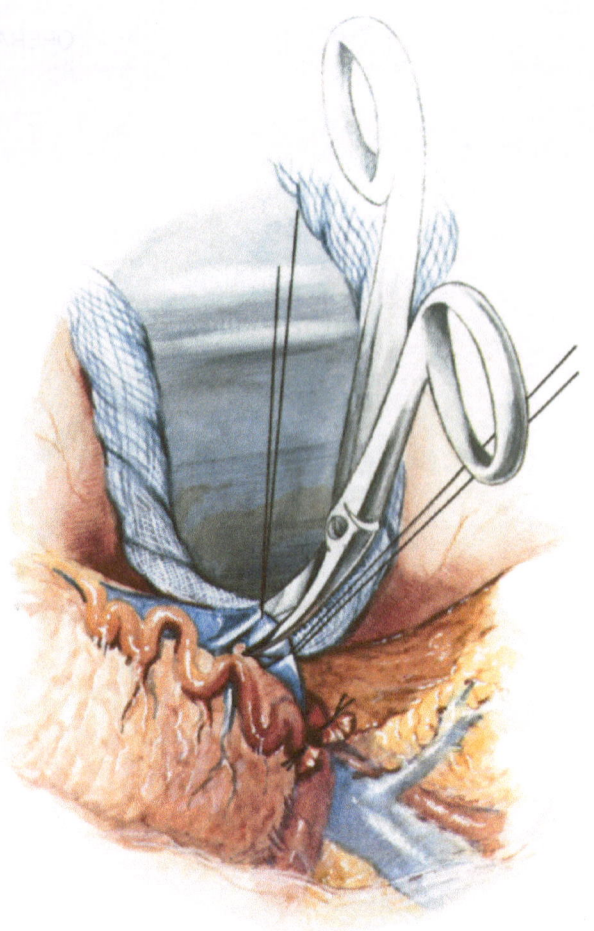

Fig. 4-40. The splenic artery and vein are ligated and divided individually.

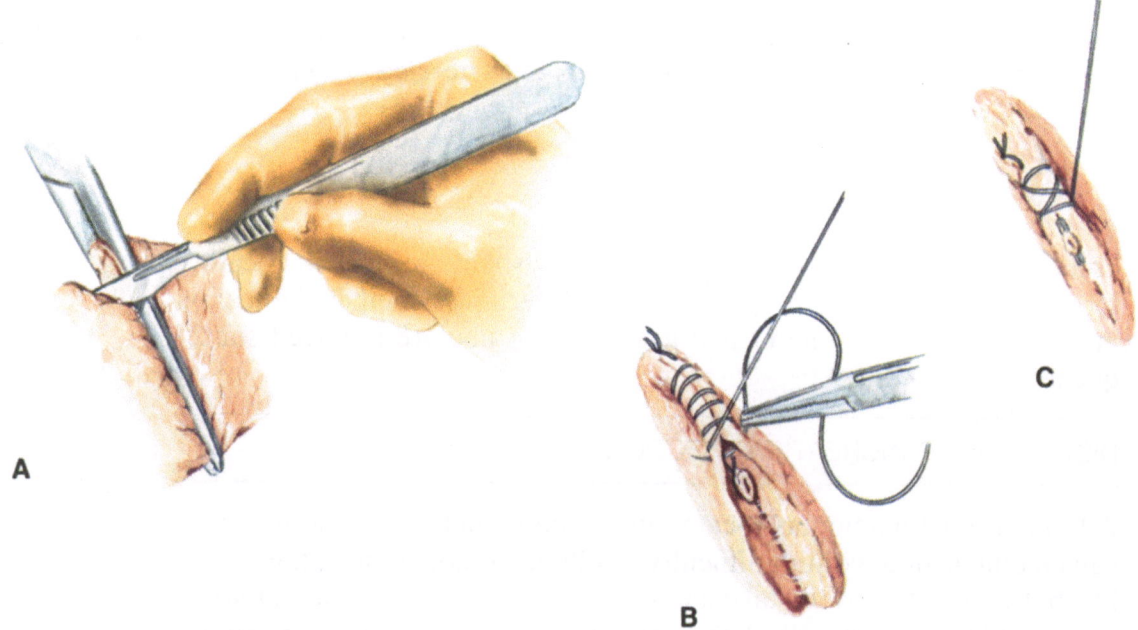

A

B

C

Fig. 4-41. The pancreas is transected **(A).** The main pancreatic duct is secured with a silk transfixion stitch or a metal clip. The cut end of the gland may be oversewn with a running silk suture **(B),** surgical staples, or individual figure-of-eight stitches **(C).**

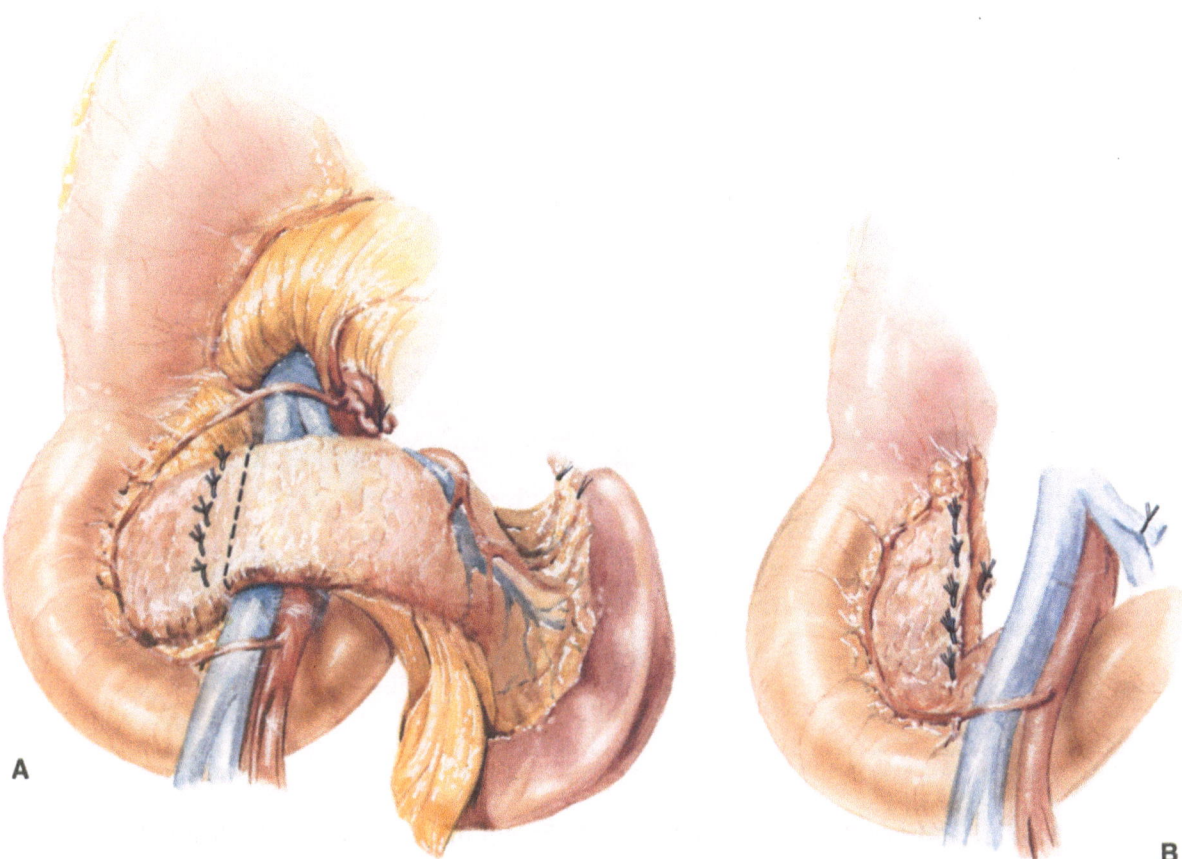

Subtotal pancreatectomy. **A.** The broken line indicates the level of transection. Deep interrupted hemostatic ligatures are placed as shown prior to division of the pancreas. Alternatively, the pancreas may be transected after a double row of surgical staples are appropriately placed. **B.** The main pancreatic duct is individually suture-ligated, and any residual bleeders or secondary ducts are transfixed with figure-of-eight stitches. If resection potentially endangers the common bile duct, a supraduodenal choledochotomy may be made and a probe or similar instrument may be used as a guide to its intrapancreatic course.

Fig. 4-42.

SUBTOTAL (80%–90%) PANCREATECTOMY

If, after *blind* distal (75%) pancreatic resection no tumor has been found and there has been no hyperglycemic rebound, subtotal pancreatectomy may be indicated (Fig. 4-42). This is also the preferred operation for pancreatic islet cell adenomatosis. Regardless of the blood glucose response after subtotal pancreatectomy, in the opinion of the authors, *blind* total pancreatectomy is not justified at the first operation.

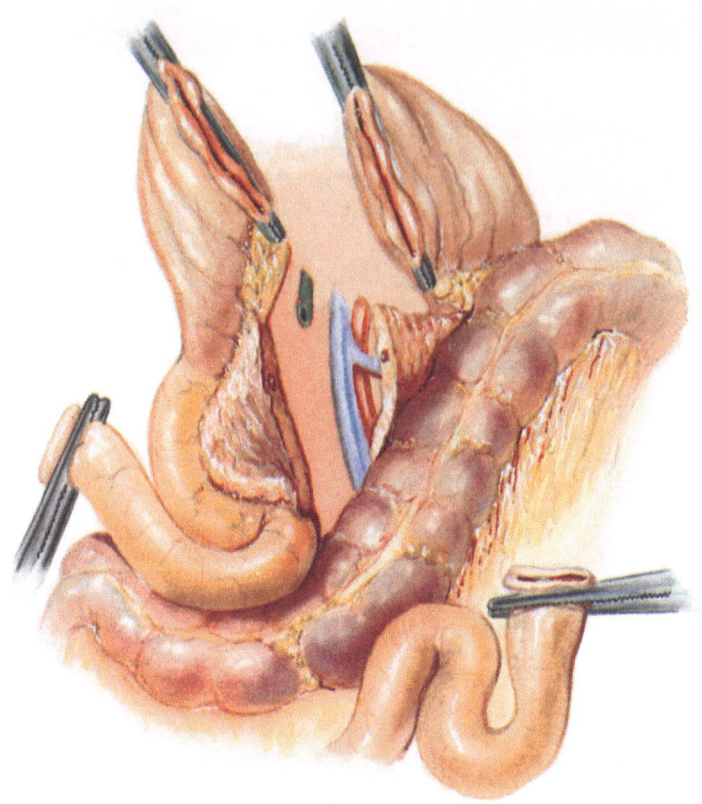

A

Fig. 4-43. **Pancreatoduodenectomy.** **A.** Extent of resection. The body and tail of the pancreas are conserved in the conventional Whipple procedure. A pylorus-preserving resection might also be considered if feasible. **B.** Completed reconstruction following pancreaticoduodenal resection. This utilizes end-to-end pancreaticojejunostomy, end-to-side choledochojejunostomy, and end-to-side gastrojejunostomy. (There are several alternative methods of reconstruction.) **C.** Completed reconstruction following total pancreatectomy. Some surgeons prefer to remove the entire pancreas, thus avoiding the potentially serious morbidity (fistula, abcess) and mortality associated with a leak at the pancreaticojejunal anastomosis. Diabetes and pancreatic insufficiency seriously detract from this procedure, although they can usually be satisfactorily controlled.

PANCREATODUODENECTOMY

This operation should be reserved for cases in which there are large invasive lesions in the head of the pancreas that are impossible to remove locally without serious injury to the common bile duct or duodenum (Fig. 4-43).

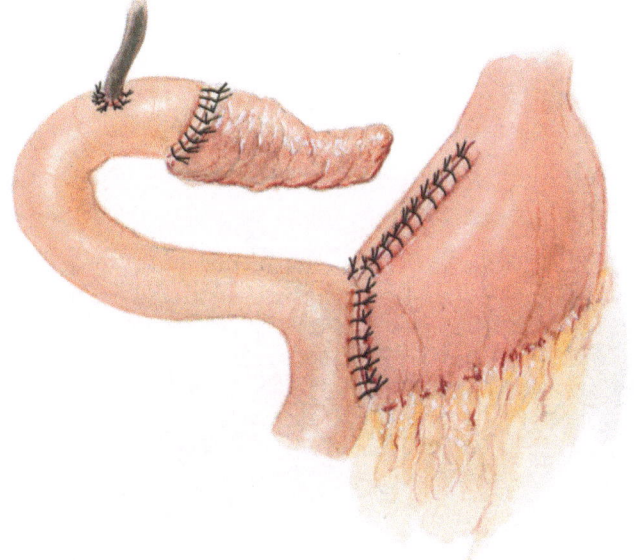

B

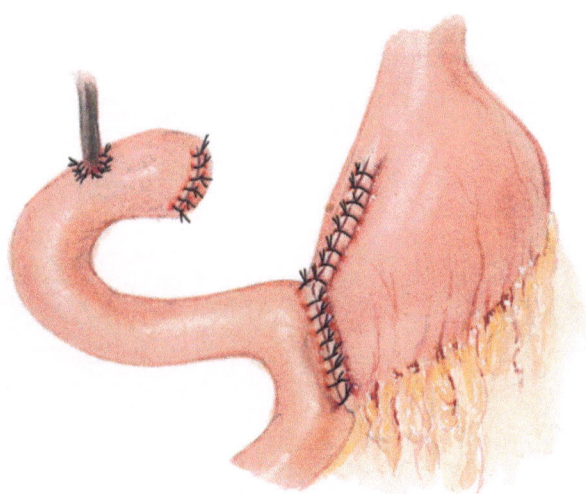

C

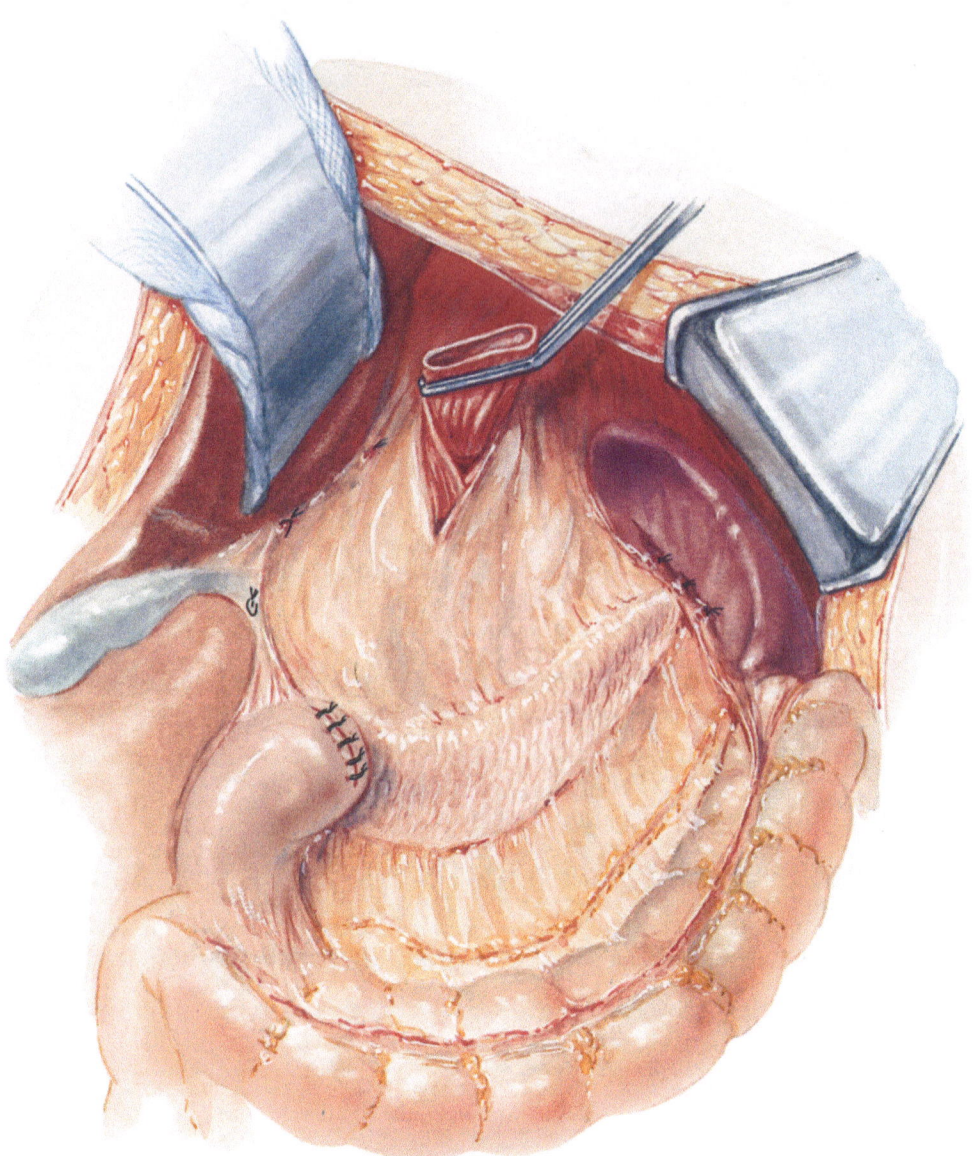

Fig. 4-44.   Mobilization and resection of the stomach. The stomach is completely mobilized by dividing the gastrocolic and gastrosplenic omenta, the right and left gastric arteries, the gastroepiploic and short gastric vessels. The duodenum is transected and closed in a conventional manner. Finally, the esophagus is transected just above the esophagogastric junction.

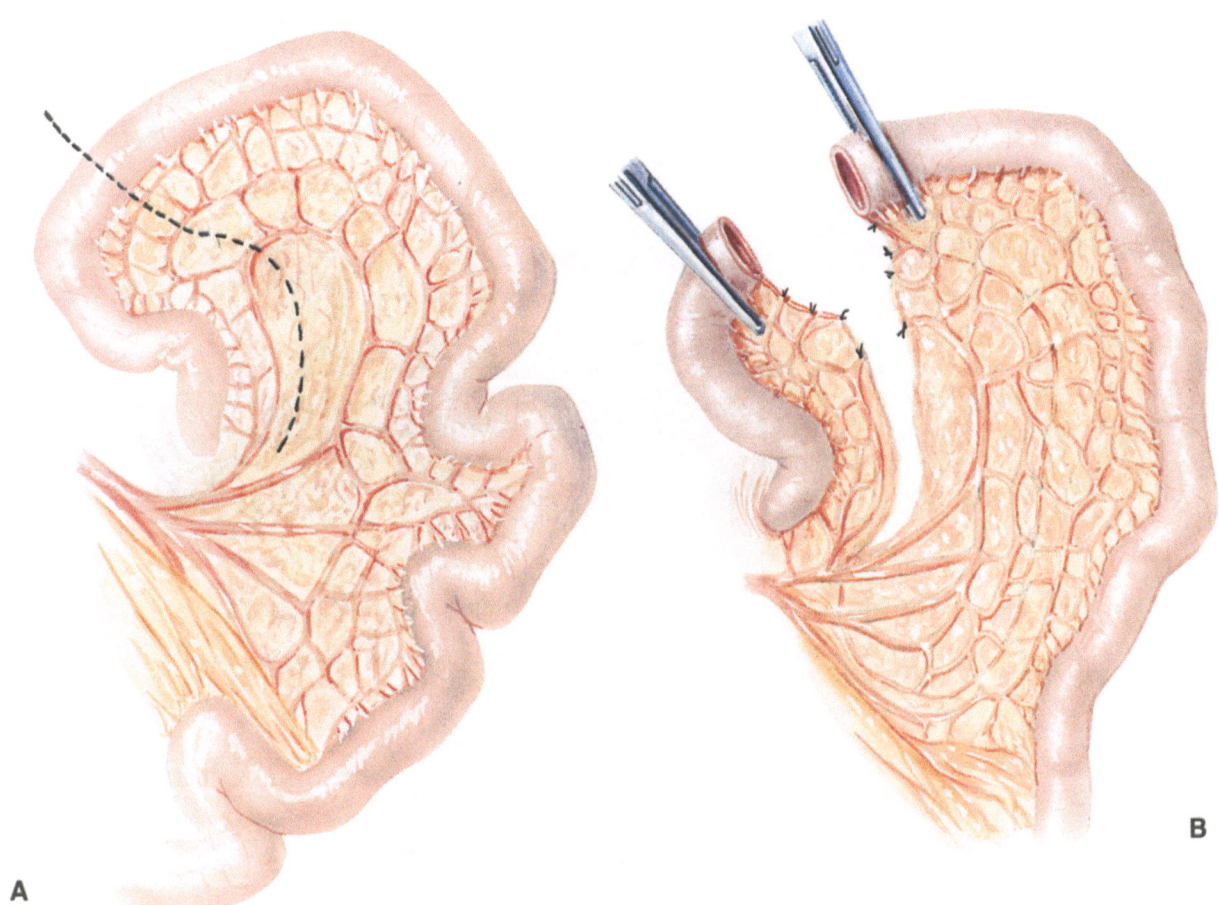

A

B

Construction of Roux-en-Y Loop.   A and B. The jejunum is transected a few inches beyond the ligament of Treitz. By incising to the base of the vascular pedicle (dotted line), adequate length is usually achieved. If necessary, progressive division of mesenteric vessels, assuring that a main arterial trunk is preserved, will allow a longer Roux limb.

Fig. 4-45.

TOTAL GASTRECTOMY FOR ZOLLINGER-ELLISON SYNDROME

A long midline or upper abdominal oblique incision is used and the abdomen is explored. The entire pancreas is exposed and examined for a gastrinoma (see Figs. 4-28 to 4-35). The greater peritoneal cavity, parapancreatic lymph node area, and liver are carefully inspected and palpated for evidence of metastasis. Enlarged lymph nodes and suspicious nodules should be biopsied and submitted for frozen section examination. (Not infrequently, tumor may be found in a lymph node in the absence of an obvious primary tumor.) To rule out the presence of a small submucosal duodenal wall tumor, duodenotomy may be necessary when a tumor is not identified in the pancreas.

Two alternative forms of reconstruction after total gastrectomy have been used with success (Figs. 4-44–4-49).

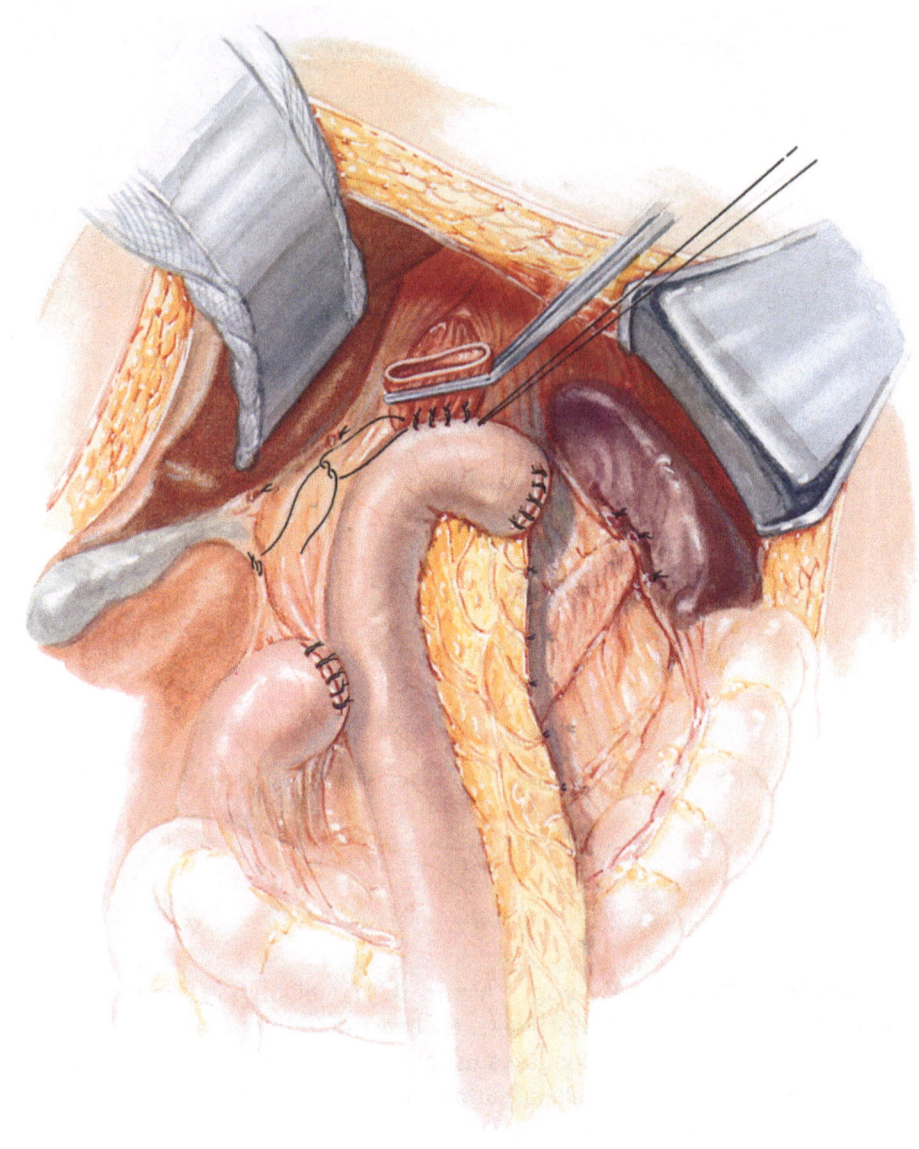

A

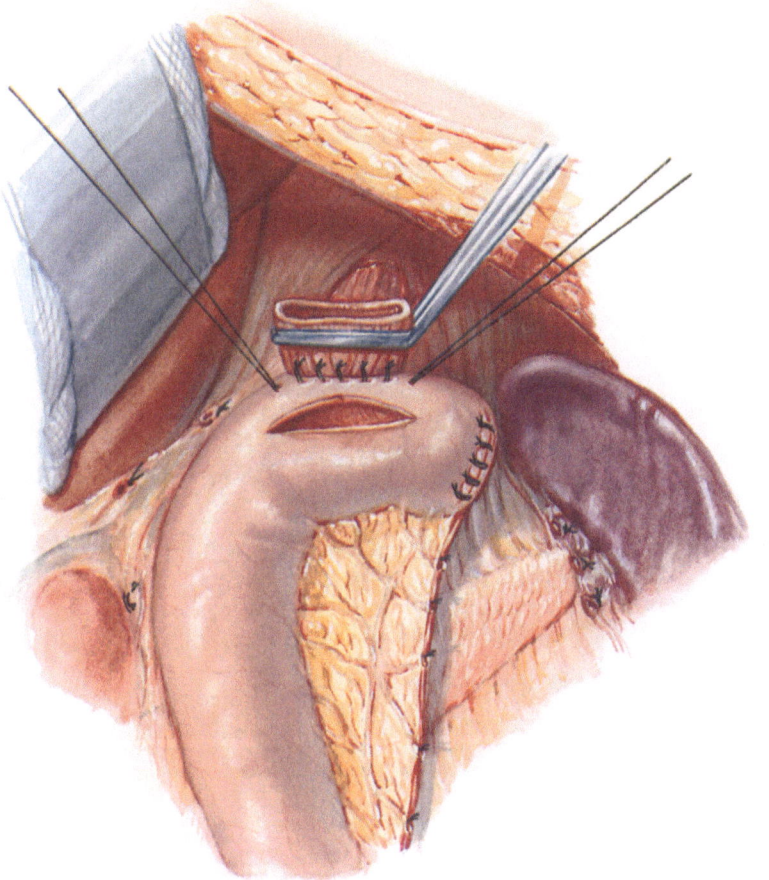

B

Esophagojejunostomy. **A** After first closing the proximal end of the jejunum, an end-to-side esophagojejunal anastomosis is constructed. The posterior
row of interrupted permanent sutures is placed somewhat obliquely in the
esophageal wall to prevent them from tearing through when tied. **B.** The posterior, outer layer is complete, and a short jejunotomy has been made which will
tend to stretch and elongate. (Continued)

Fig. 4-46.

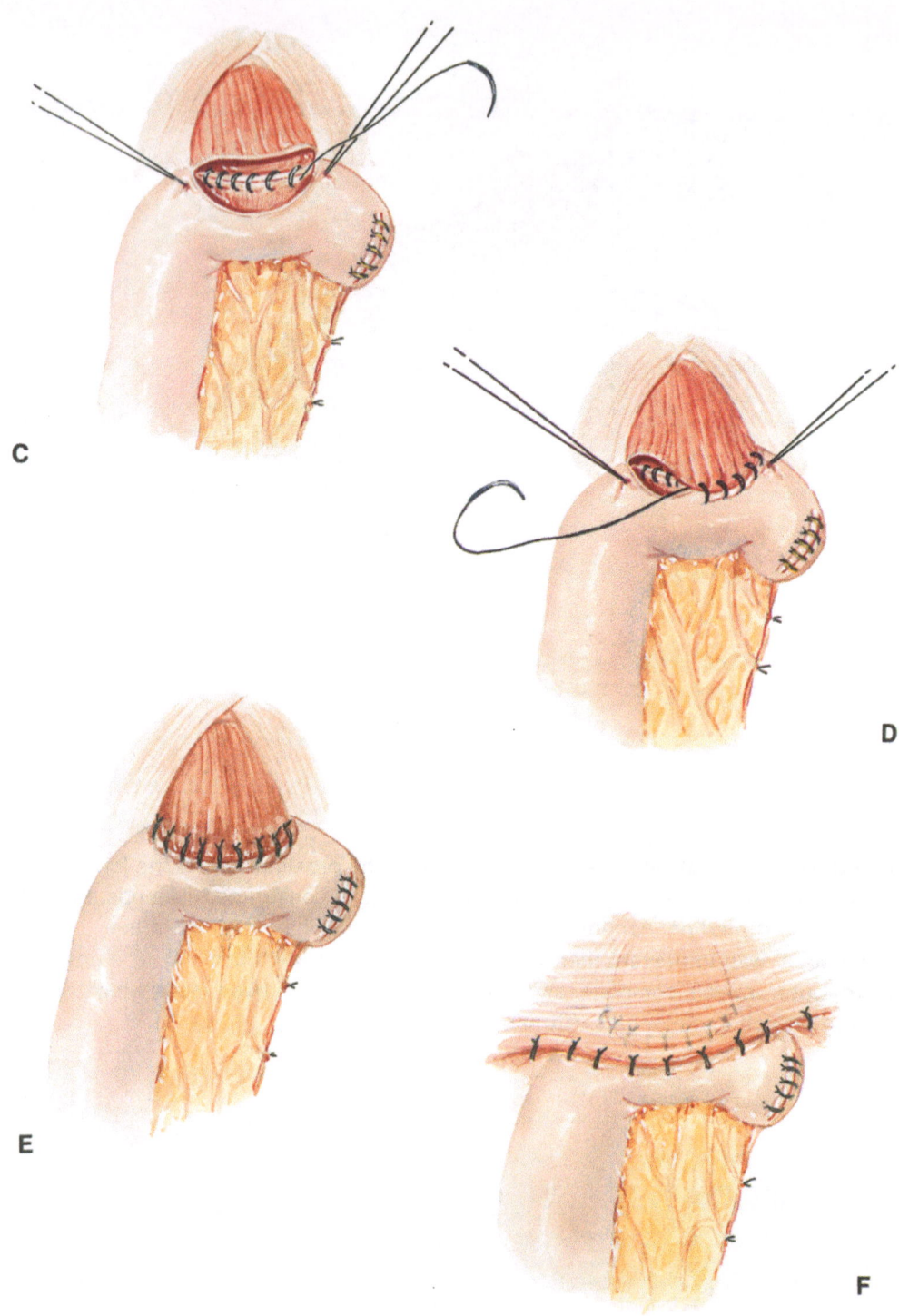

Fig. 4-46.   Esophagojejunostomy.   C and D The esophageal cuff is excised under the clamp, and the inner layers are approximated using absorbable suture.   **E and F** The anterior row of interrupted sutures is placed, and the jejunum is anchored to the diaphragm with a final row of interrupted stitches. This further supports the anastomosis and helps prevent tension on the suture line.

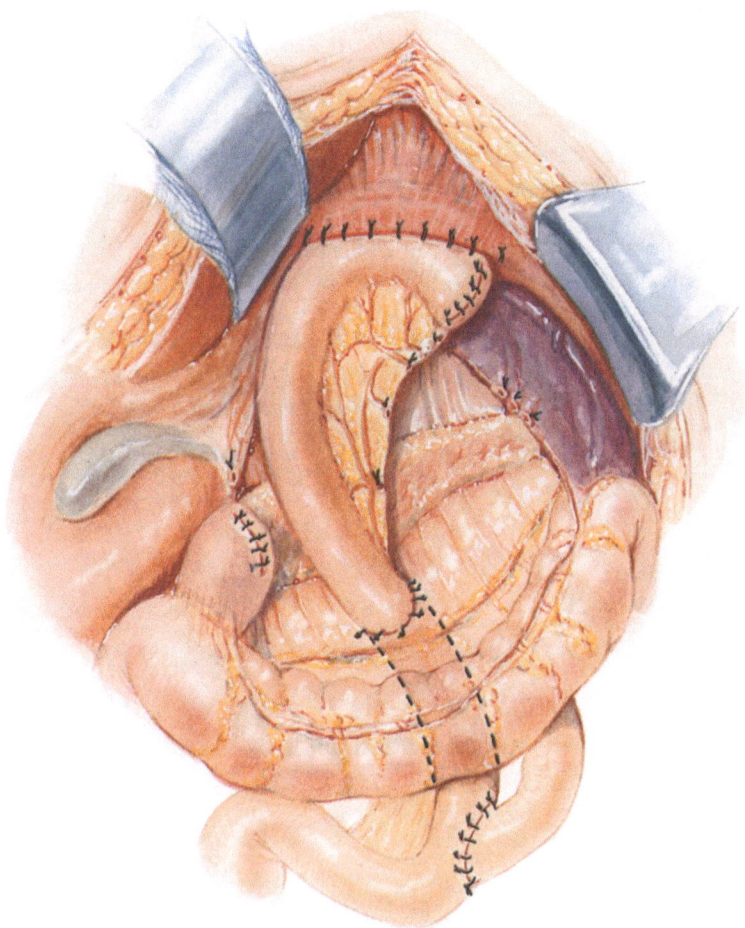

Roux-en-Y Jejunojejunostomy. The retrocolic Roux-en-Y reconstruction is completed by first closing the defect in the mesocolon around the Roux limb, then performing an end-to-side jejunojejunostomy. This anastomosis should be at least 45 cm distal to the esophagojejunostomy to prevent bile reflux esophagitis.

Fig. 4-47.

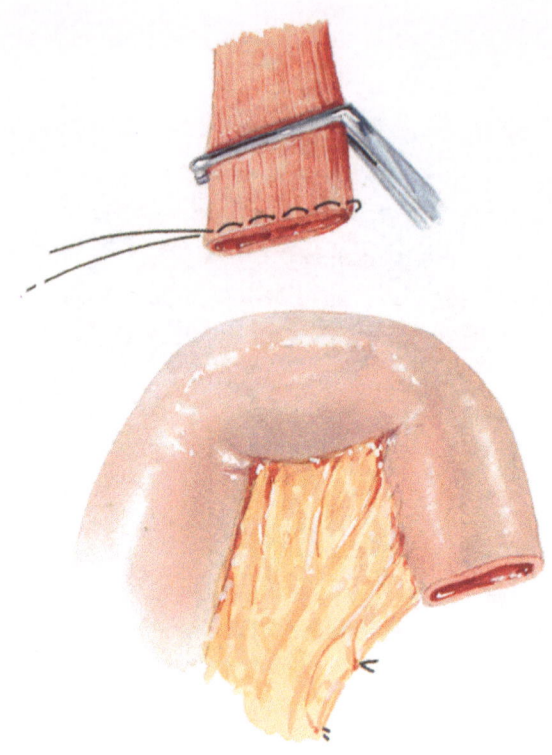

A

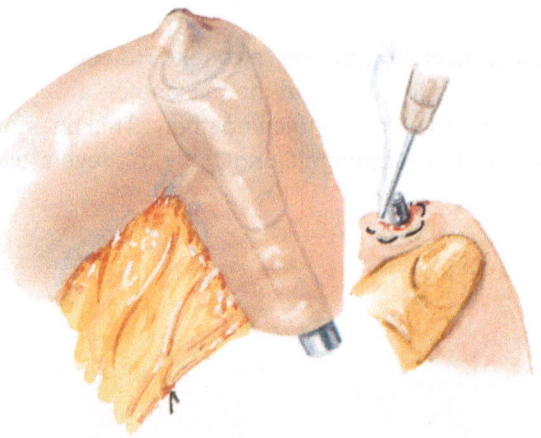

B

Fig. 4-48. **Stapled Roux-en-Y Reconstruction.** **A** The *open-ended* Roux limb is passed retrocolic to lie adjacent to the esophagus. A pursestring suture is placed in the cut end of esophagus, distal to the atraumatic bowel clamp. **B** An appropriately sized EEA intraluminal stapler has been chosen, the anvil of the cartridge removed, and the instrument passed into the cut end of the Roux limb of jejunum. The central post is moved forward enough to evaginate the antimesenteric jejunal wall. A cautery is used to create a small hole through which the central post is further advanced. A pursestring suture may be placed in the jejunum around the post, although this is usually not necessary.

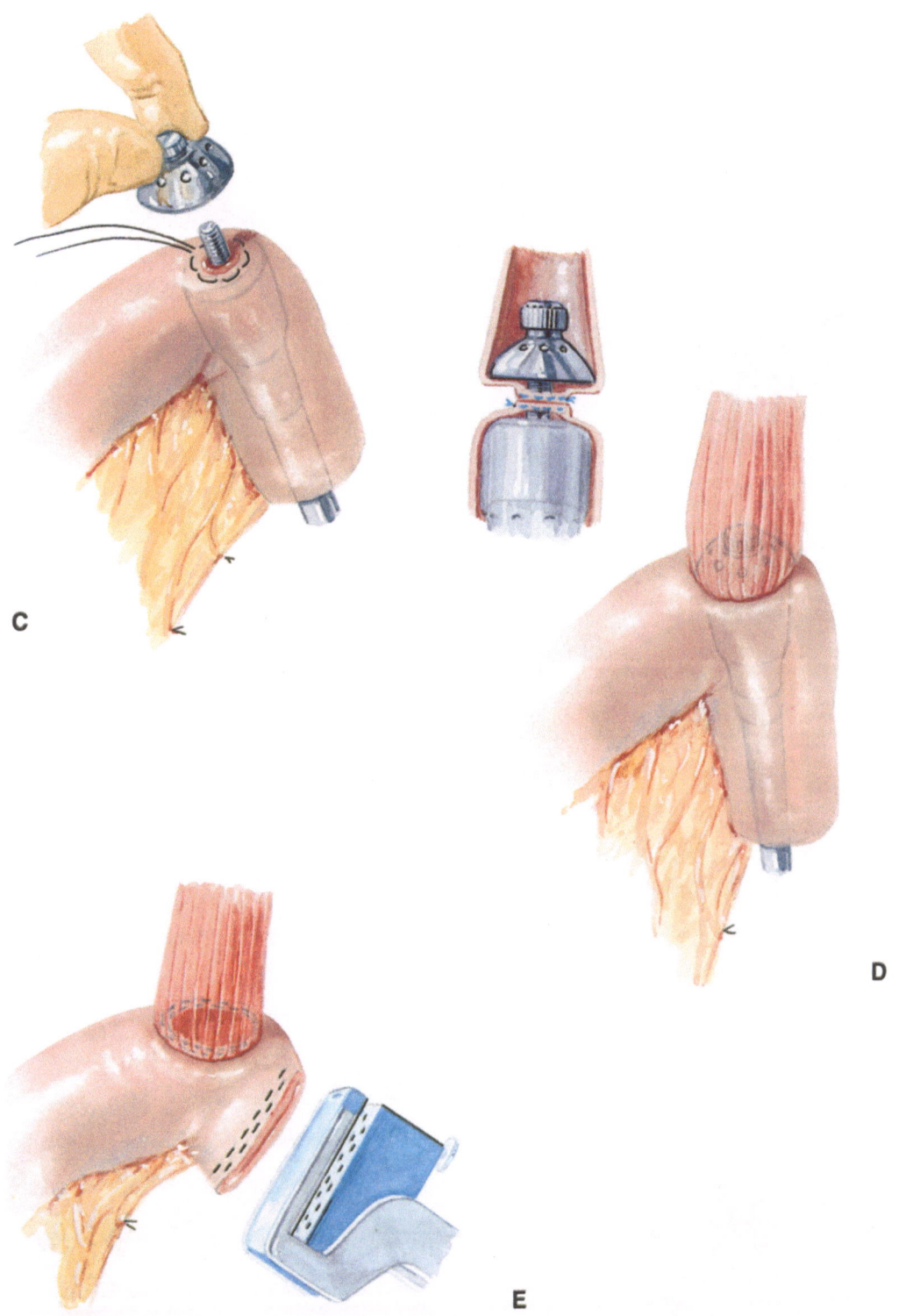

C and D The anvil is replaced on the central post, then passed into the esophagus. The pursestring suture(s) is tied and ends cut, the anvil and cartridge are closed to the proper point, and the instrument is fired. **E** Following completion of the stapled esophagojejunal anastomosis, the open end of jejunum is closed and excess excised using a TA-55 stapler.

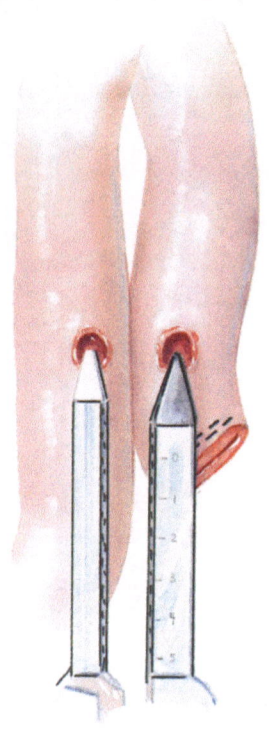

A

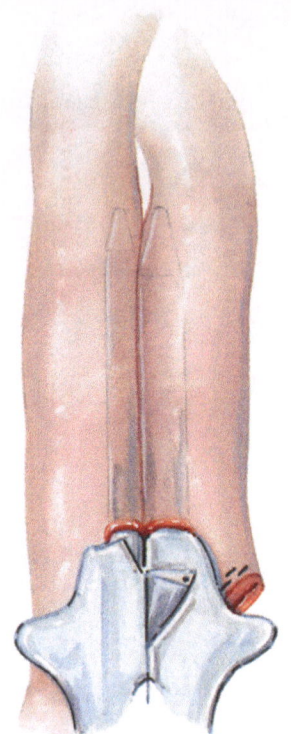

B

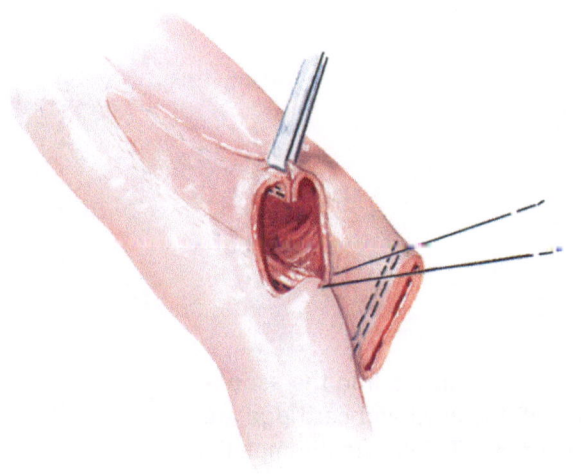

C

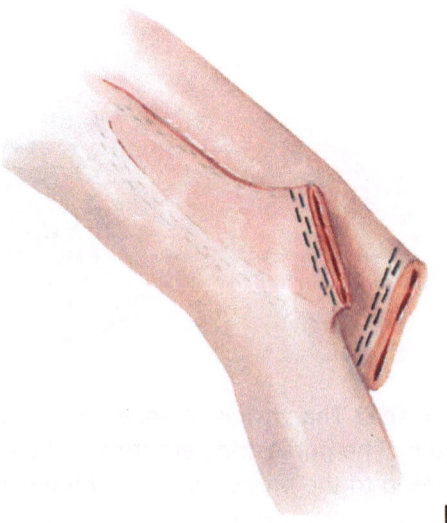

D

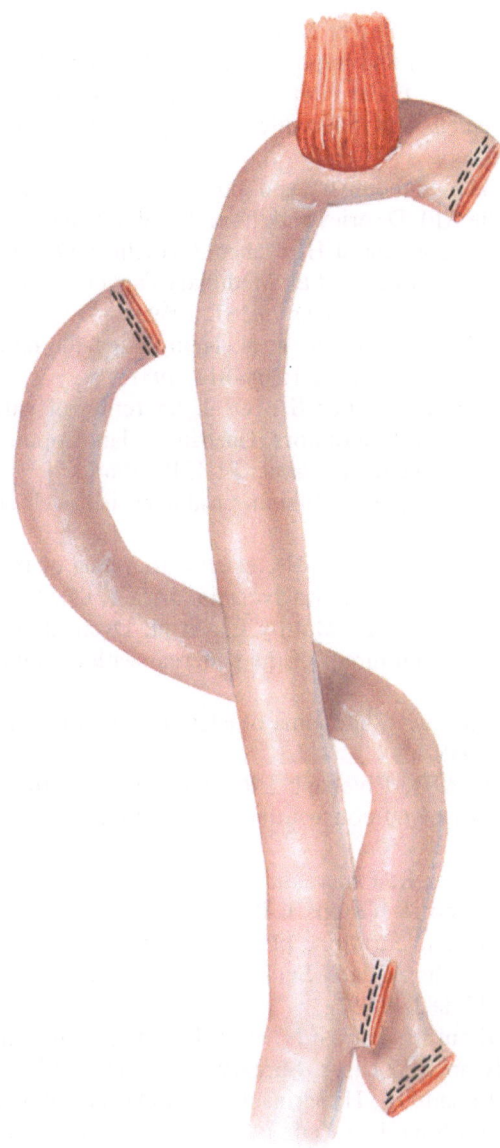

E

Stapled Roux-en-Y Jejunojejunostomy.   A and B At least 45 cm distal to   **Fig. 4-49.**
the esophagojejunostomy, a functional end-to-side jejunojejunostomy is performed. Small enterotomies are made to admit the two arms of a GI-A stapler.
The instrument is approximated and fired.   **C and D** The anastomosis is completed by *distracting* the two staple lines, then closing the now common entero-
tomy site with a TA-55 stapler. The final anastomosis has a triangular configura-
tion. **E** The final form of the stapled Roux-en-Y reconstruction includes the
stapled closure of the duodenum.

References

1. Wilder RM, Allan FH, Power MH, et al: Carcinoma of the islands of the pancreas. Hyperinsulinism and hypoglycemia. JAMA 89:348–355, 1927.
2. Bishop AE, Polak JM, Facer P, et al: Neuron specific enolase: a common marker for the endocrine cells and innervation of the gut and pancreas. Gastroenterology 83:902–915, 1982.
3. Pearse AGE: The cytochemistry and ultrastructure of polypeptide hormone-producing cells of the APUD series and the embryologic, physiologic, and pathologic implications of the concept. J Histochem Cytochem 17:303–313, 1969.
4. Szijji I, Csapo Z, Laszlo FA, et al: Medullary cancer of the thyroid gland associated with hypercorticism. Cancer 24:167, 1969.
5. Tapia FJ, Polak JM, Bloom SR, et al: Neuron-specific enolase is produced by neuroendocrine tumors. Lancet 1:808–811, 1981.
6. O'Neal LW, Pipnis DM, Luce SA, et al: Secretion of various endocrine substances by ACTH-secreting tumors. Gastrin, melanotropin, serotonin, parathormone, vasopressin, glucagon. Cancer 21:1219, 1968.
7. Miller L, Grant CS: Cholecystokinin-producing islet-cell adenoma of the pancreas. In press.
8. Wilder RM, Allan FN, Power MH, et al: Carcinoma of the islands of the pancreas, hyperinsulinism, and hypoglycemia. JAMA, 89:348–355, 1927.
9. Howland G, Campbell WR, Mattby EJ, et al: Dysinsulinism: convulsions and coma due to an islet cell tumor of the pancreas with operation and cure. JAMA, 93:674–679, 1929.
10. Whipple AO, Franz VK: Adenoma of islet cells with hyperinsulinism. Am Surg 101:1299–1335, 1935.
11. Service FJ, Dale AJD, Elveback LR, and Jiang NS: Insulinoma: clinical and diagnostic features of 60 consecutive cases. Mayo Clinic Proceedings 51:417–429, 1976.
12. Vinik AI, and Glaser B: Pancreatic endocrine tumors. In Dent TL, Eckhauser FE, Vinik AI, Turcotte JG (eds.): Pancreatic Disease: Diagnosis and Therapy. New York, Grune and Stratton, 1981, Chapter 25.
13. van Heerden JA, Edis AJ, and Service FJ: The surgical aspects of insulinomas. Ann Surg 189:677–682, 1979.
14. Stefanini P, Carboni M, Patrasi N, et al: Beta islet cell tumors of the pancreas: result of a study on 1067 cases. Surgery 75:597–609, 1974.
15. Moss NH, and Rhoads JE: Hyperinsulinism and islet cell tumors of the pancreas. In Howard JM, Jordon GL Jr, (eds.): Surgical Diseases of the Pancreas. Philadelphia, Lippincott, 1960, Chapter 21.
16. Harrison TS, Child CG, Fry WJ, et al: Current surgical management of functioning islet cell tumors of the pancreas. Ann Surg, 178:485–495, 1973.
17. Wermer P: Genetic aspects of adenomatosis of endocrine glands. Am J Med, 16:363–371, 1954.
18. Shermeta DW, Mendelsohn G, and Haller JA: Hyperinsulinemic hyperglycemia of the neonate associated with persistent fetal histology and function of the pancreas. Ann Surg, 191:182–186, 1980.
19. Harness JK, Geelhoed GW, Thompson NW, Nishigama RH, et al: Nesidioblastosis in adults: a surgical dilemma. Arch Surg, 116:575–580, 1981.
20. Greider MH, Elliot DW, and Zollinger RM: An electron microscopic study of islet cell adenomas. JAMA, 186:120, 1963.
21. Taylor CR: Immunoperoxidase techniques: theoretical and practical aspects. Arch Pathol Lab Med 102:113–121, 1978.
22. Martin ED, Potet F: Pathology of endocrine tumours of the GI tract. Clin Gastroenterol 3:511, 1974.
23. Laroche GP, Ferris DO, Priestley JT, et al: Hyperinsulinism. Arch Surg 96:765–772, 1968.

24. Marks V, Samols E: Insulinoma: natural history and diagnosis. Clin Gastroenterol 3:559, 1974.
25. Porter MR, Frantz VK: Tumors associated with hypoglycemia: pancreatic and extrapancreatic. Am J Med 944:21, 1956.
26. Fonkalsrud EW, Dilley RB, Longmire WP, et al: Insulin secreting tumors of the pancreas. Ann Surg 159:730, 1964.
27. Liepman MK: The chemotherapy of islet cell carcinoma. In Dent TL, Eckhauser FE, Vinik AI, Turcotte JG, (eds.): Pancreatic Disease: Diagnosis and Therapy. New York, Grune and Stratton, 1981, Chapter 28.
28. Koutras P, White RR: Insulin-secreting tumors of the pancreas. Surg Clin NA 52:299, 1972.
29. Stefanini P, Carboni M, Patrassi N: Surgical treatment and prognosis of insulinoma. Clin Gastroenterol 3:697, 1974.
30. Fajans SS, Floyd JC: Diagnosis and medical management of insulinomas. Ann Rev Med 30:313–329, 1979.
31. Sherman BN, Pek S, Fajans SS, Floyd JC Jr, Conn JW: Plasma proinsulin in patients with functioning pancreatic islet cell tumors. J Clin Endocrinol Metab 35:271–280, 1972.
32. Alsever RN, Roberts JP, Gerber JG, Mako MF, Rubenstein AH: Insulinoma with low circulatory insulin levels: the diagnostic value of proinsulin measurements. Ann Intern Med 82:347–350, 1975.
33. Rynearson EH: Hyperinsulinism among malingerers. Med Clin NA 31:477, 1947.
34. Couropmitree C, Freinkel N, Nagel TC, et al: Plasma C-peptide and diagnosis of factitious hyperinsulinism. Ann Intern Med 88:201, 1975.
35. Turner RC, Johnson PC: Suppression of insulin release by fish-insulin-induced hypoglycemia with reference to the diagnosis of insulinomas. Lancet 1:1483–1485, 1973.
36. Fajans SS, Conn JW: An intravenous tolbutamide test as an adjunct in the diagnosis of functioning pancreatic islet cell adenomas. J Lab Clin Med 54:811, 1959.
37. Kaplan EL, Rubenstein AH, Evans R, Lee CH, Klementschitsch P: Calcium infusion: a new provocative test for insulinomas. Ann Surg 190:501–507, 1979.
38. Kaplan EL, Lee CH: Recent advances in the diagnosis and treatment of insulinomas. Surg Clin NA 59:119–129, 1979.
39. Kahn CR, Rosen SW, Weintraub BD, Fajans SS, Gorden P: Ectopic production of chorionic gonadotropin and its subunits by islet-cell tumors. NEJM, 297:565–569, 1977.
40. Baruh S, Sherman K, Kolodny HD, et al: Fasting hypoglycemia. Med Clin NA 57:1441, 1973.
41. Fajans SS, Floyd JC Jr: Hypoglycemia: how to manage a complex case. Mod Med 41:24–31, 1973.
42. Chandalia HB, Boshell BR: Hypoglycemia associated with extrapancreatic tumors. Arch Intern Med, 129:447, 1972.
43. Daggett PR, Kurtz, Morris DV, et al: Is pre-operative localization of insulinomas necessary? Lancet February, 1981, pp 483–486.
44. Charboneau WJ, Grant CS, et al: Intraoperative ultrasonic evaluation of pancreatic insulinoma—initial experience. J Ultrasound in Med June, 1983.
45. Sigel B, Coelho JCU, Nyhus LM, et al: Detection of pancreatic tumors by ultrasound during surgery. Arch Surg 117:1058–1061, 1982.
46. Fulton RE, Sheedy PF II, McIlrath DC, et al: Preoperative localization of insulin-producing tumors of the pancreas. Am J Roentgenol 123:367–377, 1975.
47. Ingemansson S, Lunderquist A, Lundquist I, et al: Portal and pancreatic vein catheterization with radioimmunologic determination of insulin. SG&O 141:705–711, 1975.
48. Ingemansson S, Kuhl C, Larsson LI, et al: Localization of insulinomas and islet-

cell hyperplasia by pancreatic vein catheterization and insulin assay. SG&O 146:725–734, 1978.

49. Turner RC, Morris PJ, lee EC, Harris EA: Localization of insulinomas. Lancet 1:515–518, 1978.

50. Warren KW: Current management of benign and malignant pancreatic tumors. Am Surg 20:1070, 1954.

51. Thompson NW: The surgical treatment of islet cell tumors of the pancreas. In Dent TL, Eckhauser FE, Vinik AI, Turcotte JE, (eds.): Pancreatic Diseases: Diagnosis and Therapy. New York, Grune and Stratton, 1981, Chapter 26.

52. DePeyster FA: Planning the appropriate operations for islet cell tumors of the pancreas. Surg Clin NA 50:133, 1970.

53. Harrison TS, Child CG, Fry WJ, et al: Current surgical management of functioning islet cell tumors of the pancreas. Ann Surg 178:485, 1973.

54. Tutt GO, Edis AJ, Service FJ, et al: Plasma glucose monitoring during operation for insulinoma: a critical reappraisal. Surgery 88:351–356, 1980.

55. Koutras P, White RR: Insulin-secreting tumors of the pancreas. Surg Clin NA 52:299, 1972.

56. Laroche GP, Ferris DO, Priestley JT, et al: Hyperinsulinism. Arch Surg 96:763, 1968.

57. Galbut DL, Markowitz AM: Insulinoma: diagnosis, surgical management, and long-term follow-up: review of 41 cases. Am J Surg 139:682–690, 1980.

58. Fajans SS, Floyd JC Jr, Thiffault CA, et al: Further studies on diazoxide suppression of insulin release from abnormal and normal islet tissue in man. Ann NY Acad Sci 150:261–280, 1968.

59. Schein PS, Kahn R, Jordan P, et al: Streptozotocin for malignant insulinoma and carcinoid tumor. Arch Inter Med 132:555–561, 1973.

60. Moertel CG, Hanley JA, Johnson LA: Streptozotocin alone compared with streptozotocin plus fluorouracil in the treatment of advanced islet cell carcinoma. NEJM 303:1189–1194, 1980.

61. Broder LE, Carter SK: Pancreatic islet cell carcinoma II results of therapy with streptozotocin in 52 patients. Ann Intern Med 79:108–118, 1973.

62. Grampa B, Gargartini L, Grisolato PG, et al: Hypoglycaemia in infancy caused by beta cell nesidioblastosis. Am J Dis Child 128:226, 1974.

63. Telander RL: Discussion of Harness JK, Geelhoed GW, Thompson NW, et al: Nesidioblastosis in adults: a surgical dilemma. Arch Surg 116:575–580, 1981.

64. Zollinger RM, Ellison EH: Primary peptic ulcerations of the jejunum associated with islet cell tumors of the pancreas. Ann Surg 142:709–723, 1955.

65. McGuigan JE, Trudeau WL: Immuno-chemical measurement of elevated levels of gastrin in the serum of patients with pancreatic tumors of the Zollinger-Ellison variety. N Engl J Med 278:1308–1313, 1968.

66. Isenberg JI, Walsh JH, Grossman MI: The Zollinger-Ellison syndrome. Gastroenterology, 65:140–165, 1973.

67. Welbourn RB, Pearse AGE, Polak JM, et al: The APUD cells of the alimentary tract in health and disease. Med Clin North Am 58:1359, 1974.

68. Fox PS, Hofmann JW, Wilson SD, et al: Surgical management of the Zollinger-Ellison syndrome. Surg Clin North Am 54:395–407, 1974.

69. Zollinger RM, Martin EW Jr, Carey LC, et al: Observations on the postoperative tumor growth behavior of certain islet cell tumors. Ann Surg 185:525–530, 1976.

70. Creutzfeldt W, Arnold R, Creutzfeldt C, et al: Pathomorphologic, biochemical, and diagnostic aspects of gastrinomas (Zollinger-Ellison syndrome). Hum Pathol 6:47–76, 1975.

71. Martin ED, Potet F: Pathology of endocrine tumors of the gastrointestinal tract. Clin Gastroenterol 3:511, 1974.

72. Ellison EH, Wilson D: The Zollinger-Ellison syndrome. Ann Surg 110:512–530, 1964.

73. Zollinger RM: Islet cell tumors of the pancreas and alimentary tract. Am J Surg 129:102–110, 1975.
74. Bonfils S, Bades JP: The diagnosis of Z-E syndrome with special reference to the multiple endocrine adenomas. *In* Glass JGB (ed.): Progress in Gastroenterology. New York, Grune & Stratton, 1970, pp 332–355.
75. Walsh JH, Grossman MI: Gastrin. N Engl J Med 292:1324–1334, 1377–1384, 1975.
76. McCarthy DM: The place of surgery in the Zollinger-Ellison syndrome. N Engl J Med 302:1344–1347, 1980.
77. Isenberg JI, Csendes A, Walsh JH: Resting and pentagastrin-stimulated gastro-esophageal sphincter pressure in patients with Zollinger-Ellison syndrome. Gastroenterology, 61:655–658, 1971.
78. Regan PT, Malagelada JR: A reappraisal of clinical roentgenographic and endoscopic features of the Zollinger-Ellison syndrome. Mayo Clin Proc 53:19–23, 1978.
79. Modlin IM, Jaffe BM, Sank A, et al: The early diagnosis of gastrinoma. Ann Surg 196:512–517, 1982.
80. Deleu J, Tytgat H, Van Hodsenhoven GVE: Diarrhea associated with islet-cell tumors. Am J Dig Dis 9:97–108, 1964.
81. McCarthy DM: Report on the United States experience with cimetidine in the Zollinger-Ellison syndrome and other hypersecretory states. Gastroenterology, 74:453–458, 1978.
82. Go VLW, Poley JR, Hoffman AF, et al: Disturbances in fat digestion induced by acid jejunal pH due to gastric hypersecretion in man. Gastroenterology 55:705, 1968.
83. Wright HK, Hersh T, Flock MH, et al: Impaired intestinal absorption in the Zollinger-Ellison syndrome independent of gastric hypersecretion. Am J Surg 119:250–253, 1970.
84. Sircus W: Peptide-secreting tumors and peptic ulcer. Clin Gastroenterol 2:447, 1973.
85. Ballard HS, Frame B, Havstock RJ: Familial multiple endocrine adenoma–peptic ulcer complex. Medicine (Baltimore) 43:481–516, 1964.
86. Dent RI, James JH, Wang CA, et al: Hyperparathyroidism: gastric acid secretion and gastrin. Ann Surg 176:360, 1972.
87. McGuigan JE, Colwell JA, Franklin J: Effect of parathyroidectomy on hypercalcemic hypersecretory peptic ulcer disease. Gastroenterology, 66:269, 1974.
88. Turbey WJ, Passaro EW Jr: Hyperparathyroidism in the Zollinger-Ellison syndrome. Arch Surg 105:62, 1972.
89. Amberg JR, Ellison EH, Wilson SD, et al: Roentgenographic observations in the Zollinger-Ellison syndrome. JAMA 190:185, 1964.
90. Aoyagi T, Summerskill WHJ: Gastric secretion with ulcerogenic islet cell tumor: importance of basal acid output. Arch. Intern. Med 117:667–672, 1966.
91. Lewin MR, Stagg BH, Clark CG: Gastric acid secretion and diagnosis of Zollinger-Ellison syndrome. Br Med J 2:139–141, 1973.
92. Malagelada JR, Davis CS, O'Fallon WM, et al: Laboratory diagnosis of gastrinoma: a prospective evaluation of gastric analysis and fasting serum gastrin levels. Mayo Clin Proc 57:211–218, 1982.
93. Fabri PM, Johnson JA, Gower WR: What's new with G-17? Surgery 92:884–886, 1982.
94. Fabri PM, Johnson JA, Sparks J: Molecular species of gastrin in Zollinger-Ellison syndrome. A ten-year experience. Surg Forum 32:134, 1981.
95. Cowley DJ, Dymock IW, Wilson RY, et al: Zollinger-Ellison syndrome type-I: clinical and pathological correlations in a case. Gut 14:25–29, 1973.
96. Polak JM, Stagg B, Pearse AGE: Two types of Zollinger-Ellison syndrome; immunofluorescent, cytochemical and ultrastructural studies of the antral and pan-

creatic gastrin cells in different clinical states. Gut 13:501–512, 1972.

97. McGuigan JE, Wolfe MM: Secretin injection test in the diagnosis of gastrinoma. Gastroenterology 79:1324–1331, 1980.

98. Deveney CW, Deveney KS, Jaffe BM, et al: Use of calcium and secretin in the diagnosis of gastrinoma (Zollinger-Ellison syndrome). Ann Intern Med 87:680–686, 1977.

99. Malagelada JR, Glanzman SL, Go VLW: Laboratory diagnosis of gastrinoma: a prospective study of gastrin challenge tests. Mayo Clin Proc 57:219–226, 1982.

100. Korman MG, Scott DH, Hansky J, et al: Hypergastrinemia due to an excluded gastric antrum: a proposed method of differentiation from the Zollinger-Ellison syndrome. Aust NZ Med 3:266–271, 1972.

101. Ganguli PC, Pearse AGE, Polak JB, et al: Antral-gastrin cell hyperplasia in peptic ulcer disease. Lancet 1:583–586, 1974.

102. Deveney CW, Deveney KS, Way LW: The Zollinger-Ellison syndrome—23 years later. Ann Surg 188:384–393, 1978.

103. Damgaard-Peterson K, Stage JG: CT scanning in patients with Zollinger-Ellison syndrome and carcinoid syndromes. Scand J Gastroenterol [Suppl 53] 14:117–122, 1979.

104. Mills SR, Doppman JL, Dunnick NR: Evaluation of angiography in the Zollinger-Ellison syndrome. Radiology, 131:317–320, 1979.

105. Cope V, Warwick F: The role of radiology in the detection of endocrine tumors in the GI tract. Clin Gastroenterol 3:621, 1974.

106. Burcharth F, Stage FG, Stadil F, et al: Localization of gastrinomas by transhepatic portal venous catheterization and gastrin assay. Gastroenterology 77:449–450, 1978.

107. Passaro E Jr: Localization of pancreatic endocrine tumors by selective portal vein catheterization and radioimmunoassay. Gastroenterology 77 (part I):806–807, 1979.

108. Ingemansson S, Larsson LI, Lunderquist A, et al: Pancreatic vein catheterization with gastrin assay in normal patients and in patients with the Zollinger-Ellison syndrome. Am J Surg 134:558–563, 1977.

109. Glowniak JV, Shapiro B, Vinik AI, et al: Percutaneous transhepatic venous sampling of gastrin value in sporadic and familial islet cell tumors and G-cell hyperplasia. N Engl J Med 307:293–297, 1982.

110. Stremple JF, Watson CG: Serum calcium, serum gastrin, and gastric acid secretion before and after parathyroidectomy for hyperparathyroidism. Surgery 75:841–850, 1972.

111. Jaffe BM, Peskin GW, Kaplan EL: Serum levels of parathyroid hormone in the Zollinger-Ellison syndrome. Surgery 74:621, 1973.

112. Turbey WJ, Passaro EW Jr: Hyperparathyroidism in the Zollinger-Ellison syndrome. Arch Surg 105:62, 1972.

113. Brennan MF, Jensen RT, Wesley RA, et al: The role of surgery in patients with Zollinger-Ellison syndrome (ZES) managed medically. Ann Surg 196:239–245, 1982.

114. Stadil F, Stage JG: The Zollinger-Ellison syndrome. Clin Endocrinol Metab 8:433–446, 1979.

115. Zollinger RM, Ellison EC, Fabri PJ, et al: Primary peptic ulcerations of the jejunum associated with islet cell tumors. Ann Surg 192:422–430, 1980.

116. Bonfils S, Landor JH, Mignon M, et al: Results of surgical management in 92 consecutive patients with Zollinger-Ellison syndrome. Ann Surg 194:692–697, 1981.

117. Hoffman JD, Fox PS, Wilson SD: Duodenal wall tumors and the Zollinger-Ellison syndrome. Arch Surg 107:334–339, 1973.

118. Oberhelman HA Jr: Excisional therapy for ulcerogenic tumors of the duodenum. Arch Surg 104:447–453, 1972.

119. Wolfe MM, Alexander RW, McGuigan JE: Extrapancreatic, extraintestinal gastrinoma: Effective treatment by surgery. N Engl J Med 306:1533–1536, 1982.

120. Richardson CT, Feldman M, McClelland RN: Effect of vagotomy in Zollinger-Ellison syndrome. Gastroenterology 77:682–686, 1979.

121. McClelland RN: Discussion of Brennan MF, Jensen RT, Wesley RA, et al: The role of surgery in patients with Zollinger-Ellison syndrome (ZES) managed medically. Ann Surg 196:239–245, 1982.

122. Friesen SR: Discussion of Brennan MF, Jensen RT, Wesley RA, et al: The role of surgery in patients with Zollinger-Ellison syndrome (ZES) managed medically. Ann Surg 196:239–245, 1982.

123. Moertel CG, Hanley JA, Johnson LA: Streptozocin alone compared with streptozocin plus fluorouracil in the treatment of advanced islet cell carcinoma. N Engl J Med 303:1189–1194, 1980.

124. Verner JV, Morrison AB: Islet cell tumor and a syndrome of refractory watery diarrhea and hypokalemia. Am J Med, 25:374–380, 1958.

125. Modlin IM: Endocrine tumors of the pancreas. Surg Gynecol Obstet 149:751–769, 1979.

126. Kraft AR, Tompkins RK, Zollinger RM: Recognition and management of the diarrheal syndrome caused by nonbeta islet cell tumors of the pancreas. Am J Surg 119:163–170, 1970.

127. Cooperman AM, DeSantis D, Winkelman E, et al: Watery diarrhea syndrome: Two unusual cases and further evidence that VIP is a humoral mediator. Ann Surg 187:325–328, 1978.

128. Said SI, Faloona GR: Elevated plasma and tissue levels of vasoactive intestinal polypeptide in the watery diarrhea syndrome due to pancreatic, bronchogenic and other tumors. N Engl J Med 293:155–160, 1975.

129. Long RG, Bryant MG, Mitchell SJ, et al: Clinicopathological study of pancreatic and ganglioneuroblastoma tumours secreting vasoactive intestinal polypeptide (vipomas). Br Med J 282:1767–1771, 1981.

130. Verner JV, Morrison AB: Endocrine pancreatic islet disease with diarrhea. Arch Inter Med 133:492–500, 1974.

131. Modlin IM, Bloom SR, Mitchell S, et al: VIP: the cause of the watery diarrhea syndrome. *In* Grossman M, Speranza V, Basso N, et al (eds): Proceedings of the International Symposium on Gastrointestinal Hormones and Pathology of the Digestive System. New York, Plenum, 1978, pp 195–202.

132. Fahrenbrug J, Schaffalitsky de Mackadell OB: Verner-Morrison syndrome and vasoactive intestinal polypeptide (VIP). Scand J Gastroenterol [Suppl 14] 53:57, 1979.

133. Ebeid A, Mujray PD, Fischer JE: Vasoactive intestinal peptide and the watery diarrhea syndrome. Ann Surg 187:411–416, 1978.

134. Visser PA, Friesen SR: Uncommon tumors of the APUD system. Surg Clin North Am 59:143–158, 1979.

135. Krejs GJ, Fordtran JS, Bloom SR, et al: Effect of VIP infusion on water and ion transport in the human jejunum. Gastroenterology 78:722–727, 1980.

136. Kingham JGC, Dick R, Bloom SR, et al: Vipoma: localization by percutaneous transhepatic portal venous sampling. Br Med J 2:1682–1683, 1978.

137. Jaffe BM: The diarrheogenic syndrome: Verner-Morrison, WDHA syndromes. *In* Friesen SR (ed): Surgical Endocrinology: Clinical Syndromes. Philadelphia, Lippincott, 1978, ch 15.

138. Nagorney DM, Bloom SR, Polak JA, et al: Resolution of recurrent Verner-Morrison syndrome by resection of metastatic vipoma. Surgery 93:348–353, 1978.

139. Kahn CR, Lev AG, Gardner JD, et al: Pancreatic cholera: beneficial effects of treatment with streptozocin. N Engl J Med 292:941–945, 1975.

140. Montenegro-Rodas F, Samaan NA: Glucagonoma tumors and syndrome. Curr Probl Cancer 1981.
141. Becker SW, Kahn D, Rothman S: Cutaneous manifestations of internal malignant tumors. Arch Dermatol Syph 45:1069–1080, 1942.
142. McGavran MH, Unger RH, Recant L, et al: A glucagon-secreting α-cell carcinoma of the pancreas. N Engl J Med 274:1408, 1966.
143. Mallinson CN, Bloom SR, Warin AP, et al: A glucagonoma syndrome. Lancet 2:15, 1974.
144. Danforth DN Jr, Triche T, Doppman JL, et al: Elevated plasma proglucagon-like component with a glucagon secreting tumor: effect of streptozotocin. N Engl J Med 295:242–245, 1976.
145. Pearse AGE, Polak JM: Endocrine tumours of neural crest origin: neurolophomas, apudomas, and the APUD concept. Med Biol 52:3, 1974.
146. Prinz RA, Dorsch TR, Lawrence AM: Clinical aspects of glucagon-producing islet-cell tumors. Am J Gastroenterol 76:125–131, 1981.
147. Leichter SB: Clinical and metabolic aspects of glucagonoma. Medicine (Baltimore) 59:100–113, 1980.
148. Higgins GA, Recant L, Fischman AB: The glucagonoma syndrome: surgically curable diabetes. Am J Surg 137:142–148, 1979.
149. Wilkinson SD: Necrolytic migratory erythema with pancreatic carcinoma. Proc R Soc Med 64:25–26, 1971.
150. Unger RH, Orci L: Physiology and pathophysiology of glucagon. Physiol Rev 56:778, 1976.
151. Unger RH, Orci L: Glucagon: secretion, transport, metabolism physiologic regulation of secretion, and derangements in diabetes. *In* DeGroot LG, et al (eds): Endocrinology. New York, Grune & Stratton, 1979.
152. Cho KJ, Wilcox CW, Reuter SR: Glucagon-producing islet cell tumor of the pancreas. Am J Roentgenol Radium Ther Nucl Med 129:159–161, 1977.
153. Ingemansson S, Halst J, Larsson L, et al: Localization of glucagonomas by catheterization of the pancreatic veins and with glucagon assay. Surg Gynecol Obstet 145:509–516, 1977.
154. Montenegro F, Lawrence GD, Macron W, et al: Metastatic glucagonoma: improvement after surgical debulking. Am J Surg 139:424–427, 1980.
155. Prinz RA, Badrinath D, Banerji M, et al: Operative and chemotherapeutic management of malignant glucagon-producing tumors. Surgery 90:713–719, 1981.
156. Friesen SR: Tumors of the endocrine pancreas. N Engl J Med 306:580–590, 1982.
157. Larsson L-I, Holst JJ, Kühl C, et al: Pancreatic somatostatinoma: clinical features and physiological implications. Lancet 1:666–668, 1977.
158. Gerich JE, Patton GS: Somatostatin, physiology, and clinical applications. Med Clin North Am 62:375–391, 1978.
159. Krejs GJ, Orci L, Coneon JM, et al: Somatostatinoma syndrome: biochemical, morphologic, and clinical features. N Engl J Med 301:285–292, 1979.
160. Ganda OP, Weig GC, Soeldner J, et al: "Somatostatinoma": a somatostatin-containing tumor of the endocrine pancreas. N Engl J Med 296:963–967, 1977.

Index

Page numbers in italics refer to figures; those followed by a t refer to tables.

319